CANCER ETIOLOGY, DIAGNOSIS AND TREATMENTS

FREE RADICALS

THE ROLE OF ANTIOXIDANTS AND PRO-OXIDANTS IN CANCER DEVELOPMENT

Cancer Etiology, Diagnosis and Treatments

Additional books in this series can be found on Nova's website
under the Series tab.

Additional e-books in this series can be found on Nova's website
under the e-book tab.

CANCER ETIOLOGY, DIAGNOSIS AND TREATMENTS

FREE RADICALS

THE ROLE OF ANTIOXIDANTS AND PRO-OXIDANTS IN CANCER DEVELOPMENT

BILL STONE
EDITOR

New York

For permission to use material from this book please contact us:
Telephone 631-231-7269; Fax 631-231-8175
Web Site: http://www.novapublishers.com

Library of Congress Cataloging-in-Publication Data

ISBN: 978-1-63117-177-2

Library of Congress Control Number: 2014930031

Published by Nova Science Publishers, Inc. † New York

Contents

Preface

This book is focused on the role that pro-oxidants and antioxidants have on cancer development. The impact of reactive oxygen species (ROS) and antioxidant agents on cancer has been intensively investigated since considerable evidence suggests that these factors are central to the development of more effective cancer chemotherapeutic agents and chemoprevention strategies. This book presents a detailed overview of these immensely important health-related topics and will, hopefully, stimulate further research and development.

The first Chapter by Drs. Aysegul Cort and Tomris Ozben provides a nuanced review of the role that antioxidants and pro-oxidants play in cancer development and therapy. This Chapter emphasizes the importance of ROS and oxidative stress in modulating normal cellular signal transduction mechanisms. Of particular interest is how these signals are altered in cancer cells, which often have a higher level of intrinsic oxidative stress than normal cells. An understanding of how oxidative stress modulates the pathways determining cell fate (e.g., proliferation, differentiation, apoptosis and necrosis) is essential for the rationale design of future chemotherapies. A detailed introduction is provided into the varieties of endogenous (enzymatic and non-enzymatic) and exogenous antioxidants (e.g.,. vitamin C, vitamin E, carotenoids, and polyphenols). In the case of exogenous antioxidants, the authors describe their specific molecular functions, the evidence for and against their anticancer effects as well as possible interactions with traditional chemopreventive agents.

The second chapter, by Drs. Décio Sabbatini Barbosa, Danielle Venturini, Francis Fregonesi Brinholi, Andressa Keiko Matsumoto, Carine Coneglian de Farias, Chiara Cristina Bortolasci, Kamila Landucci Bonifácio and Luciana Higachi, addresses a question that is of key importance for many healthcare providers, i.e., is there an actual health benefit from antioxidant supplementation during cancer treatment? A related and equally important question is whether or not antioxidant supplementation could alter the efficacy of cancer chemotherapy. This is a very comprehensive chapter with many specific cancers and antioxidants discussed in detail. Among the exogenous antioxidants discussed are polyphenols, alpha-tocopherol, ascorbate, carotenoids, selenium, resveratrol, curcumin, green tea compounds and quercetin. Among the endogenous antioxidant enzymes discussed are superoxide dismutase (SOD), catalase (CAT) and glutathione peroxidase (GPX). The relationship of antioxidants to oxidative stress and DNA damage is thoroughly detailed. This is an excellent chapter for those readers wanting to get an overview of the "big picture."

Chapter 3, by Sharon E. Campbell, Aashish S. Morani, William L. Stone, Koyamangalath Krishnan and Victoria P. Palau, is completely focused on vitamin E and cancer. Vitamin E is the primary lipid-soluble antioxidant and its role in cancer is perhaps the most studied of all antioxidants. Dr. Campbell emphasizes the fact that vitamin E is not a single compound but is at least four tocopherols (alpha-, beta-, delta- and gamma-tocopherol) and four corresponding tocotrienols. Much of the literature on vitamin E fails to distinguish between the different isoforms and this has created a "vitamin E muddle." This chapter is meticulous in reviewing the relationship between each vitamin E isoform and it role in cancer biology and in modulating signal transduction pathways. All-rac-alpha-tocopheryl acetate (an ester of synthetic alpha-tocopherol) is the most studied of all vitamin E isoforms yet the evidence reviewed in this chapter suggests some of the "non-alpha-tocopherol" isoforms of vitamin E might be far superior chemopreventive agents. It is, perhaps, premature to dismiss the potential chemopreventive properties of vitamin E supplements but it is an optimal time to focus on isoforms other than all-rac-alpha-tocopheryl acetate. As detailed in this chapter, it is very clear that the ability of some vitamin E isoforms to modulate cancer-relevant signal transduction pathways is not just a function of antioxidant potency.

Chapter 4 by Drs. Ying Qu, Xiaojiang Cui and Ninghui Cheng also describes a single antioxidant system, i.e., the endogenous glutaredoxin (Grx) system which plays a key role in modulating many cancer cell phenotypes such as uncontrolled growth, the epithelial–mesenchymal transition, migration/invasion, and chemo-resistance. Grx proteins, in conjunction with glutathione and glutathione reductase are able to reduce disulfide bonds formed in target proteins by oxidative stress. Moreover, Grxs are involved in DNA synthesis and are overexpressed in a number of cancers, e.g., pancreatic, breast, colon and lung cancer tissues. The cancer-relevant signaling pathways modulated by Grxs are discussed in detail. A recurrent theme in this book revolves around the concept that cancer cells often express a high level of intrinsic oxidative stress that makes them particularly susceptible to apoptosis induced by therapies causing an additional layer of oxidative stress. This chapter explores, therefore, how potential inhibitors of Grxs antioxidant activity in cancer cells could be promising candidates for novel chemotherapeutic agents.

Chapters 5 and 6 are significant since they both illustrate the promise that pro-oxidant therapies present for treating of cancer. Pancreatic cancer is one of the most aggressive types of major cancers and causes more than 1% of all U.S. mortality. Chapter 5 by Drs. John A. Cieslak and Joseph J. Cullen describe the advances that have been made in utilizing high dose intravenous ascorbate (vitamin C) for the treatment of pancreatic cancer. Dietary ascorbate, and ascorbate at normal physiological levels, is considered a powerful water-soluble antioxidant. Intravenous ascorbate at pharmacological levels can, however, act as a pro-oxidant. As is often the case for cancer cells, pancreatic cancer cells exhibit an enhanced sensitivity to pro-oxidant induced cell death compared to normal cells. The authors describe the results of Phase I trials, which strongly suggest that pharmacological ascorbate in pancreatic cancer patients is both safe and has potential efficacy. This is clearly one of the more promising clinical applications of cancer redox therapy.

Chapter 6 describes original research by Drs. William L. Stone, Yu Lin Jiang, Christopher McGoldrick, Marianne Brannon and Koymangalath Krishnan and the research here exploits the high level of cancer cell intrinsic oxidative stress for the design of prodrugs that are selectively activated by a novel cancer esterase to activate a pro-oxidant drug with the ability to deplete intracellular glutathione (GSH). GSH is the primary intracellular antioxidant and its depletion can cause oxidative stress induced apoptosis. The novel cancer esterase targeted was acylamino-acid-releasing enzyme (AARE), which is over expressed in some tumors and cancer cell lines. A bioinformatics approach was used to predict the three dimensional structure of AARE. Protein-ligand docking studies were then used for the rationale design of a prototype prodrug, which was subsequently synthesized and purified. As proof-of-concept, the novel prodrug was found to deplete GSH *in vitro* in the presence of AARE. This preclinical study also suggests that it might be possible to select cancer patients who might be responders to the novel chemotherapeutic prodrug, i.e., those having cancer cells overexpressing AARE and a high level of intrinsic oxidative stress.

Chapters 7 and 8 are both devoted to specific cancers, i.e., colorectal cancer (CRC) and prostate cancer respectively. In the Chapter 7, Dr. Martina Perše provides a detailed review of the role antioxidant defenses play in the pathogenesis of colorectal cancer (CRC). Antioxidant defenses are logically divided into three levels (i.e., protective, reduction/neutralization and reparative) and the role of each level is carefully delineated in molecular detail. After providing a picture of the antioxidant defense “landscape”, Dr. Perse explains how the failure of antioxidant systems has potential carcinogenic consequences. An emphasis is placed on *in vivo* results generated using transgenic mice models, thereby assuring a degree of preclinical relevance. It is certainly significant that mice deficient in some (but not all) key antioxidant enzymes can develop an increased tumor burden with age or a phenotype such as inflammation, which is associated with increased cancer risk.

Dr. Perse next provides a brief but necessary description of the specific antioxidant and pro-oxidant mechanisms unique to the large intestine. One major factor is the presence of intestinal microflora and their potential role in promoting oxidative stress and inflammation. As detailed by Dr. Perse, the leap to clinically relevant information on the role of antioxidants and pro-oxidants in human CRC is not straightforward. While very recent genetic data suggests an association of CRC with several single-nucleotide polymorphisms (SNPs) in genes involved in antioxidative protective system, the results of several large-scale, placebo-controlled intervention studies show that supplementation with antioxidant micronutrients did not reduce the occurrence of CRC. Potential reasons for this apparent paradox are provided in this Chapter. Finally, Dr. Perse provides insights into the challenges and new approaches that need to be addressed to test hypothesis that modulating antioxidants and pro-oxidants can be of help in preventing CRC.

Chapter 8 by Drs. Trevor Memmott, Evita Weagel, Chris Hamilton, Richard A. Robison, and Kim L. O’Neill is focused on the role of oxidative stress imbalance in the development of prostate cancer, which is the second leading cause of cancer deaths in men. This chapter first provides an excellent overview of the steps from benign prostate hyperplasia to prostatic intraepithelial neoplasia to prostate cancer as well as the roles played by ROS and oxidative stress at each stage of this progression. Similarly the involvement of hypoxia and hormones are detailed as well as the molecular aspects of prostate cancer such as oncogenes, tumor suppressor genes and mitochondrial mutations. The molecular mechanisms whereby ROS promote aggressive prostate cancer phenotypes are outlined and an understanding of these mechanisms is essential in the design of more effective therapeutic agents.

Both Chapter 9 and chapter 10 are concerned with the analytical techniques used to measure oxidative stress or antioxidant capacity. Clearly these measurements are of central importance to this book and to the whole field of redox cancer biology. Chapter 9 presents original research by Drs. Matthew E. Pamenter and Sameh S. Ali that describes a novel technique to measure the production of specific ROS in cultured cells by the use spin-trap reagents and electron paramagnetic resonance (EPR). Despite being the "gold" standard for measuring ROS, EPR has not been exploited to probe specific ROS production in cellular systems. Chapter 9 remedy's this situation and the authors provide a detailed set of experimental procedures that will be of immense practical use to researchers in the general area of free radical biology.

Chapter 10 by Drs. Vanessa Fuchs-Tarlovsky and Jessica Calderon-Cuevas deals with the fundamental question of how dietary antioxidants alter measureable oxidative stress parameters in human plasma and how these parameters correlate with various cancers. These issues are very important to the functional food industry and to the advice that oncologists and nutritionists provide to the general public and cancer patients.

In: Free Radicals
Editor: Bill Stone
ISBN: 978-1-63117-177-2

Chapter I

Free Radicals: The Role of Antioxidants and Pro-Oxidants in Cancer Development and Therapy

Aysegul Cort and Tomris Ozben *
Antalya Turkey Department of Clinical Biochemistry Faculty of Medicine Akdeniz University, Antalya, Turkey

Abstract

Oxidative stress is defined as an imbalance between the presence of relatively high levels of free radicals and reactive metabolites and their elimination by protective mechanisms, referred to as antioxidants. This impaired balance causes damage to important biomolecules such as proteins, lipids, and DNA in the cells, with potential impact on the whole organism. Oxidative stress can induce various biological responses, including a transient growth arrest and adaptation, gene transcription, and initiation of signal transduction pathways. These events determine whether a cell will undergo necrosis, senescence, apoptosis, or will survive and proliferate. The extent of these responses depends on the cellular genetic background, and the intensity and duration of the oxidative stress. It is known that high levels of oxidative stress are toxic, but low levels may elicit cellular proliferation indicating cell responses to reactive oxygen species (ROS) are dose-dependent. Cancer cells evolve in oxidative circumstances depending on cell type and tumor evolution stage. Cancer cells are under increased oxidative stress compared to normal cells due to oncogen-induced transformation, increased metabolic activity, mitochondrial malfunction, altered energy metabolism due to malnutrition; an excessive production of proinflamatory cytokines, which in turn may increase ROS production. Some chemotherapeutic agents and radiation therapy generate ROS in patients during cancer therapy. Therapies which generate an oxidative burst in tumors proved to be efficient in killing some type of cancer cells. ROS levels should reach to a level above a threshold in order to induce tumor cell death. Accumulation of intrinsic ROS with therapy-generated ROS and inhibition of ROS elimination by antioxidants

* Dept. of Clinical Biochemistry Faculty of Medicine Akdeniz University 07070 Antalya Turkey
Email: ozben@akdeniz.edu.tr

represent a powerful mechanism for killing cancer cells. Because of toxic side effects and potential mutagenic effect, caution should be taken in using ROS-generating agents. The therapeutic strategies involving induction of cancer cell death selectively offer promise in a variety of clinical settings.

Keywords: cancer, reactive oxygen species, antioxidants

Abbreviations

5-FU:	Fluorouracil
Akt:	Protein kinase B
AP-1:	Activator protein 1
APAF:	Apoptosis-inducing factors
APL:	Acute promyelocitic leukemia
ASK1:	Apoptosis signal-regulating kinase 1
Bcl-2:	B-cell lymphoma 2
CAT:	Catalase
CDKs:	Cyclin dependent kinases
CREB:	cAMP response element-binding protein
Cyt-c:	Cytochrome c
EGCG:	Epigallocatechin-3-gallate
EGFR:	Epidermal growth factor receptor
ERK:	Extracellular-signal-regulated kinase
FADD:	Fas-associated protein with death domain
FLIP:	FLICE inhibitory protein
GCL:	γ-glutamylcysteine ligase
GGT:	γ-glutamyl-transpeptidase
GPx:	Glutathione peroxidase
GSH:	Glutathione
HIF-1α:	Hypoxia-inducible factor 1-alpha
HTLV-1:	Human T-lymphotropic virus 1
JNK:	C-Jun NH2-teminal Kinase
KEAP1:	Kelch-like ECH-associated protein 1
MAPK:	Mitogen-activated protein kinase
MEK:	MAPK kinases
MMP-9:	Matrix metallopeptidase 9
mTOR:	Mammalian target of rapamycin
NAC:	N-acetyl cysteine
NF-κB:	Nuclear factor-κB
Nrf2:	Nuclear factor (erythroid-derived 2)-like 2
PI3K:	Phosphoinositide 3-kinase
RNS:	Reactive nitrogen species
ROS:	Reactive Oxygen Species
SAPKs:	Stress activated protein kinase
SELECT:	Selenium and vitamin E cancer prevention trial

SOD:	Superoxide dismutase
SOx:	Oxidation of these Cys residues
STAT:	Signal transducer and activator of transcription
TAC:	Total antioxidant capacity
TNF:	Tumor necrosis factor
UV:	Ultraviolet
VEGF:	Vascular endothelial growth factor

Introduction

Reactive Oxygen Species (ROS) are produced during normal cellular function in aerobic organisms due to their reliance on oxidative processes for life. It is fascinating how such simple molecules are able to regulate life and death. ROS are generally perceived as toxicants that induce various deleterious effects, like cell dysfunction, death or malignant transformation. ROS are generated during irradiation by UV light, X-rays and gamma rays; products of metal-catalyzed reactions; present as pollutants in the atmosphere; produced by neutrophils and macrophages during inflammation; by-products of mitochondria-catalyzed electron transport reactions and other mechanisms [1]. Beneficial effects of ROS involve physiological roles in the function of a number of cellular signalling systems. Lower concentrations of ROS induce a mitogenic response. In contrast, at high concentrations, ROS are important mediators of damage to cell structures, including membrane lipids, proteins and nucleic acids [2]. In order to protect from the harmful effects of ROS, aerobic organisms developed powerful antioxidant mechanisms to adapt to live in an oxidative environment. Oxidative damage accumulates during the life cycle, and radical-related damage to DNA, proteins and lipids play a key role in the development of cancer despite the presence of the antioxidant defence system of the cells to counteract oxidative damage from ROS. In this chapter, we discuss the role of ROS in the pathogenesis of cancer and the relevance of antioxidants in preventing ROS induced damage to cellular structures and their role in cellular signalling cascades.

Cancer cells adapt to survive under high levels of oxidative stress and produce high levels of intrinsic ROS which may exert selective enrichment of the population of cells that are capable of stress adaptation [3]. Cells surviving under high oxidative stress are likely to have acquired adaptive mechanisms to counteract the potential toxic effects of elevated ROS and promote cell-survival pathways.

ROS modulate activities and expression of many transcription factors and signalling proteins that are involved in stress response and cell survival through multiple mechanisms (Figure 1). The expression of signalling proteins are tightly controlled through the rate of gene transcription. A number of transcription factors, such as nuclear factor-κB (NF-κB), AP-1, HIF-1α and p53, contain redox-sensitive cysteine residues at their DNA-binding site. Oxidation of these Cys residues (SOx) may disrupt the transactivation activity and inhibit the expression of the target genes. RAS and Akt, can be directly modified by oxidation of their Cys, Tyr and Met amino acids, resulting in alterations of their functions. Certain proteins can be functionally modulated by their interacting proteins, which are redox sensitive.

Modification of such interacting proteins by ROS causes dissociation of the protein complex leading to a functional change in the protein components.

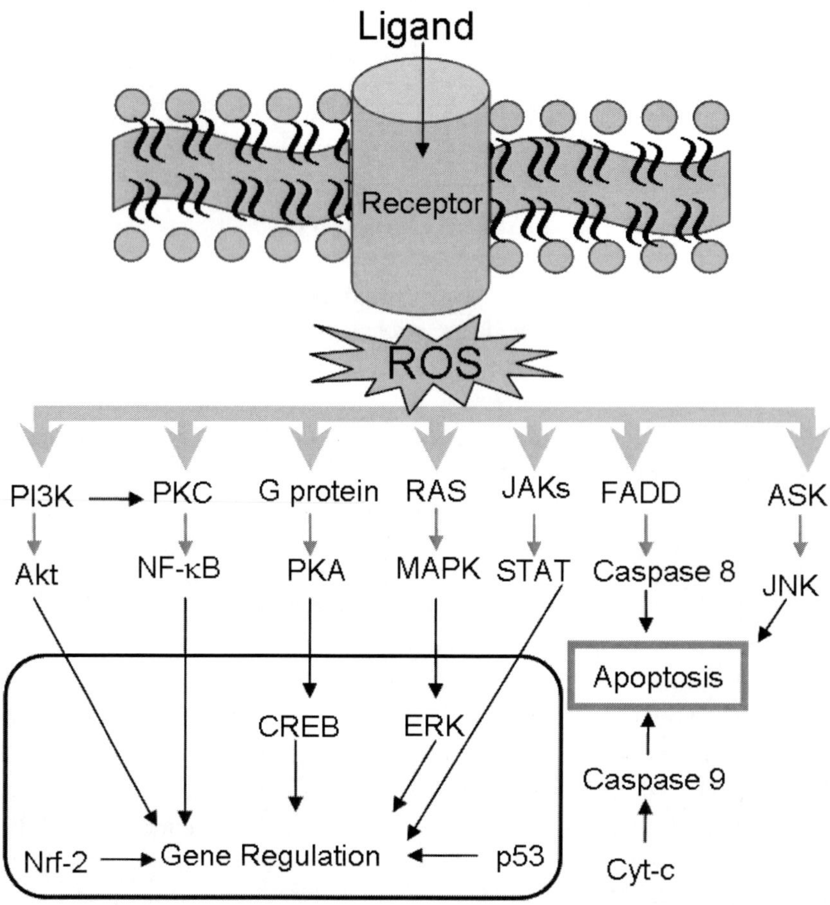

Figure 1. ROS affected signalling pathways. PI3K: Phosphoinositide 3-kinase, Akt: Protein kinase B, CREB: cAMP response element-binding protein, ERK: Extracellular-signal-regulated kinase, STAT: Signal transducer and activator of transcription, FADD: Fas-associated protein with death domain.

Generation of ROS during Cancer Therapy

ROS are responsible for triggering cell death and reversing chemo-resistance in tumors [4]. Drugs generating ROS enhance the antitumour effect of anticancer therapy and can be used as an alternative cancer treatment. This approach is currently under heavy investigation in cancer research. Intracellular ROS function to trigger initiation of downstream signaling events in regulating apoptosis, cell cycle and cell differentiation [5]. Numerous *in vitro* studies [6, 7, 8] have demonstrated that a wide range of anticancer agents induce programmed cell death (apoptosis) in malignant cells by generating ROS which is considered as an important therapeutic interventional approach in cancer. Oxidative stress has been shown to decrease the lethal dose of several types of antineoplastic agents and induce cancer cell apoptosis. Conventional chemotherapy drugs, such as doxorubicin, etoposide, cisplatin or paclitaxel, can induce apoptosis by activating p53 expression and ceramide pathway or affecting Bcl-2-like proteins, or interfering with the redox or energy balance of the cell [9]. Cancer cells produce higher levels of ROS than normal cells, and this contributes to cancer progression [10, 11, 12]. It was reported that ROS selectively sensitized oncogenically transformed cells to β-phenylethyl isothiocyanate-induced cell death [13]. Increasing ROS generation in cancer cells could be a strategy for cancer therapy. Hagen et al. reported that the mitochondria plays a significant role in ROS-mediated cell death [14]. A strategy to sensitize cancer cells to drug-induced apoptosis is to combine a ROS-generating drug with inhibitors of mitochondrial respiration in order to enhance ROS production and cell death [15].

ROS in Apoptosis

ROS involves both mitochondria and death receptor mediated apoptosis. Activation of the Fas receptor, belonging to the TNF/NGF receptor family, results in a signal transduction pathway involving ROS mainly derived from NADPH oxidase as an upstream event of Fas activation and apoptosis induction. This assumption was proved based on the fact that antioxidants blocked Fas receptor-mediated apoptosis [16]. Fas receptor-induced ROS generate ceramide. ROS have also been shown to be involved in induction of both Fas receptor and Fas ligand genes. Fas induced ROS response is required for Yes/EGFR/Fas interactions as upstream events of Fas-tyrosine phosphorylation, which is a signal for subsequent recruitment of Fas-associated death domain and caspase 8 and apoptosis induction [17]. Additionally, FasL-induced ROS mediate the ubiquitination and subsequent degradation by proteasome of FLICE inhibitory protein (FLIP) to further enhance Fas activation [18] (Figure 2).

Mitochondria-mediated apoptosis is initiated by releasing soluble mitochondrial intermembrane proteins such as cytochrome c and apoptosis-inducing factors (APAF) which activate downstream caspases and nucleases, ultimately leading to apoptotic cell death. The activation of apoptosis is regulated through several proapoptotic second messengers, such as ROS, nitric oxide, lipid messenger, ceramide, calcium, and proapoptotic Bcl-2 family members (e.g., Bax, Bid, and Bad). It is also regulated through a number of inhibitors, such as antiapoptotic Bcl-2 family members. C-Jun NH2-teminal Kinase (JNK), also termed as stress activated protein kinase (SAPKs) is a major signaling molecule mediating ROS-induced opening of mitochondria permeability transition pore complex [19].

All the MAPK pathway family members are activated and regulated through phosphorylation cascades by upstream kinases which are called as MAPK kinases (MEK) and further upper level MAPKK kinases (MAP3K, MEKK). Two MEK family members, MEK4 and MEK7, have been implicated in phosphorylation of JNKs. A number of different MAP3Ks can activate MKK4 and MKK7, suggesting that a wide range of stimuli can activate MAPK pathway. These include MEKK1, 2, 3, and 4, MLK, and ASK1 (apoptosis signal-regulating kinase 1). MEKK4 can also activate p38 MAPK pathway by inducing MKK3 or MKK6. Research into the molecular mechanisms of oxidative stress-mediated activation of JNK and p38 pathways has focused on redox-sensitive proteins such as thioredoxin and glutaredoxin. It is well known that ROS oxidizes thioredoxin which dissociates from ASK1 for its activation, resulting in the activation of JNK and p38 pathways [20]. Recent studies have suggested that ROS-mediated ASK1 activation is involved in cancer [21]. After activation by ROS, JNK translocates close to mitochondria membrane and activates pore-destabilizing proteins (Bax/Bak) or inhibits pore-stabilizing proteins (Bcl-2 and Bcl-xl), leading to opening of permeability transition pore complex. A recent study reported that Piperlongumine, a natural alkaloid, selectively killed glioblastoma cells via accumulating ROS which caused activation of JNK and p38 [22].

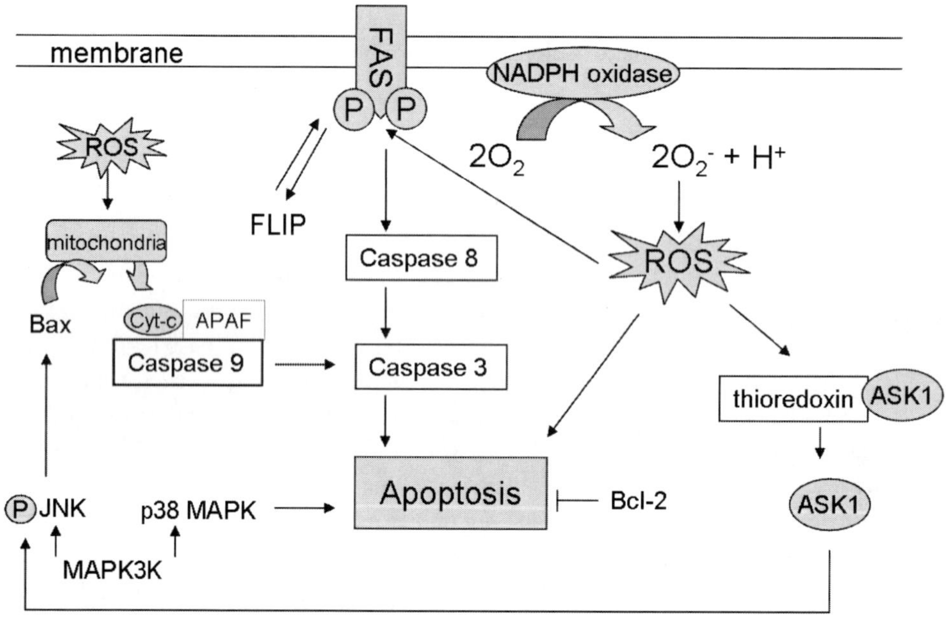

Figure 2. ROS induced apoptosis. ASK1: Apoptosis signal-regulating kinase 1.

ROS in Autophagy

Autophagy is a regulated lysosomal pathway involved in the degradation and recycling of cytoplasmic materials [23]. The autophagic process is essential not only to maintain homeostasis, differentiation and development, but is critical for cell survival during periods of nutrient deprivation or stress. It is activated during amino-acid deprivation and has been reported to associate with cancer [24, 25]. Autophagy is initiated with formation of a crescent-shaped isolation membrane/phagophore which is a closed double-membrane structure, called autophagosom by the surrounding of cytoplasmic constituents. Under starvation conditions, cells form ROS, specifically H_2O_2, which is essential for autophagosome formation and autophagic degradation. Phosphatidyl inositol 3 kinase dependent oxidative signal leads to inhibition of Atg4 cysteine protease as a direct target for oxidation by H_2O_2 and inhibits Atg4 delipidating activity, whereas the initial processing of LC3 (priming) by Atg4 is not altered [26]. Expression of this regulatory mutant prevented formation of autophagosomes in cells which characterizes a molecular mechanism for redox regulation of the autophagic process [27]. Beclin-1 is upregulated in response to ROS in cancer cells. It was reported that increasing expression of Beclin-1 in a breast cancer cell line promoted formation of autophagosomal vesicles and suppressed tumor growth *in vitro* and in a nude mouse model [28]. Mice heterozygous for disruption of beclin-1 gene developed spontaneous lung and liver tumors as well as B-cell lymphomas [29, 30]. Involvement of both Bcl-XL and Bax in the autophagic process suggest that ROS may have synergetic effects in apoptosis and autophagy [31]. ROS induce autophagy through inhibition of mTOR [32]. PTEN activated autophagy via downregulation of PI3K–Akt–mTOR signaling is inhibited by ROS [33]. Increased ROS activates the ASK1–JNK/p38 pathway suggesting a connection between ROS-induced autophagy and apoptosis. AMP-activated protein kinase is required for ROS-triggered autophagy [26]. Mitochondrial ROS generation activates p38 and p53 in cancer cells [34]. ROS generation causes oxidative DNA damage leading to genome instability or genetic replication mutations. Expression of p53 participates in gene repair or cell death program via apoptosis and autophagy [35, 36, 37]. Chen et al. demonstrated that oxidative stress caused autophagy-induced cell death in transformed and cancer cell lines [15]. Blocking autophagosome accumulation by chemical inhibitors or knocking down of autophagy genes effectively blocked ROS-induced cell death. Similarly, blocking ROS generation also effectively blocked autophagy and cell death. It was reported that ROS are involved in caspase-independent cell death in macrophage cells [38]. ROS scavengers block autophagic cell death but not ROS induced apoptosis. Thorpe et al. reported that autophagy genes were upregulated in response to oxidative stress in yeast Saccharomyces cerevisiae [39]. Oxidative stress was demonstrated to trigger a lysosomal-dependent necrotic cell death [38]. In a recent work, it was found that growth of advanced pancreatic cancer required ongoing autophagy in part to suppress accumulation of cytotoxic ROS levels [40]. Cells under oxidative stress undergo cell death through multiple pathways including apoptosis, autophagy or necrosis [27]. Targeting ROS generation could selectively induce autophagic cell death in cancer cells. Oxidative stress induces autophagy and leads to oxidative stress-induced cell death that might be selectively applied towards transformed and cancer cells. This may lead to the development of therapeutic drugs that will selectively target cancer cells to undergo autophagy-induced cell death independent of apoptosis.

Mitochondrial ROS act as a tumor suppressor by activating pro-autophagic genes and blocking anti-autophagic genes in carcinogenesis. In contrast, ROS also play a pro-tumor role under certain circumstances. Mitochondrial ROS play multifaceted roles as the ‘molecular switch’ for regulation of several autophagic pathways. Developing and discovering potential novel cancer drug targeting ROS-modulated autophagy is a promising new field in the fight against cancer.

ROS in Cell Cycle

Normal cell cycle consists of four phases: (a) A presynthetic phase (G1 phase); (b) DNA synthesis (S); (c) Post-DNA synthesis (G2); (d) Mitosis (M) during which G2 cells divides into two daughter cells. Cell cycle is regulated by intrinsic molecular mechanisms. These mechanisms induce or block progression through the cycle and depend primarily on cyclins and cyclin dependent kinases (CDKs) produced in cells [41]. Oxidative stress reduces the rate of cell proliferation by inhibiting transition of cells from the G0 to the G1 phase, prolonging the G1 phase, slowing progression through the S phase by inhibiting DNA synthesis, inhibiting cell cycle progression through the restriction point, and causing arrest at cell cycle checkpoints [42]. 4-Hydroxyalkenals are cytotoxic aldehyde products of lipid peroxidation. When oxidized by aldehydes, CDKs lose their activity. Inhibition of CDKs prevents passage through the restriction point and causes checkpoint arrest which inhibits cell cycle progression, reduces rate of cell proliferation, inhibits transition of cells from G0 to G1 phase, prolongs G1 phase, and slows progression through S phase by inhibiting DNA synthesis. Oxidative stress interferes with the cytotoxic effects of antineoplastic agents on cancer cells by interfering with cell cycle. Tumor cells in G0 are unaffected by chemotherapy and can usually reenter the division cycle after chemotherapy is completed. Tumor cells can also repair damage caused by drugs that do not require ongoing DNA synthesis [43, 44].

High or sustained levels of ROS might contribute to the development of cancer [45], as shown by the inhibitory effects of antioxidants on tumor formation [46]. This effect of ROS on cancer development might be due to the role of ROS on cell proliferation, in addition to ROS induced inhibition of apoptosis or ROS mediated mutagenesis. The effect of ROS on cell proliferation depends the level of ROS present [47], low ROS level results in correct cell cycle progression whereas high level leads to uncontrolled cell proliferation, such as in cancer [48]. Second messengers such as p21 and MAPK, involved in cell proliferation, are regulated by ROS. Furthermore, ROS were shown to be important modulators of ubiquitination and phosphorylation of cell cycle associated enzymes. Evidence is accumulating regarding the central role of ROS in the regulation of cell cycle progression. In addition, ROS have recently been found to activate growth factor receptors in the absence of the growth factor receptor ligands, thereby further controlling cell proliferation [49].

ROS in Cell Differentiation

Stem cells are characterized by their ability to both self-renew to maintain the stem cell pool and also differentiate to give rise to fresh specialized tissues. Molecular mechanisms underlying cell-fate decision to renew or differentiate are not completely understood, but recent studies indicate that mitochondrial ROS (mROS) play a significant role [50]. mROS are important for human cell differentiation as well as human pluripotent stem cells were shown to repress uncoupling protein 2 during differentiation, a process that generally increases production of mROS [51]. Mitochondrial mass and oxygen consumption were also shown to increase during differentiation of human embryonic stem cells [52] as well as during differentiation of induced pluripotent stem cells [53]. Reduction of mROS by knockdown of the complex III protein (Rieske Iron Sulfur Protein) or mitochondrial-targeted antioxidants inhibit differentiation of human mesenchymal stem cells to adipocytes [54]. Owusu-Ansah et al. discovered that scavenging ROS by overexpression of GTPx-1 retards differentiation of Drosophila multipotent hematopoietic progenitors, while increasing ROS by depletion of the mitochondrial complex I protein ND75 or deletion of SOD2 increased differentiation [55].

ROS in Inflammation

Chronic inflammation is associated with a high cancer risk [56]. Epidemiological and experimental data suggest a link between inflammation and cancer [57, 58] and anti-inflammatory therapies show efficacy in cancer prevention and treatment [59]. Free radicals and aldehydes produced during chronic inflammation induce deleterious gene mutation and post-translational modifications of key cancer related proteins. These molecules include transcription factors such as NF-κB, controlling the expression of cancer genes (e.g., suppressor genes and oncogenes) and key inflammatory enzymes such as inducible nitric oxide synthase and cyclooxygenase-2. Toll-like receptors; ROS and reactive nitrogen species (RNS); pro and anti-inflammatory cytokines; metals; antioxidant enzymes; peroxisome proliferator-activated receptor ligands; kinases; growth factors; and tumor suppressor proteins, p53 and retinoblastoma proteins are generated during inflammatory processes. All of them are potential targets for cancer chemoprevention and treatment. Mediators of these targets have strong potential for use as chemopreventive agents in inflammation-mediated carcinogenesis. Inflammatory bowel diseases such as Crohn disease and ulcerative colitis are associated with increased risk of colon adenocarcinoma [60, 61, 62], and chronic pancreatitis is related to an increased rate of pancreatic cancer [63]. Successful applications include the use of tumor necrosis factor-α inhibitors for Crohn disease [64] and interferon-α for hepatitis [65].

Antioxidants in many natural foods target the inflammatory cascade. These include red wine [66, 67], raw fruits and vegetables [68, 69]. Many other antioxidants such as green tea [70], curcumin [71], and garlic [72] have strong anti-inflammatory properties. Chronic inflammation is associated with immunosuppression, which is a risk factor for cancer. Current treatment strategies for diseases reactive species are frequently aimed to treat or prevent causes of inflammation. Although these strategies have led to some progress in combating with diseases overloading reactive species and associated cancers, exposure often occurs again after eradication, treatment to eradicate the causes fail, or the treatment has long-term side effects. Therefore, identification of molecules and pathways involved in chronic inflammation and cancer is critical to develop agents that might prevent progression of reactive species overload disease and cancer associated with disease progression.

Antioxidants

Minimum levels of ROS are kept due to antioxidant defense allowing useful roles of ROS to perform cell signaling and redox regulation. Antioxidants are usually present at low concentrations compared to oxidizable substrates and thereby significantly delay or prevent the oxidation of substrates. Antioxidants at physiological levels prevent or quench free radical formation or chelate redox metals. Antioxidants work in aqueous and/or membrane domains and effect gene expression in a positive way. Cellular redox homeostasis is maintained by the endogenous antioxidant defense system, which includes antioxidant enzymes such as superoxide dismutase (SOD), catalase (CAT), glutathione peroxidase (GPx), glutathione (GSH), proteins, and low-molecular-weight scavengers, such as uric acid, coenzyme Q, and lipoic acid. Oxidatively damaged nucleic acids are repaired by specific enzymes, oxidized proteins are removed by proteolytic systems, and oxidized lipids are repaired by phospholipases, peroxidases, and acyl transferases [73]. Antioxidants, like vitamin C and E, carotenoids, and polyphenols (e.g., flavonoids) are the main exogenous antioxidants. Clinical studies imply that eating a diet rich in fruits, vegetables, whole grains, legumes, and omega-3 fatty acids helps humans in disease prevention [74]. Large amounts of antioxidant nutrients can also act as pro-oxidants and increases oxidative stress [75, 76].

Vitamin E and its members tocopherols and tocotrienols have strong association with prevention of cancer and inhibition of tumor growth both *in vitro* and *in vivo* [77, 78]. It was demonstrated that vitamin E has an effective role in preventing chemotherapy resistance in cancer cells and a protective role in acute interstitial disease [79]. γ-Tocopheryl quinone induced endoplasmatic reticulum stress and mutagenesis *in vitro* whereas α-tocopheryl quinone had no such an effect [80, 81]. γ-Tocopherol is nitrated to form the 5-nitro-γ-tocopherol and thereby traps RNS more effectively than α-tocopherol. It was demonstrated that nitrogen dioxide induced single-strand DNA break in V79 lung cells, however, this reaction was efficiently inhibited by γ-tocopherol. Separate or combined consumption of selenium and vitamin E (all-rac-α-tocopheryl acetate) in the selenium and vitamin E cancer prevention trial (SELECT) showed no benefit in decreasing bladder cancer incidence. During the course of trial, a modest number of men were diagnosed with incident bladder cancer. The results of this trial are disappointing, considering previous evidence that increased selenium and vitamin E were inversely associated with the bladder cancer risk [82]. Vitamin C is the most potent antioxidant in extracellular fluids and scavenges superoxide, hydrogen peroxide, hydroxyl radical, and peroxyl radicals, efficiently. Ascorbic acid also protects membranes against peroxidation by enhancing the activity of tocopherol [83]. It was reported that vitamin C included antioxidant mixture (vitamin C, E and selenium) given concurrently with chemotherapy (cisplatin-induced toxicity) did not cause any significant benefit in cancer patients [84]. Fuchs-Tarlovsky et al. demonstrated that supplementing cervical cancer patients with antioxidants (vitamin C, E, beta-carotene, and selenium) during treatment with cisplatinum and radiotherapy maintained hemoglobin levels above 12 g/dL, as well as increased quality of life compared with the placebo group [85]. Carotenoids inhibit free-radical reactions. Survival rates of the patients on chemotherapy supplemented with vitamin A increased in comparison with those not given vitamin A [86]. In the current meta-analysis, authors found that the administration of beta-carotene supplements alone had no overall preventive effect on both cancer incidence and mortality. In addition, no association was found within subgroup meta-analyses based on the type of prevention (primary or secondary), methodological quality of the studies, and dose of beta-carotene. However, beta-carotene supplementation alone was found to have a significant association with an increased risk of urothelial cancer, especially bladder cancer, and with a marginally increased risk of cancer among current smokers. The finding of a marginally increased cancer risk among current smokers was similar to those of the previous meta-analysis. Potential biological mechanisms have been proposed responsible for the increased risk of cancer among smokers receiving beta-carotene supplementation. Beta-carotene may act as a pro-oxidant in the presence of chronic oxidative stress such as smoking and carotenoids increase oxidative stress caused by cigarette smoking and promote toxic effects in tissues. Meta-analysis showed no increase in lung cancer risk among smokers receiving beta-carotene supplementation [87]. Two meta-analyses were reported regarding the relationship between beta-carotene supplements and lung cancer risk: one study concluded that beta-carotene supplementation was not associated with an increased incidence of lung cancer [88], and the other study reported that beta-carotene supplementation was significantly associated with an increased incidence of lung cancer, and this association was stronger in current smokers [89]. Jeon et al searched 848 articles published in the last 14 years and selected 6 randomized controlled trials among these studies for their meta-analysis, including 40,544 total participants, 20,290 in beta-carotene supplement groups, and 20,254 in placebo groups. They found no evidence of an overall primary or secondary preventive effect of beta-carotene supplements on cancer incidence and mortality. In contrast, beta-carotene supplements increased the risk of cancer incidence marginally. They conclude that the potential effects of beta-carotene supplementation, either beneficial or harmful need to be investigated further in larger clinical trials [90]. Yeon et al. reported that antioxidant vitamins such as vitamin A, β-carotene, vitamin C, and vitamin E increased significantly plasma total antioxidant capacity (TAC), and in contrast, 8-OHdG level was negatively associated with vitamin A and β-carotene intake. Furthermore, antioxidants were reported to decrease oxidative DNA damage in cultured cells and in humans [91]. They concluded that fruit and vegetable consumption, and associated increase in TAC, are important for the prevention of breast cancer.

N-acetyl cysteine (NAC) administration to cancer patients has been based on the assumption that NAC can increase glutathione production, leading to decreased oxidative stress related cytotoxicity [92]. In our previous study, NAC diminished oxidative stress induced by bleomycin and H_2O_2 leading to decreased apoptosis in testicular germ tumor cells. On the basis of our findings, we proposed that concurrent use of NAC with bleomycin should be avoided, or at least followed carefully during conventional treatment of testicular cancer patients [8]. Co-incubation with NAC couldn't reverse Bleomycin and H_2O_2 induced increase in Caspase-8 activity in NCCIT cells, indicating that NAC does not protect NCCIT cells from Bleomycin- and H_2O_2-induced death receptor (extrinsic) pathway of apoptosis [93]. We conclude that NAC mediated suppression of Bleomycin-and H_2O_2-induced apoptosis in NCCIT cells involves mainly inactivation of signalling molecules in the mitochondrial pathway of apoptosis. NAC had no effect on the death receptor pathway of apoptosis induced by Bleomycin and H_2O_2 incubation in NCCIT cells. Quercetin is a flavonoid with anticancer properties. It was reported that quercetin inhibited ROS production in lipopolysaccharide-stimulated monocytic leukemia cell line [94]. Quercetin inhibited the activity of taxol (without altering the microtubule targeting of taxol) to induce G2/M arrest in colorectal cancer cells [95]. It was concluded that long-term exposure of cancer cells to quercetin prevents cell proliferation and survival, and the interference of quercetin with cell-cycle progression diminishes the efficacy of microtubule-targeting drugs such as taxol to arrest cells at G2/M [95]. Amifostine was shown to protect normal, but not malignant cells against radicals and anticancer drugs. Amifostine provided significant protection against mucositis in paclitaxel treated ovarian cancer patients [96]. Amifostine reduced frequency of severe esophagitis after chemotherapy and radiotherapy in non-small-cell lung cancer [97].

Curcumin (diferuloylmethane) is the chief component of the spice turmeric and is isolated from *Curcuma longa*. Curcumin is responsible for the yellow color of the spice as well as the majority of turmeric's therapeutic effects [98]. Curcumin was reported to have anticancer activities both *in vitro* in many cancer cell lines and *in vivo* models. Several reports documented its antiproliferative effect on cultured cells such as on colon cancer [99] and breast cancer cells [100]. Curcumin was reported to suppress cell proliferation and inflammation, induce apoptosis, sensitize tumor cells to cancer therapies, and suppress invasion, angiogenesis, and metastasis of cancer cells [101]. Cort et al. reported that curcumin presented synergistic anticancer activity with bleomycin in human malignant testicular germ cells [102]. In another study, curcumin decreased oxidative stress in germ cells induced by bleomycin, without decreasing chemotherapeutic effect of bleomycin. It can be concluded that curcumin has certain inhibitory effects on oxidative stress and its concomitant use with bleomycin should be followed closely during the treatment of testicular cancer [103]. It was reported that concurrent use of tannic acid or procyanidins recovered cardiotoxicity induced by doxorubicin. Tannic acid ameliorated doxorubicin-induced cardiotoxicity and potentiated its anticancer activity in both *in vitro* and *in vivo* animal models of mammary tumor [104]. In an *in vitro* cytotoxic study, procyanidins protected cardiomyocytes from doxorubicin-induced cardiotoxicity via suppression of oxidative stress [105]. Green tea polyphenols especially epigallocatechin-3-gallate (EGCG), have preventive effects against cancer by inhibiting growth factor signaling, key cellular enzymes, gene transcription, and induction of tumor suppressor genes. EGCG is a strong radical scavenger and a metal chelator. It was reported that EGCG decreased hepatic levels of lipid peroxides and protein carbonyls and increased hepatic levels of antioxidants and antioxidant enzymes. Green tea catechins increased survival time and decreased tumor load in mice with multiple mammary adenocarcinoma [106].

Resveratrol found in grapes, nuts, fruits, and red wine, is a potent antioxidant with cancer-preventive properties [107]. Resveratrol is a chemosensitizing agent and can act as a chemotherapeutic adjuvant particularly due to its effect, on cell cycle arrest, cyclins and Cdks modulations, and apoptosis induction in some cancer models [108, 109]. Aires et al. reported that pretreatment of human colon carcinoma cells with resveratrol induced DNA damages synergized with irinotecan's active metabolite SN38 and also with oxaliplatin to induce cancer cells death [110]. Rath et al proposed a new novel strategy in the therapeutic use of nutrient synergy as an effective way to control the critical processes of cancer, including metastasis, angiogenesis, cell proliferation, and apoptosis. The nutrient synergy proposed by research group consisted of a mixture of: ascorbic acid, l-lysine, l-proline, l-arginine, NAC, EGCG, selenium, copper and manganese [111]. Their claim was to control all types of cancers by optimum therapeutic dosage of certain essential nutrients especially in combination. The use of nutrient synergy was found to be effective in a variety of cancer cell types, including solid tumors, leukemias, HTLV-1 (Human T-lymphotropic virus 1) virus-derived leukemia, breast and prostate cancers [112, 113]. The pro-apoptotic effect of nutrient synergy on cancer cells was indicated by the up-regulation of p53, p21, and Bax protein expression and decrease in Bcl-2, as well as cell cycle arrest, up-regulation of TGF-beta, and the decline in TGF-alpha cytokine expression [114]. The nutrient synergy inhibited proliferation and induced apoptosis in both HTLV-1-infected and noninfected cell lines [115]. Treatment with a diet containing lysine, proline, arginine, ascorbic acid, and green tea extract to athymic nude mice implanted with human melanoma A2058 cells strongly suppressed tumor growth with inhibition of MMP-9 (Matrix metallopeptidase 9) and VEGF (Vascular endothelial growth factor) secretion [116]. Roomi et al. reported the therapeutic potential of a novel nutrient mixture (consisting of ascorbic acid, lysine, proline, and green tea extract) in the treatment of hepatocellular carcinoma *in vitro* as well as *in vivo* [117]. Mukhtar et al. proposed a certain phytococktail, in which various natural and synthetic products were mixed in concentrations that could easily be consumed by humans [118]. Long lasting cancer chemopreventive effects in humans might be achieved by the use different agents in the cocktails via acting on different molecular pathways. Table 1 shows the effects of antioxidants on toxicity induced by chemotherapeutic agents.

Transcription factor Nuclear factor (erythroid-derived 2)-like 2 (Nrf2) which regulates physiological antioxidant pathways and activates cytoprotective genes [119]. Transcription of

Nrf2 induced by several oncogenes, mediates a ROS detoxification program required for tumour initiation. Kelch-like ECH-associated protein 1 (KEAP1)–NRF2 pathway is used as an adaptive mechanism by tumours to keep their ROS status. KEAP1 is a repressor protein that promotes NRF2 degradation. High ROS levels are balanced by this pathway. Mutations in NRF2 or KEAP1 are seen in lung, head-and-neck, and bladder cancers [120]; these mutations enhance NRF2 activity and are associated with resistance to standard chemotherapy and poor survival from cancer [121]. Treatment of C57bl/6J mice with EGCG increased gene expression of γ-glutamyltransferase, glutamate cysteine ligase, and hemeoxygenase-1 in an Nrf2-antioxidant response element-dependent manner [122]. Similar results were reported in the tumor cells of colon cancer xenograft-bearing nude mice treated with dietary EGCG [123]. EGCG mediated hemeoxygenase-1 and SOD enhancement were inhibited by siRNA disruption of Nrf2 in human mammary epithelial cells. It was concluded that Nrf2 has a role in the EGCG-mediated induction of endogenous antioxidant systems [120]. Nrf2 transcription is regulated by the K-Ras oncogene through a Mek–Erk–Jun pathway, and causes a reduction in ROS in primary fibroblasts. This effect depends on the levels of oncogene activation: expression of K-Ras at 'endogenous' levels, close to those observed as tumour cells develop from normal cells, reduces ROS levels, whereas huge increases in K-Ras expression induce cellular stress and increase ROS levels. It was shown that antioxidants are induced in the early stages of K-Ras-driven pancreatic-cancer development in mice. Transcriptional activation of Nrf2 is part of the tumorigenic activity of oncogenes and therefore contributes to the development of other malignancies such as lung cancer. It is concluded that a stress-response program is turned on early in tumour development; and oncogene activity is coupled with the transcriptional induction of Nrf2. Nrf2-mediated adaptation to ROS stress is crucial for early stages of tumour development, and if blocked may slow cancer progression.

Redox metabolism, homeostasis of ROS and their detoxification, is critical in cell signalling and regulation of apoptosis. An increase in the generation of ROS, or a reduction in their detoxification, such as depletion of glutathione, induces apoptosis through depolarisation and permeabilisation of the mitochondrial membrane. The content of GSH in some tumor cells is typically associated with higher levels of GSH-related enzymes, such as γ-glutamylcysteine ligase (GCL) and γ-glutamyl-transpeptidase (GGT) activities, as well as a higher expression of GSH-transporting export pumps. Depleting GSH by inhibiting GCL, a key enzyme of GSH biosynthesis is a hot topic in this research field [124]. A key mechanism for GSH's cell proliferative role in DNA synthesis is related to the maintenance of reduced glutaredoxin or thioredoxin, which is required for the activity of ribonucleotide reductase, the rate-limiting enzyme in DNA synthesis. GSH levels are associated with cellular proliferation and metastatic activity of cancer cells [125]. A high percentage of tumor cells with high GSH content were shown to survive in the presence of oxidative stress, thereby representing the main task force in metastatic invasion [126]. Maintenance of high intracellular levels of GSH are critical for the growth of metastatic cells.

Mitogenesis and cell proliferation induced by ROS such as H_2O_2 and superoxide anion in has been demonstrated in several mammalian cell types [127]; and a reduction in cellular oxidants via supplementation with antioxidants such as superoxide dismutase, catalasc, β-carotene, and flavonoids inhibits cell proliferation *in vitro* [128]. However, high concentrations of ROS can trigger apoptotic or necrotic cell death [129, 130, 131].

Due to the critical role of ROS in initiating or promoting malignant phenotypes of tumor cells, treating ROS-induced diseases such as cancer with antioxidants has been accepted as a therapeutic approach [132]. Indeed, dietary antioxidants such as green tea polyphenols and curcumin have been recommended for cancer prevention [133, 102]. However, usage of antioxidant supplementation is currently receiving much attention because of epidemiological studies linking the use of some antioxidants with increased mortality in primarily higher-risk populations and lack of strong efficacy data for protection against cancer, at least in populations with adequate baseline dietary consumption [4] [134]. In addition to dietary antioxidant therapy, several other strategies have emerged to reverse cancerous phenotype through reducing oxidant stress. Three studies reported possible drug interactions with the administration of high dose nutraceuticals [135].

The first study concluded that a possible drug interaction occurred between the chemotherapy regime and magnesium and calcium infusions [136]. The second study with glutamine indicated a reduced cytotoxicity from the paclitaxel administered [137]. The third clinical study with vitamin B6 showed a significant decrease in the response rate with cisplatin [138].

Pro-Oxidants

Pro-oxidants are chemicals that induce oxidative stress, usually through the formation of ROS or by inhibiting antioxidant systems [139]. Antioxidants scavenge directly initiating pro-oxidant species. Antioxidant systems effectively keep the level of pro-oxidants below a critical threshold in a healthy cell. Free radicals are considered as pro-oxidants, and antioxidants also might have pro-oxidant behaviour. β-Carotene possesses pro-oxidant properties in several cell models. Its pro-oxidant effects include oxidative damage to the cell structures (DNA, lipids and proteins) or, a modulation of redox-sensitive genes and transcription factors.

The presence of antioxidants may limit the pro-oxidant character of the carotenoid [140]. Vitamin C is considered as a potent antioxidant and pro-oxidant. Pro-oxidant character happens when it combines with iron and copper reducing Fe^{3+} to Fe^{2+}, which in turn reduces hydrogen peroxide to hydroxyl radicals. The pro-oxidant activity induced by ascorbic acid is comparable to that observed for many other anticancer drugs, such as arsenic trioxide, which is currently being used for treatment of acute promyelocitic leukemia (APL) and is also being evaluated for treating solid tumors. Pathi et al. demonstrated that ascorbate-induced cell death is associated with its pro-oxidant activity [141]. α-Tocopherol is also known to be a useful and powerful antioxidant but in high concentrations it acts as a pro-oxidant. When it reacts with a free radical, it becomes a radical itself, and if there is not enough ascorbic acid for its regeneration, it will remain in this highly reactive state. Flavonoids can act as pro-oxidants, although each one responds differently to the environment in which it is inserted. Dietary phenolics can also act as pro-oxidants in systems that contain redox-active metals. The presence of O_2 and transition metals like iron and copper catalyze the redox cycling of phenolics and may lead to the formation of ROS and phenoxyl radicals which damage DNA, lipids and other biological molecules. Phenolic acids, are considered as antioxidants but under certain conditions behave as pro-oxidants [142]. Under certain conditions (high concentrations of phenolic antioxidants, high pH, presence of iron) phenolic antioxidants initiate an auto-oxidation process and behave like pro-oxidants.

Table1. Effects of antioxidants on toxicity induced by chemotherapeutic agents

Compound	*In vitro* and *in vivo* studies demonstrating the effects of compounds on toxicity in different types of cancers	Therapeutic efficacy of drug
Vitamin E	Potentiates the apoptotic effects of paclitaxel and doxorubicin in hepatocellular carcinoma [143] and bladder cancer [144], lung cancer [145[. Increases intracellular accumulation of doxorubicin in multidrug resistance tumor cells [146]. Synergistic anticancer response with chemotherapeutic agents in breast cancer [147].	Increased
Vitamin C	Phenylaminonaphthoquinones with ascorbate [148] induce cell cycle arrest in human bladder cancer cell. Ascorbic acid does not block the anticancer effects of paclitaxel [149]. Vitamin C enhances the antitumor activity of 5-FU (Fluorouracil), cisplatin and bleomycin in esophageal cancer [87] and bleomycin in breast cancer [139]. Ascorbic acid suppresses photodynamic therapy induced cell death in sarcoma cancer cells[150]. Vitamins A, C and E increased irinotecan-induced DNA lesions in lymphocytes cells [151]	Increased
Vitamin A	Increased sensitization to doxorubicin, paclitaxel, and radiation in breast [152] and lung [153] cancers, glioblastoma [154]. Synergistic effect when combined with cisplatin in nasopharyngeal cancer [155].	Increased
Flavonoids	Synergistic effect with taxol in prostate cancer [156]. Apigenin and luteolin potentiate anti-proliferative effect of chemotherapeutic drugs in pancreatic cancer [157]. Xanthohumol increases sensitization to doxorubicin and radiotherapy in breast cancer [158]. EGCG inhibits bladder cancer cell invasion [159] . Tectorigenin chemosensitize paclitaxel-induced cytotoxicity in ovarian cancer [160].	Increased
Polyphenols	Resveratrol [161] induces apoptosis associated with mitochondrial dysfunction in bladder carcinoma cells. Tea polyphenols and cisplatin synergistically induced apoptosis in breast cancer cells [162].	Increased

There is a considerable amount of evidence to suggest the pro-oxidative potential of polyphenols, hepatic, intestinal and renal toxicities of high doses of polyphenols and potential DNA damaging effects and leukemiogenic activities of flavonoids. It was demonstrated that the EGCG, is unstable under cell culture conditions and undergoes oxidative polymerization with co-generation of H_2O_2. The oxidative stress generated may have implications regarding potential toxicity of these compounds. Treatment of rat hepatocytes with EGCG reduced cell viability by increased production of ROS and depletion of reduced glutathione [111].

Although consumption of polyphenols has been suggested to have beneficial biological effects in cancer chemoprevention, there is considerable evidence suggesting that such compounds are not without risk of adverse effects. The effective final concentrations of ROS in cancer cells are important for the pro-oxidant cancer therapy. For patients presenting a low ROS level in cancer cells, higher doses of agents might be required. However, some advanced tumors that have developed an enhanced anti-oxidant system to adapt to increased oxidative stress might embrace a low level of ROS and high chemo-resistance. Clearly, more research is needed to better understand the effects of antioxidants, whether positive or negative, particularly in the context of dose, timing, duration, and susceptibility of consumers to disease.

Conclusıon

The probability that antioxidants interfere with the conventional cancer treatments, which are designed to prevent the mortality of cancer patients, is a complex issue. Although numerous chemotherapy drugs induce the formation of ROS, their anticancer effects do not, in general, depend on the formation of these free radicals [163, 164]. They act by blocking the synthesis of DNA precursors, damaging the integrity of DNA, or interfering with DNA replication, separation of the two double helixes after replication, or the function of the mitotic spindle [165, 166, 167]. Antioxidant supplementation may in certain circumstances aid the prevention of free radical induced side effects without inhibiting the positive effects of the chemotherapy and provide a safe and effective means of enhancing the response to cancer chemotherapy. The cancer cells should divide rapidly for the cytotoxic effect of pro-oxidant anticancer agents. Excess ROS in cancer cells slows or arrests cell growth and interferes with the effectiveness of chemotherapy since anticancer drugs are effective only when there is rapid cell proliferation. Antioxidant supplementation during chemotherapy may overcome the growth-inhibiting effects of oxidative stress and maintain responsiveness to anti-neoplastic agents [168].

Tumour cells can bypass normal responses to cellular stress by switching on programs driven by oncogenic mutations and changes in metabolism that allow sustained growth even in conditions where nutrients and oxygen are scarce. This state is accompanied by the generation of potentially toxic by-products, including ROS. Although, high ROS levels are harmful to normal cells, they may help tumour development by inducing DNA damage and accelerating the rate of cancer-causing mutations; activating inflammatory pathways; and stabilizing the hypoxia-inducible factor a key regulator of energy metabolism. These cancer-promoting actions of ROS can be prevented by antioxidants such as Resveratrol [169], EGCG [170]. Additional studies are required to define whether such supplements can either increase or decrease cancer risk depending on the presence of specific predisposing oncogenic lesions. As for the implications of these findings for cancer treatment, large clinical trials are needed to clarify to demonstrate if the cancer cells become more vulnerable to death by oxidative stress [120].

Antioxidants can reduce or prevent many side effects of anticancer drugs, and the protective effects of some supplements are not always due to their antioxidant properties. The antioxidant status of cancer patients plays an important role in their response to chemotherapy. However, supportive nutritional therapy with antioxidants during chemotherapy reduces the level of ROS generated by cancer treatment, overcomes growth-inhibiting effects of oxidative stress and disturbs responsiveness to antineoplastic agents [171]. There is considerable data suggesting that antioxidants enhance effectiveness of conventional treatments and decrease some of the serious side effects of radiation and chemotherapy. Consequently, antioxidant supplementation may in some circumstances help to prevent free radical-induced side effects without inhibiting the positive effects of the chemotherapy and provide a safe and effective means of enhancing response to cancer chemotherapy. Frequently, the effects of antioxidants with chemotherapy and radiation were found to be synergistic [102].

Patients tolerated standard treatment better, had less weigth loss, had better life quality, and lived longer than patients receiving no supplements. The data accumulated so far supports the concurrent use of chemotherapy with dietary antioxidants [172]. Whether or not an antioxidant supplement would be helpful, harmful, or neutral depends on the specific antioxidant and its dose and timing, the chemotherapy drugs being used, the type of cancer being treated and the type of diet the patient is consuming. Clinical data relying on good randomized clinical trials are relatively rare in the field. Well designed randomized controlled trials are needed to fully elucidate the impact of single antioxidants and antioxidant combinations in conventional cancer therapy.

In several studies, antioxidant supplementation has resulted in increased survival times, increased tumor response, or both, as well as less toxicities than controls [173, 174]. There is no evidence of antioxidant interference with chemotherapy mechanisms in current literature. In contrast, antioxidants may even improve tumor response or patient survival [175]. Large clinical trials are needed to clarify the effects of antioxidants on chemotherapy and its side effects.

References

[1] Cadenas E. Biochemistry of oxygen toxicity. *Annu. Rev. Biochem.,* 1989;58:79-110.

[2] Valko M, Rhodes CJ, Moncol J, Izakovic M, Mazur M. Free radicals, metals and antioxidants in oxidative stress-induced cancer. *Chem. Biol. Interact.,* 2006 Mar 10;160(1):1-40.

[3] Trachootham D, Alexandre J, Huang P. Targeting cancer cells by ROS-mediated mechanisms: a radical therapeutic approach? *Nat. Rev Drug. Discov.,* 2009 Jul;8(7): 579-91.

[4] Wang J, Yi J. Cancer cell killing via ROS: to increase or decrease, that is the question. *Cancer Biol. Ther.,* 2008 Dec;7(12):1875-84.

[5] Fleury C, Mignotte B, Vayssiere JL. Mitochondrial reactive oxygen species in cell death signaling. *Biochimie,* 2002 Feb-Mar;84(2-3):131-41.

[6] Cort A, Timur M, Ozdemir E, Kucuksayan E, Ozben T. Synergistic anticancer activity of curcumin and bleomycin: an in vitro study using human malignant testicular germ cells. *Mol. Med. Report.,* 2012 Jun;5(6):1481-6.

[7] Yen CY, Chiu CC, Haung RW, Yeh CC, Huang KJ, Chang KF, et al. Antiproliferative effects of goniothalamin on Ca9-22 oral cancer cells through apoptosis, DNA damage and ROS induction. *Mutat. Res.*, 2012 Sep 18;747(2):253-8.
[8] Cort A, Ozdemir E, Timur M, Ozben T. Effects of N-acetyl-L-cysteine on bleomycin induced oxidative stress in malignant testicular germ cell tumors. *Biochimie,* 2012 Dec;94(12):2734-9.
[9] Renschler MF. The emerging role of reactive oxygen species in cancer therapy. *Eur. J. Cancer,* 2004 Sep;40(13):1934-40.
[10] Pelicano H, Carney D, Huang P. ROS stress in cancer cells and therapeutic implications. *Drug Resist. Updat.,* 2004 Apr;7(2):97-110.
[11] Schumacker PT. Reactive oxygen species in cancer cells: live by the sword, die by the sword. *Cancer Cell,* 2006 Sep;10(3):175-6.
[12] Waris G, Ahsan H. Reactive oxygen species: role in the development of cancer and various chronic conditions. *J. Carcinog.,* 2006;5:14.
[13] Trachootham D, Zhou Y, Zhang H, Demizu Y, Chen Z, Pelicano H, et al. Selective killing of oncogenically transformed cells through a ROS-mediated mechanism by beta-phenylethyl isothiocyanate. *Cancer Cell,* 2006 Sep;10(3):241-52.
[14] Hagen T, D'Amico G, Quintero M, Palacios-Callender M, Hollis V, Lam F, et al. Inhibition of mitochondrial respiration by the anticancer agent 2-methoxyestradiol. *Biochem. Biophys. Res, Commun.,* 2004 Sep 24;322(3):923-9.
[15] Chen Y, McMillan-Ward E, Kong J, Israels SJ, Gibson SB. Oxidative stress induces autophagic cell death independent of apoptosis in transformed and cancer cells. *Cell Death Differ.,* 2008 Jan;15(1):171-82.
[16] Simon HU, Haj-Yehia A, Levi-Schaffer F. Role of reactive oxygen species (ROS) in apoptosis induction. *Apoptosis,* 2000 Nov;5(5):415-8.
[17] Reinehr R, Becker S, Eberle A, Grether-Beck S, Haussinger D. Involvement of NADPH oxidase isoforms and Src family kinases in CD95-dependent hepatocyte apoptosis. *J. Biol. Chem.,* 2005 Jul 22;280(29):27179-94.
[18] Wang X, Zhang J, Xu T. Cyclophosphamide as a potent inhibitor of tumor thioredoxin reductase in vivo. *Toxicol. Appl. Pharmacol.,* 2007 Jan 1;218(1):88-95.
[19] Benhar M, Engelberg D, Levitzki A. ROS, stress-activated kinases and stress signaling in cancer. *EMBO Rep.,* 2002 May;3(5):420-5.
[20] Son YO, Hitron JA, Cheng S, Budhraja A, Zhang Z, Lan Guo N, et al. The dual roles of c-Jun NH2-terminal kinase signaling in Cr(VI)-induced apoptosis in JB6 cells. *Toxicol. Sci.,* 2011 Feb;119(2):335-45.
[21] Ahn J, Won M, Choi JH, Kim YS, Jung CR, Im DS, et al. Reactive oxygen species-mediated activation of the Akt/ASK1/p38 signaling cascade and p21(Cip1) downregulation are required for shikonin-induced apoptosis. *Apoptosis,* 2013 Jul;18(7):870-81.
[22] Liu JM, Pan F, Li L, Liu QR, Chen Y, Xiong XX, et al. Piperlongumine selectively kills glioblastoma multiforme cells via reactive oxygen species accumulation dependent JNK and p38 activation. *Biochem. Biophys. Res. Commun.,* 2013 Jun 22.
[23] Levine B, Yuan J. Autophagy in cell death: an innocent convict? *J. Clin. Invest.,* 2005 Oct;115(10):2679-88.
[24] Cuervo AM. Autophagy: in sickness and in health. *Trends Cell Biol.,* 2004 Feb;14 (2):70-7.

[25] Shintani T, Klionsky DJ. Autophagy in health and disease: a double-edged sword. *Science,* 2004 Nov 5;306(5698):990-5.

[26] Huang J, Lam GY, Brumell JH. Autophagy signaling through reactive oxygen species. *Antioxid. Redox. Signal.,* 2011 Jun;14(11):2215-31.

[27] Scherz-Shouval R, Shvets E, Fass E, Shorer H, Gil L, Elazar Z. Reactive oxygen species are essential for autophagy and specifically regulate the activity of Atg4. *EMBO J.,* 2007 Apr 4;26(7):1749-60.

[28] Liang XH, Jackson S, Seaman M, Brown K, Kempkes B, Hibshoosh H, et al. Induction of autophagy and inhibition of tumorigenesis by beclin 1. *Nature,* 1999 Dec 9;402(6762):672-6.

[29] Qu X, Yu J, Bhagat G, Furuya N, Hibshoosh H, Troxel A, et al. Promotion of tumorigenesis by heterozygous disruption of the beclin 1 autophagy gene. *J. Clin. Invest.,* 2003 Dec;112(12):1809-20.

[30] Yue Z, Jin S, Yang C, Levine AJ, Heintz N. Beclin 1, an autophagy gene essential for early embryonic development, is a haploinsufficient tumor suppressor. *Proc. Natl. Acad. Sci. USA,* 2003 Dec 9;100(25):15077-82.

[31] Ling LU, Tan KB, Lin H, Chiu GN. The role of reactive oxygen species and autophagy in safingol-induced cell death. *Cell Death Dis.,* 2011;2:e129.

[32] Gibson SB. A matter of balance between life and death: targeting reactive oxygen species (ROS)-induced autophagy for cancer therapy. *Autophagy,* 2010 Oct;6(7):835-7.

[33] Azad MB, Chen Y, Gibson SB. Regulation of autophagy by reactive oxygen species (ROS): implications for cancer progression and treatment. *Antioxid. Redox. Signal,* 2009 Apr;11(4):777-90.

[34] Liu B, Cheng Y, Zhang B, Bian HJ, Bao JK. Polygonatum cyrtonema lectin induces apoptosis and autophagy in human melanoma A375 cells through a mitochondria-mediated ROS-p38-p53 pathway. *Cancer Lett.,* 2009 Mar 8;275(1):54-60.

[35] Rigoulet M, Yoboue ED, Devin A. Mitochondrial ROS generation and its regulation: mechanisms involved in H(2)O(2) signaling. *Antioxid. Redox. Signal.,* 2011 Feb 1;14(3):459-68.

[36] Dalby KN, Tekedereli I, Lopez-Berestein G, Ozpolat B. Targeting the prodeath and prosurvival functions of autophagy as novel therapeutic strategies in cancer. *Autophagy,* 2010 Apr;6(3):322-9.

[37] Li ZY, Yang Y, Ming M, Liu B. Mitochondrial ROS generation for regulation of autophagic pathways in cancer. *Biochem. Biophys. Res. Commun.,* 2011 Oct 14;414(1): 5-8.

[38] Brunk UT, Dalen H, Roberg K, Hellquist HB. Photo-oxidative disruption of lysosomal membranes causes apoptosis of cultured human fibroblasts. *Free Radic. Biol. Med.,* 1997;23(4):616-26.

[39] Thorpe GW, Fong CS, Alic N, Higgins VJ, Dawes IW. Cells have distinct mechanisms to maintain protection against different reactive oxygen species: oxidative-stress-response genes. *Proc. Natl. Acad. Sci. USA,* 2004 Apr 27;101(17):6564-9.

[40] Yang S, Wang X, Contino G, Liesa M, Sahin E, Ying H, et al. Pancreatic cancers require autophagy for tumor growth. *Genes Dev.,* 2011 Apr 1;25(7):717-29.

[41] Boonstra J, Post JA. Molecular events associated with reactive oxygen species and cell cycle progression in mammalian cells. *Gene,* 2004 Aug 4;337:1-13.

[42] Diaz-Moralli S, Tarrado-Castellarnau M, Miranda A, Cascante M. Targeting cell cycle regulation in cancer therapy. *Pharmacol. Ther.,* 2013 May;138(2):255-71.

[43] Conklin KA. Cancer chemotherapy and antioxidants. *J. Nutr.,* 2004 Nov;134(11): 3201S-4S.

[44] Conklin KA. Chemotherapy-associated oxidative stress: impact on chemotherapeutic effectiveness. *Integr. Cancer Ther.,* 2004 Dec;3(4):294-300.

[45] Ralph SJ, Rodriguez-Enriquez S, Neuzil J, Moreno-Sanchez R. Bioenergetic pathways in tumor mitochondria as targets for cancer therapy and the importance of the ROS-induced apoptotic trigger. *Mol. Aspects Med.,* 2010 Feb;31(1):29-59.

[46] Zhang Y, Zhao W, Zhang HJ, Domann FE, Oberley LW. Overexpression of copper zinc superoxide dismutase suppresses human glioma cell growth. *Cancer Res.,* 2002 Feb 15;62(4):1205-12.

[47] Deshpande SS, Irani K. Oxidant signalling in carcinogenesis: a commentary. *Hum. Exp. Toxicol.,* 2002 Feb;21(2):63-4.

[48] Verbon EH, Post JA, Boonstra J. The influence of reactive oxygen species on cell cycle progression in mammalian cells. *Gene,* 2012 Dec 10;511(1):1-6.

[49] Inoguchi T, Sonta T, Tsubouchi H, Etoh T, Kakimoto M, Sonoda N, et al. Protein kinase C-dependent increase in reactive oxygen species (ROS) production in vascular tissues of diabetes: role of vascular NAD(P)H oxidase. *J. Am. Soc. Nephrol.,* 2003 Aug;14(8 Suppl 3):S227-32.

[50] Sena LA, Chandel NS. Physiological roles of mitochondrial reactive oxygen species. *Mol. Cell,* 2012 Oct 26;48(2):158-67.

[51] Zhang J, Khvorostov I, Hong JS, Oktay Y, Vergnes L, Nuebel E, et al. UCP2 regulates energy metabolism and differentiation potential of human pluripotent stem cells. *EMBO J.,* 2011 Dec 14;30(24):4860-73.

[52] Cho YM, Kwon S, Pak YK, Seol HW, Choi YM, Park do J, et al. Dynamic changes in mitochondrial biogenesis and antioxidant enzymes during the spontaneous differentiation of human embryonic stem cells. *Biochem. Biophys. Res. Commun.,* 2006 Oct 6;348(4):1472-8.

[53] Prigione A, Adjaye J. Modulation of mitochondrial biogenesis and bioenergetic metabolism upon in vitro and in vivo differentiation of human ES and iPS cells. *Int. J. Dev. Biol.,* 2010;54(11-12):1729-41.

[54] Tormos KV, Anso E, Hamanaka RB, Eisenbart J, Joseph J, Kalyanaraman B, et al. Mitochondrial complex III ROS regulate adipocyte differentiation. *Cell Metab.,* 2011 Oct 5;14(4):537-44.

[55] Owusu-Ansah E, Banerjee U. Reactive oxygen species prime Drosophila haematopoietic progenitors for differentiation. *Nature,* 2009 Sep 24;461(7263):537-41.

[56] Hofseth LJ, Ying L. Identifying and defusing weapons of mass inflammation in carcinogenesis. *Biochim. Biophys. Acta.,* 2006 Jan;1765(1):74-84.

[57] Grivennikov SI, Greten FR, Karin M. Immunity, inflammation, and cancer. *Cell,* 2010 Mar 19;140(6):883-99.

[58] Grivennikov SI, Karin M. Inflammation and oncogenesis: a vicious connection. *Curr. Opin. Genet. Dev.,* 2010 Feb;20(1):65-71.

[59] Gonda TA, Tu S, Wang TC. Chronic inflammation, the tumor microenvironment and carcinogenesis. *Cell Cycle,* 2009 Jul 1;8(13):2005-13.

[60] Ekbom A, Helmick C, Zack M, Adami HO. Increased risk of large-bowel cancer in Crohn's disease with colonic involvement. *Lancet,* 1990 Aug 11;336(8711):357-9.

[61] Ekbom A, Helmick C, Zack M, Adami HO. Ulcerative colitis and colorectal cancer. A population-based study. *N. Engl. J. Med.,* 1990 Nov 1;323(18):1228-33.

[62] Gillen CD, Walmsley RS, Prior P, Andrews HA, Allan RN. Ulcerative colitis and Crohn's disease: a comparison of the colorectal cancer risk in extensive colitis. *Gut,* 1994 Nov;35(11):1590-2.

[63] Ekbom A, McLaughlin JK, Nyren O. Pancreatitis and the risk of pancreatic cancer. *N. Engl. J. Med.,* 1993 Nov 11;329(20):1502-3.

[64] Hanauer SB, Sandborn WJ, Rutgeerts P, Fedorak RN, Lukas M, MacIntosh D, et al. Human anti-tumor necrosis factor monoclonal antibody (adalimumab) in Crohn's disease: the CLASSIC-I trial. *Gastroenterology,* 2006 Feb;130(2):323-33; quiz 591.

[65] Feld JJ, Hoofnagle JH. Mechanism of action of interferon and ribavirin in treatment of hepatitis C. *Nature,* 2005 Aug 18;436(7053):967-72.

[66] Estruch R, Sacanella E, Badia E, Antunez E, Nicolas JM, Fernandez-Sola J, et al. Different effects of red wine and gin consumption on inflammatory biomarkers of atherosclerosis: a prospective randomized crossover trial. Effects of wine on inflammatory markers. *Atherosclerosis,* 2004 Jul;175(1):117-23.

[67] Luceri C, Caderni G, Sanna A, Dolara P. Red wine and black tea polyphenols modulate the expression of cycloxygenase-2, inducible nitric oxide synthase and glutathione-related enzymes in azoxymethane-induced f344 rat colon tumors. *J. Nutr.,* 2002 Jun;132(6):1376-9.

[68] Wannamethee SG, Lowe GD, Rumley A, Bruckdorfer KR, Whincup PH. Associations of vitamin C status, fruit and vegetable intakes, and markers of inflammation and hemostasis. *Am. J. Clin. Nutr.,* 2006 Mar;83(3):567-74; quiz 726-7.

[69] Sanchez-Moreno C, Cano MP, de Ancos B, Plaza L, Olmedilla B, Granado F, et al. High-pressurized orange juice consumption affects plasma vitamin C, antioxidative status and inflammatory markers in healthy humans. *J. Nutr.,* 2003 Jul;133(7):2204-9.

[70] Peng G, Dixon DA, Muga SJ, Smith TJ, Wargovich MJ. Green tea polyphenol (-)-epigallocatechin-3-gallate inhibits cyclooxygenase-2 expression in colon carcinogenesis. *Mol. Carcinog.,* 2006 May;45(5):309-19.

[71] Maheshwari RK, Singh AK, Gaddipati J, Srimal RC. Multiple biological activities of curcumin: a short review. *Life Sci.,* 2006 Mar 27;78(18):2081-7.

[72] Ide N, Lau BH. Garlic compounds minimize intracellular oxidative stress and inhibit nuclear factor-kappa b activation. *J. Nutr.,* 2001 Mar;131(3s):1020S-6S.

[73] Poljsak B, Suput D, Milisav I. Achieving the Balance between ROS and Antioxidants: When to Use the Synthetic Antioxidants. *Oxid. Med. Cell Longev.,* 2013;2013:956792.

[74] Willett WC. The Mediterranean diet: science and practice. *Public Health Nutr.,* 2006 Feb;9(1A):105-10.

[75] Podmore ID, Griffiths HR, Herbert KE, Mistry N, Mistry P, Lunec J. Vitamin C exhibits pro-oxidant properties. *Nature,* 1998 Apr 9;392(6676):559.

[76] Palozza P. Pro-oxidant actions of carotenoids in biologic systems. *Nutr. Rev.,* 1998 Sep;56(9):257-65.

[77] Ju J, Picinich SC, Yang Z, Zhao Y, Suh N, Kong AN, et al. Cancer-preventive activities of tocopherols and tocotrienols. *Carcinogenesis,* 2010 Apr;31(4):533-42.

[78] Yang CS, Suh N. Cancer prevention by different forms of tocopherols. *Top Curr. Chem.,* 2013;329:21-33.

[79] Zarogoulidis P, Cheva A, Zarampouka K, Huang H, Li C, Huang Y, et al. Tocopherols and tocotrienols as anticancer treatment for lung cancer: future nutrition. *J. Thorac. Dis.,* 2013 Jun;5(3):349-52.

[80] Wang X, Thomas B, Sachdeva R, Arterburn L, Frye L, Hatcher PG, et al. Mechanism of arylating quinone toxicity involving Michael adduct formation and induction of endoplasmic reticulum stress. *Proc. Natl. Acad. Sci. USA,* 2006 Mar 7;103(10):3604-9.

[81] Cornwell DG, Williams MV, Wani AA, Wani G, Shen E, Jones KH. Mutagenicity of tocopheryl quinones: evolutionary advantage of selective accumulation of dietary alpha-tocopherol. *Nutr. Cancer,* 2002;43(1):111-8.

[82] Lotan Y, Goodman PJ, Youssef RF, Svatek RS, Shariat SF, Tangen CM, et al. Evaluation of vitamin E and selenium supplementation for the prevention of bladder cancer in SWOG coordinated SELECT. *J. Urol.,* 2012 Jun;187(6):2005-10.

[83] Proteggente AR, Pannala AS, Paganga G, Van Buren L, Wagner E, Wiseman S, et al. The antioxidant activity of regularly consumed fruit and vegetables reflects their phenolic and vitamin C composition. *Free Radic. Res.,* 2002 Feb;36(2):217-33.

[84] Weijl NI, Elsendoorn TJ, Lentjes EG, Hopman GD, Wipkink-Bakker A, Zwinderman AH, et al. Supplementation with antioxidant micronutrients and chemotherapy-induced toxicity in cancer patients treated with cisplatin-based chemotherapy: a randomised, double-blind, placebo-controlled study. *Eur. J. Cancer,* 2004 Jul;40(11):1713-23.

[85] Fuchs-Tarlovsky V, Bejarano-Rosales M, Gutierrez-Salmean G, Casillas MA, Lopez-Alvarenga JC, Ceballos-Reyes GM. [Effect of antioxidant supplementation over oxidative stress and quality of life in cervical cancer]. *Nutr. Hosp.,* 2011 Jul-Aug;26(4):819-26.

[86] Israel L, Hajji O, Grefft-Alami A, Desmoulins D, Succari M, Cals MJ, et al. [Vitamin A augmentation of the effects of chemotherapy in metastatic breast cancers after menopause. Randomized trial in 100 patients]. *Ann. Med. Interne,* (Paris). 1985;136(7): 551-4.

[87] Abdel-Latif MM, Raouf AA, Sabra K, Kelleher D, Reynolds JV. Vitamin C enhances chemosensitization of esophageal cancer cells in vitro. *J. Chemother,* 2005 Oct;17(5): 539-49.

[88] Gallicchio L, Boyd K, Matanoski G, Tao XG, Chen L, Lam TK, et al. Carotenoids and the risk of developing lung cancer: a systematic review. *Am. J. Clin. Nutr.,* 2008 Aug; 88 (2): 372-83.

[89] Tanvetyanon T, Bepler G. Beta-carotene in multivitamins and the possible risk of lung cancer among smokers versus former smokers: a meta-analysis and evaluation of national brands. *Cancer,* 2008 Jul 1;113(1):150-7.

[90] Jeon YJ, Myung SK, Lee EH, Kim Y, Chang YJ, Ju W, et al. Effects of beta-carotene supplements on cancer prevention: meta-analysis of randomized controlled trials. *Nutr. Cancer,* 2011 Nov;63(8):1196-207.

[91] Yeon JY, Suh YJ, Kim SW, Baik HW, Sung CJ, Kim HS, et al. Evaluation of dietary factors in relation to the biomarkers of oxidative stress and inflammation in breast cancer risk. *Nutrition,* 2011 Sep;27(9):912-8.

[92] Lin PC, Lee MY, Wang WS, Yen CC, Chao TC, Hsiao LT, et al. N-acetylcysteine has neuroprotective effects against oxaliplatin-based adjuvant chemotherapy in colon cancer patients: preliminary data. *Support Care Cancer,* 2006 May;14(5):484-7.

[93] Cort A, Timur M, Dursun E, Kucuksayan E, Aslan M, Ozben T. Effects of N-acetylcystein on bleomycin-induced apoptosis in malignant testicular germ cell tumors. *J. Physiol. Biochem.,* 2012 Dec;68(4):555-62.

[94] Zhang M, Swarts SG, Yin L, Liu C, Tian Y, Cao Y, et al. Antioxidant properties of quercetin. *Adv. Exp. Med. Biol.,* 2011;701:283-9.

[95] Samuel T, Fadlalla K, Turner T, Yehualaeshet TE. The flavonoid quercetin transiently inhibits the activity of taxol and nocodazole through interference with the cell cycle. *Nutr. Cancer,* 2010;62(8):1025-35.

[96] Lorusso D, Ferrandina G, Greggi S, Gadducci A, Pignata S, Tateo S, et al. Phase III multicenter randomized trial of amifostine as cytoprotectant in first-line chemotherapy in ovarian cancer patients. *Ann. Oncol.,* 2003 Jul;14(7):1086-93.

[97] Komaki R, Lee JS, Kaplan B, Allen P, Kelly JF, Liao Z, et al. Randomized phase III study of chemoradiation with or without amifostine for patients with favorable performance status inoperable stage II-III non-small cell lung cancer: preliminary results. *Semin. Radiat. Oncol.,* 2002 Jan;12(1 Suppl 1):46-9.

[98] Duvoix A, Blasius R, Delhalle S, Schnekenburger M, Morceau F, Henry E, et al. Chemopreventive and therapeutic effects of curcumin. *Cancer Lett.,* 2005 Jun 8;223(2):181-90.

[99] Hanif R, Qiao L, Shiff SJ, Rigas B. Curcumin, a natural plant phenolic food additive, inhibits cell proliferation and induces cell cycle changes in colon adenocarcinoma cell lines by a prostaglandin-independent pathway. *J. Lab. Clin. Med.,* 1997 Dec;130(6): 576-84.

[100] Ramachandran C, You W. Differential sensitivity of human mammary epithelial and breast carcinoma cell lines to curcumin. *Breast Cancer Res. Treat.,* 1999 Apr;54(3): 269-78.

[101] Aggarwal BB, Kumar A, Bharti AC. Anticancer potential of curcumin: preclinical and clinical studies. *Anticancer Res.,* 2003 Jan-Feb;23(1A):363-98.

[102] Cort A, Timur M, Ozdemir E, Kucuksayan E, Ozben T. Synergistic anticancer activity of curcumin and bleomycin: an in vitro study using human malignant testicular germ cells. *Mol. Med. Rep.,* 2012 Jun;5(6):1481-6.

[103] Cort A, Ozdemir E, Timur M, Ozben T. Effects of curcumin on bleomycininduced oxidative stress in malignant testicular germ cell tumors. *Mol. Med. Rep.,* 2012 Oct;6 (4):860-6.

[104] Tikoo K, Sane MS, Gupta C. Tannic acid ameliorates doxorubicin-induced cardiotoxicity and potentiates its anti-cancer activity: potential role of tannins in cancer chemotherapy. *Toxicol. Appl. Pharmacol.,* 2011 Mar 15;251(3):191-200.

[105] Li W, Xu B, Xu J, Wu XL. Procyanidins produce significant attenuation of doxorubicin-induced cardiotoxicity via suppression of oxidative stress. *Basic Clin. Pharmacol. Toxicol.,* 2009 Mar;104(3):192-7.

[106] Lambert JD, Elias RJ. The antioxidant and pro-oxidant activities of green tea polyphenols: a role in cancer prevention. *Arch. Biochem. Biophys.,* 2010 Sep 1;501(1) :65-72.

[107] Jang M, Cai L, Udeani GO, Slowing KV, Thomas CF, Beecher CW, et al. Cancer chemopreventive activity of resveratrol, a natural product derived from grapes. *Science,* 1997 Jan 10;275(5297):218-20.

[108] Harikumar KB, Kunnumakkara AB, Sethi G, Diagaradjane P, Anand P, Pandey MK, et al. Resveratrol, a multitargeted agent, can enhance antitumor activity of gemcitabine in vitro and in orthotopic mouse model of human pancreatic cancer. *Int. J. Cancer,* 2010 Jul 15;127(2):257-68.

[109] Colin D, Gimazane A, Lizard G, Izard JC, Solary E, Latruffe N, et al. Effects of resveratrol analogs on cell cycle progression, cell cycle associated proteins and 5fluoro-uracil sensitivity in human derived colon cancer cells. *Int. J. Cancer,* 2009 Jun 15;124(12):2780-8.

[110] Aires V, Limagne E, Cotte AK, Latruffe N, Ghiringhelli F, Delmas D. Resveratrol metabolites inhibit human metastatic colon cancer cells progression and synergize with chemotherapeutic drugs to induce cell death. *Mol. Nutr. Food Res.,* 2013 Jul;57(7): 1170-81.

[111] Tabrez S, Priyadarshini M, Urooj M, Shakil S, Ashraf GM, Khan MS, et al. Cancer chemoprevention by polyphenols and their potential application as nanomedicine. *J. Environ. Sci. Health C Environ. Carcinog. Ecotoxicol. Rev.,* 2013;31(1):67-98.

[112] Roomi MW, Ivanov V, Kalinovsky T, Niedzwiecki A, Rath M. Anti-tumor effect of ascorbic acid, lysine, proline, arginine, and epigallocatechin gallate on prostate cancer cell lines PC-3, LNCaP, and DU145. *Res. Commun. Mol. Pathol. Pharmacol.,* 2004; 115-116:251-64.

[113] Roomi MW, Roomi NW, Ivanov V, Kalinovsky T, Niedzwiecki A, Rath M. Modulation of N-methyl-N-nitrosourea induced mammary tumors in Sprague-Dawley rats by combination of lysine, proline, arginine, ascorbic acid and green tea extract. *Breast Cancer Res.,* 2005;7(3):R291-5.

[114] Harakeh S, Diab-Assaf M, Niedzwiecki A, Khalife J, Abu-El-Ardat K, Rath M. Apoptosis induction by Epican Forte in HTLV-1 positive and negative malignant T-cells. *Leuk. Res.,* 2006 Jul;30(7):869-81.

[115] Harakeh S, Abdel-Massih RM, Gil PR, Sperling RA, Meinhardt A, Niedwiecki A, et al. The effect of PEG-coated gold nanoparticles on the anti-proliferative potential of Specific Nutrient Synergy. *Nanotoxicology,* 2010 Jun;4(2):177-85.

[116] Roomi MW, Ivanov V, Netke S, Kalinovsky T, Niedzwiecki A, Rath M. In vivo and in vitro antitumor effect of ascorbic acid, lysine, proline and green tea extract on human melanoma cell line A2058. *In Vivo.* 2006 Jan-Feb;20(1):25-32.

[117] Roomi MW, Roomi NW, Kalinovsky T, Niedzwiecki A, Rath M. In vivo and In vitro effect of a nutrient mixture on human hepatocarcinoma cell line SK-HEP-1. *Exp. Oncol., 2010* Jul;32(2):84-91.

[118] Mukhtar H, Ahmad N. Cancer chemoprevention: future holds in multiple agents. *Toxicol. Appl. Pharmacol.,* 1999 Aug 1;158(3):207-10.

[119] Sporn MB, Liby KT. NRF2 and cancer: the good, the bad and the importance of context. *Nat. Rev. Cancer,* 2012 Aug;12(8):564-71.

[120] Perera RM, Bardeesy N. Cancer: when antioxidants are bad. *Nature,* 2011 Jul 7;475(7354):43-4.

[121] Wang XJ, Sun Z, Villeneuve NF, Zhang S, Zhao F, Li Y, et al. Nrf2 enhances resistance of cancer cells to chemotherapeutic drugs, the dark side of Nrf2. *Carcinogenesis,* 2008 Jun;29(6):1235-43.

[122] Shen G, Xu C, Hu R, Jain MR, Nair S, Lin W, et al. Comparison of (-)-epigallocatechin-3-gallate elicited liver and small intestine gene expression profiles between C57BL/6J mice and C57BL/6J/Nrf2 (-/-) mice. *Pharm. Res.,* 2005 Nov;22 (11):1805-20.

[123] Yuan JH, Li YQ, Yang XY. Inhibition of epigallocatechin gallate on orthotopic colon cancer by upregulating the Nrf2-UGT1A signal pathway in nude mice. *Pharmacology,* 2007;80(4):269-78.

[124] Traverso N, Ricciarelli R, Nitti M, Marengo B, Furfaro AL, Pronzato MA, et al. Role of glutathione in cancer progression and chemoresistance. *Oxid. Med. Cell Longev.,* 2013;2013:972913.

[125] Carretero J, Obrador E, Anasagasti MJ, Martin JJ, Vidal-Vanaclocha F, Estrela JM. Growth-associated changes in glutathione content correlate with liver metastatic activity of B16 melanoma cells. *Clin. Exp. Metastasis.,* 1999;17(7):567-74.

[126] Carretero J, Obrador E, Esteve JM, Ortega A, Pellicer JA, Sempere FV, et al. Tumoricidal activity of endothelial cells. Inhibition of endothelial nitric oxide production abrogates tumor cytotoxicity induced by hepatic sinusoidal endothelium in response to B16 melanoma adhesion in vitro. *J. Biol. Chem.,* 2001 Jul 13;276 (28):25775-82.

[127] D'Souza RJ, Phillips HM, Jones PW, Strange RC, Aber GM. Interactions of hydrogen peroxide with interleukin-6 and platelet-derived growth factor in determining mesangial cell growth: effect of repeated oxidant stress. *Clin. Sci.,* (Lond). 1993 Dec;85(6):747-51.

[128] Alliangana DM. Effects of beta-carotene, flavonoid quercitin and quinacrine on cell proliferation and lipid peroxidation breakdown products in BHK-21 cells. *East Afr. Med. J.,* 1996 Nov;73(11):752-7.

[129] Chang MC, Chan CP, Wang YJ, Lee PH, Chen LI, Tsai YL, et al. Induction of necrosis and apoptosis to KB cancer cells by sanguinarine is associated with reactive oxygen species production and mitochondrial membrane depolarization. *Toxicol. Appl. Pharmacol.,* 2007 Jan 15;218(2):143-51.

[130] Dypbukt JM, Ankarcrona M, Burkitt M, Sjoholm A, Strom K, Orrenius S, et al. Different pro-oxidant levels stimulate growth, trigger apoptosis, or produce necrosis of insulin-secreting RINm5F cells. The role of intracellular polyamines. *J. Biol. Chem.,* 1994 Dec 2;269(48):30553-60.

[131] Halliwell B. Oxidative stress and cancer: have we moved forward? *Biochem. J.,* 2007 Jan 1;401(1):1-11.

[132] Kong Q, Lillehei KO. Antioxidant inhibitors for cancer therapy. *Med. Hypotheses,* 1998 Nov;51(5):405-9.

[133] Siddiqui IA, Adhami VM, Saleem M, Mukhtar H. Beneficial effects of tea and its polyphenols against prostate cancer. *Mol. Nutr. Food Res.,* 2006 Feb;50(2):130-43.

[134] Seifried HE, Anderson DE, Fisher EI, Milner JA. A review of the interaction among dietary antioxidants and reactive oxygen species. *J. Nutr. Biochem.,* 2007 Sep;18(9): 567-79.

[135] Schloss JM, Colosimo M, Airey C, Masci PP, Linnane AW, Vitetta L. Nutraceuticals and chemotherapy induced peripheral neuropathy (CIPN): A systematic review. *Clin. Nutr.,* 2013 Apr 13.

[136] Hochster HS, Grothey A, Childs BH. Use of calcium and magnesium salts to reduce oxaliplatin-related neurotoxicity. *J. Clin. Oncol.,* 2007 Sep 1;25(25):4028-9.

[137] Smyth JF, Bowman A, Perren T, Wilkinson P, Prescott RJ, Quinn KJ, et al. Glutathione reduces the toxicity and improves quality of life of women diagnosed with ovarian cancer treated with cisplatin: results of a double-blind, randomised trial. *Ann. Oncol.,* 1997 Jun;8(6):569-73.

[138] Maestri A, De Pasquale Ceratti A, Cundari S, Zanna C, Cortesi E, Crino L. A pilot study on the effect of acetyl-L-carnitine in paclitaxel- and cisplatin-induced peripheral neuropathy. *Tumori,* 2005 Mar-Apr;91(2):135-8.

[139] Puglia CD, Powell SR. Inhibition of cellular antioxidants: a possible mechanism of toxic cell injury. *Environ. Health Perspect.,* 1984 Aug;57:307-11.

[140] Palozza P, Serini S, Di Nicuolo F, Piccioni E, Calviello G. Pro-oxidant effects of beta-carotene in cultured cells. *Mol. Aspects Med.,* 2003 Dec;24(6):353-62.

[141] Pathi SS, Lei P, Sreevalsan S, Chadalapaka G, Jutooru I, Safe S. Pharmacologic doses of ascorbic acid repress specificity protein (Sp) transcription factors and Sp-regulated genes in colon cancer cells. *Nutr. Cancer,* 2011;63(7):1133-42.

[142] Carocho M, Ferreira IC. A review on antioxidants, pro-oxidants and related controversy: natural and synthetic compounds, screening and analysis methodologies and future perspectives. *Food Chem. Toxicol.,* 2013 Jan;51:15-25.

[143] Rajendran P, Li F, Manu KA, Shanmugam MK, Loo SY, Kumar AP, et al. gamma-Tocotrienol is a novel inhibitor of constitutive and inducible STAT3 signalling pathway in human hepatocellular carcinoma: potential role as an antiproliferative, pro-apoptotic and chemosensitizing agent. *Br. J. Pharmacol.,* 2011 May;163(2):283-98.

[144] Kanai K, Kikuchi E, Mikami S, Suzuki E, Uchida Y, Kodaira K, et al. Vitamin E succinate induced apoptosis and enhanced chemosensitivity to paclitaxel in human bladder cancer cells in vitro and in vivo. *Cancer Sci.,* 2010 Jan;101(1):216-23.

[145] Lim SJ, Choi MK, Kim MJ, Kim JK. Alpha-tocopheryl succinate potentiates the paclitaxel-induced apoptosis through enforced caspase 8 activation in human H460 lung cancer cells. *Exp. Mol. Med.,* 2009 Oct 31;41(10):737-45.

[146] Tang J, Fu Q, Wang Y, Racette K, Wang D, Liu F. Vitamin E reverses multidrug resistance in vitro and in vivo. *Cancer Lett.,* 2013 Aug 9;336(1):149-57.

[147] Sylvester PW, Ayoub NM. Tocotrienols Target PI3K/Akt Signaling in Anti-Breast Cancer Therapy. *Anticancer. Agents Med. Chem.,* 2013 Sep;13(7):1039-47.

[148] Felipe KB, Benites J, Glorieux C, Sid B, Valenzuela M, Kviecinski MR, et al. Antiproliferative effects of phenylaminonaphthoquinones are increased by ascorbate and associated with the appearance of a senescent phenotype in human bladder cancer cells. *Biochem. Biophys. Res. Commun.,* 2013 Apr 19;433(4):573-8.

[149] Park JH, Davis KR, Lee G, Jung M, Jung Y, Park J, et al. Ascorbic acid alleviates toxicity of paclitaxel without interfering with the anticancer efficacy in mice. *Nutr. Res.,* 2012 Nov;32(11):873-83.

[150] Frank J, Flaccus A, Schwarz C, Lambert C, Biesalski HK. Ascorbic acid suppresses cell death in rat DS-sarcoma cancer cells induced by 5-aminolevulinic acid-based photodynamic therapy. *Free Radic. Biol. Med.,* 2006 Mar 1;40(5):827-36.

[151] Kontek R, Drozda R, Sliwinski M, Grzegorczyk K. Genotoxicity of irinotecan and its modulation by vitamins A, C and E in human lymphocytes from healthy individuals and cancer patients. *Toxicol. In Vitro,* 2010 Mar;24(2):417-24.

[152] Croker AK, Allan AL. Inhibition of aldehyde dehydrogenase (ALDH) activity reduces chemotherapy and radiation resistance of stem-like ALDHhiCD44(+) human breast cancer cells. *Breast Cancer Res. Treat,* 2012 May;133(1):75-87.

[153] Arrieta O, Gonzalez-De la Rosa CH, Arechaga-Ocampo E, Villanueva-Rodriguez G, Ceron-Lizarraga TL, Martinez-Barrera L, et al. Randomized phase II trial of All-trans-retinoic acid with chemotherapy based on paclitaxel and cisplatin as first-line treatment in patients with advanced non-small-cell lung cancer. *J. Clin. Oncol.,* 2010 Jul 20;28 (21):3463-71.

[154] Karmakar S, Banik NL, Ray SK. Combination of all-trans retinoic acid and paclitaxel-induced differentiation and apoptosis in human glioblastoma U87MG xenografts in nude mice. *Cancer,* 2008 Feb 1;112(3):596-607.

[155] Hung SH, Lee FP, Su CH, Tseng H. Effect of all-trans retinoic acid on the growth of two nasopharyngeal cancer cell lines and its treatment potential in combination with cisplatin. *Eur. Arch. Otorhinolaryngol.,* 2013 Feb;270(2):695-704.

[156] Ping SY, Hour TC, Lin SR, Yu DS. Taxol synergizes with antioxidants in inhibiting hormal refractory prostate cancer cell growth. *Urol. Oncol.,* 2010 Mar-Apr;28(2):170-9.

[157] Johnson JL, Gonzalez de Mejia E. Interactions between dietary flavonoids apigenin or luteolin and chemotherapeutic drugs to potentiate anti-proliferative effect on human pancreatic cancer cells, in vitro. *Food Chem. Toxicol.,* 2013 Jul 18.

[158] Kang Y, Park MA, Heo SW, Park SY, Kang KW, Park PH, et al. The radio-sensitizing effect of xanthohumol is mediated by STAT3 and EGFR suppression in doxorubicin-resistant MCF-7 human breast cancer cells. *Biochim. Biophys. Acta.,* 2013 Mar;1830(3) :2638-48.

[159] Qin J, Wang Y, Bai Y, Yang K, Mao Q, Lin Y, et al. Epigallocatechin-3-gallate inhibits bladder cancer cell invasion via suppression of NF-kappaBmediated matrix metalloproteinase-9 expression. *Mol. Med. Rep.,* 2012 Nov;6(5):1040-4.

[160] Yang YI, Lee KT, Park HJ, Kim TJ, Choi YS, Shih Ie M, et al. Tectorigenin sensitizes paclitaxel-resistant human ovarian cancer cells through downregulation of the Akt and NFkappaB pathway. *Carcinogenesis,* 2012 Dec;33(12):2488-98.

[161] Lin X, Wu G, Huo WQ, Zhang Y, Jin FS. Resveratrol induces apoptosis associated with mitochondrial dysfunction in bladder carcinoma cells. *Int. J. Urol.,* 2012 Aug;19(8): 757-64.

[162] Periasamy VS, Alshatwi AA. Tea polyphenols modulate antioxidant redox system on cisplatin-induced reactive oxygen species generation in a human breast cancer cell. *Basic Clin. Pharmacol. Toxicol.,* 2013 Jun;112(6):374-84.

[163] Valko M, Izakovic M, Mazur M, Rhodes CJ, Telser J. Role of oxygen radicals in DNA damage and cancer incidence. *Mol. Cell Biochem.,* 2004 Nov;266(1-2):37-56.

[164] Valko M, Leibfritz D, Moncol J, Cronin MT, Mazur M, Telser J. Free radicals and antioxidants in normal physiological functions and human disease. *Int. J. Biochem. Cell Biol., 2007*;39(1):44-84.

[165] Valdez BC, Murray D, Nieto Y, Li Y, Wang G, Champlin RE, et al. Synergistic cytotoxicity of the DNA alkylating agent busulfan, nucleoside analogs and

suberoylanilide hydroxamic acid in lymphoma cell lines. *Leuk Lymphoma,* 2012 May;53(5):973-81.

[166] Ledermann JA, Gabra H, Jayson GC, Spanswick VJ, Rustin GJ, Jitlal M, et al. Inhibition of carboplatin-induced DNA interstrand cross-link repair by gemcitabine in patients receiving these drugs for platinum-resistant ovarian cancer. *Clin. Cancer Res.,* 2010 Oct 1;16(19):4899-905.

[167] LaPointe NE, Morfini G, Brady ST, Feinstein SC, Wilson L, Jordan MA. Effects of eribulin, vincristine, paclitaxel and ixabepilone on fast axonal transport and kinesin-1 driven microtubule gliding: implications for chemotherapy-induced peripheral neuropathy. *Neurotoxicology,* 2013 Jul;37:231-9.

[168] Ozben T. Oxidative stress and apoptosis: impact on cancer therapy. *J. Pharm. Sci.,* 2007 Sep;96(9):2181-96.

[169] Bishayee A. Cancer prevention and treatment with resveratrol: from rodent studies to clinical trials. *Cancer Prev. Res.,* (Phila). 2009 May;2(5):409-18.

[170] Yang CS, Wang X, Lu G, Picinich SC. Cancer prevention by tea: animal studies, molecular mechanisms and human relevance. *Nat. Rev. Cancer,* 2009 Jun;9(6):429-39.

[171] Conklin KA. Dietary antioxidants during cancer chemotherapy: impact on chemotherapeutic effectiveness and development of side effects. *Nutr. Cancer,* 2000;37(1):1-18.

[172] Block KI, Koch AC, Mead MN, Tothy PK, Newman RA, Gyllenhaal C. Impact of antioxidant supplementation on chemotherapeutic efficacy: a systematic review of the evidence from randomized controlled trials. *Cancer Treat Rev.,* 2007 Aug;33(5):407-18.

[173] Lissoni P, Chilelli M, Villa S, Cerizza L, Tancini G. Five years survival in metastatic non-small cell lung cancer patients treated with chemotherapy alone or chemotherapy and melatonin: a randomized trial. *J. Pineal. Res.,* 2003 Aug;35(1):12-5.

[174] Cerea G, Vaghi M, Ardizzoia A, Villa S, Bucovec R, Mengo S, et al. Biomodulation of cancer chemotherapy for metastatic colorectal cancer: a randomized study of weekly low-dose irinotecan alone versus irinotecan plus the oncostatic pineal hormone melatonin in metastatic colorectal cancer patients progressing on 5-fluorouracil-containing combinations. *Anticancer Res.,* 2003 Mar-Apr;23(2C):1951-4.

[175] Fuchs-Tarlovsky V. Role of antioxidants in cancer therapy. *Nutrition,* 2013 Jan;29(1):15-21.

In: Free Radicals
Editor: Bill Stone

ISBN: 978-1-63117-177-2

Chapter II

Is There an Actual Benefit in Antioxidant Supplementation on Cancer Treatment?

Décio Sabbatini Barbosa*, Danielle Venturini, Francis Fregonesi Brinholi, Andressa Keiko Matsumoto, Carine Coneglian de Farias, Chiara Cristina Bortolasci, Kamila Landucci Bonifácio and Luciana Higachi
Department of Pathology, Clinical Analysis and Toxicology,
State University of Londrina, Londrina, Brazil

Abstract

Despite advances in cancer research, there is still a long way before we get convincing answers to many questions. The scope of this chapter is to discuss if there is an actual benefit in a cancer treatment with the concomitant use of antioxidants and its possible adverse effects. Oxidative stress (OS) is defined as an imbalance between endogenous antioxidant mechanisms and reactive oxygen/nitrogen species (ROS/RNS) due to a deficiency in antioxidant substances, an excessive production of free radicals or both. OS is a key component in linking environmental toxicity to the multistage carcinogenic process and starts even before cancer treatment begins. Free radicals or ROS have a well-established role in the initiation of cancer through effects on DNA damage that result in mutations, leading to the activation of oncogenes and loss of tumor suppressor gene function and, ironically, these same ROS are formed in cancer treatment. So, a great problem is that the functional OS generated for treatment destroys not only mutagenic cells, but healthy tissues. Antioxidant supplementation has been shown to decrease OS, but there is still controversy with respect to cancer treatment. Much debate has arisen about whether antioxidant supplementation alters the efficacy of cancer chemotherapy. Some have argued that antioxidants scavenge the ROS integral to the activity of certain chemotherapy drugs, thereby diminishing treatment efficacy. Others suggest that antioxidants may mitigate toxicity and thus allow for uninterrupted treatment schedules and a reduced need for lowering chemotherapy doses. In addition, there are several controversial publications with respect to cancer treatment. Some studies suggest that antioxidant supplementation may affect cancer treatment outcome, but they are still limited in the quality and number of patients used. In contrast, other papers that show that antioxidant supplementation during chemotherapy administration reduced the toxic effects of ROS produced during cancer treatment. Consumption of fruits and vegetables has been associated with a low incidence and mortality of cancer. It is not known which dietary constituents are responsible for this association, but it is often assumed that antioxidants play a significant role in this respect. The meta-analysis of randomized controlled trials indicates that there is no clinical evidence supporting an overall primary and secondary preventive effect of antioxidant supplements on cancer. Therefore, therapies using novel antioxidant molecules (or old but in different doses) are in course to clarify critical questions about their safety and efficacy in cancer treatment.

Keywords: cancer, antioxidant, oxidative stress

Abbreviations

8-hydroxy-2-deoxyguanosine	8-OH-dG
Activator protein 1	Ap-1
Base excision repair	BER
Caspase-3	CASP3
Caspase-9	CASP9
Catalase	CAT
Copper	Cu^{+}
Copper/zinc superoxide dismutase	Cuznsod
Cuznsod	SOD1
Cyclooxygenase 2	Cox2
epigallocatechin-3-gallate	EGCG
Ferrous	Fe^{2+}
Flavonoids	FOH
Glutathione	GSH
Glutathione disulfide	GSSG
Glutathione peroxidase	Gpx
Hepatitis B virus	HBV
Hepatitis C virus	HCV
Hydrogen atoms to lipid	$L^{\bullet}$
Hydrogen peroxide	H_2O_2
Hydroperoxides	ROOH
Hydroxyl radical	$^{\bullet}OH$
Interleukines	IL
Lipid hydroperoxide	LOOH
Lipid peroxidation	Lpo
Lipid peroxyl	$LOO^{\bullet}$
Lipids	LH
Malondialdehyde	Mda
Manganese superoxide dismutase	Mnsod

Mitochondrial DNA	mtDNA
Nuclear factor kappa	Nf-kβ
Nucleotide excision repair	NER
Oxidative stress	OS
Peroxynitrite	$OONO^-$
Reactive nitrogen species	RNS
Reactive oxygen species	ROS
Selenate	SeO_4^{-2}
Selenite	SeO_3^{-2}
Selenium metallic form	Se^0
Selenocysteine	Secys
Selenomethionine	Seme
Superoxide anion	$O_2^{\bullet-}$
Superoxide dismutase	SOD
Surveillance, Epidemiology and End Results	SEER
Thioredoxin	Trx
Thioredoxin reductases	Trxr

Introduction

Cancer Epidemiology

Several factors may affect the interpretation of cancer incidence, mortality, and survival statistics. According the Surveillance, Epidemiology and End Results (SEER) Program, an authoritative source of information on cancer incidence and survival in the United States, we can quote: survival rates for all cancers combined, early detection/screening, changes in diagnostic criteria, technological advances in diagnostic procedures, evolution of stage classifications, interpreting relative survival, comparison with other databases, errors in data collection and comparison of this report with previous reports [1]. However, several immigrant studies have documented that cancer rates in successive generations of immigrants shift in the direction of the prevailing rates in the host country, suggesting that the international variations in cancer rates for most cancers largely reflect differences in environmental risk factors (including lifestyle and culture) rather than genetic differences [2].

It was estimated that there were about 12.7 million new cancer cases and 7.6 million cancer deaths in 2008 worldwide [3]. Overall incidence rates (per 100,000) for 1998-2002 among the 45 select cancer registries worldwide vary by nearly 6-fold in men, from 86.3 in Algeria to 453.3 in U.S. blacks, and by nearly 4-fold in women, from 80.3 in Algeria to 302.3 in U.S. non-Hispanic whites. However, regional variations in overall cancer rates may mask important differences in cancer types. The most frequently diagnosed cancers by sex vary considerably across countries. The most commonly diagnosed cancer among men is lung cancer in most parts of Eastern Europe and Asia; prostate cancer in North America, Australia, Western and Northern Europe, and South America; liver cancer in parts of West Africa; Kaposi sarcoma in central parts of Africa; cancer of the esophagus in East Africa; and bladder cancer in Egypt. Among women, the most frequently diagnosed cancer is breast cancer in most parts of the world, including Australia, Western Asia, North Africa, North America, and parts of South America; cervical cancer in Central America, parts of South America, Sub-Saharan Africa, and India; liver cancer in Mongolia and Vietnam; and lung cancer in China and North Korea [4]. In this context, we briefly describe the international incidence for some common cancers, including: lung cancer, colorectal cancer, breast cancer, prostate cancer, stomach and liver cancer.

Lung cancer is the leading cause of cancer deaths in men and the second leading cause of cancer deaths in women, with about 1.6 million new lung cancer cases in 2008 [3]. In men, the highest lung cancer incidence rates are reported in the United States (blacks) and in Eastern European countries, and the lowest rates are found in Africa, Central and South America, and South Central Asia. In women, the highest lung cancer rates are reported in North America and parts of Europe, including the United Kingdom and Denmark, and the lowest rates are found in Africa, South Central Asia, and Latin America. International variations in lung cancer rates and trends largely reflect differences in the stage and degree of the tobacco epidemic [5,6] because smoking accounts for about 80% of global lung cancer deaths in men and 50% of the deaths in women [7,8].

Colorectal cancer is the third most common cancer in men and the second in women. Worldwide, 1.2 million new colorectal cancer cases were expected to occur in 2008. Generally, the highest incidence rates among both men and women are reported in Eastern European countries (Czech Republic and Slovakia), Japan (Miyagi), New Zealand, Australia, Germany, and U.S. blacks, whereas the lowest rates are found in Africa, Central and South America, and South Central Asia (India and Pakistan). U.S. Hispanic and Asian men and women have lower incidence rates than U.S. white or black men and women, but they have higher rates than their counterparts in Latin America and Asia; exceptions to these patterns are the substantially high rates in Japan (Miyagi) and Singapore [4]. While colorectal cancer incidence rates are stabilizing or declining in historically high-risk areas (United States, New Zealand, Canada), they are rapidly increasing in several historically low-risk countries, including Japan, Korea, China, and Eastern European countries (Slovakia, Slovenia, and Czech Republic). The increase in the incidence rates in several Asian and Eastern European countries and Spain is thought to reflect changes in dietary and lifestyle factors associated with westernization, including smoking and obesity [9]. The decrease in the incidence rate in the United States in the most recent time period largely reflects detection and removal of precancerous lesions through colorectal cancer screening [10].

Breast cancer is the most commonly diagnosed cancer and the leading cause of cancer death in women worldwide, with an estimated 1.4 million new breast cancer cases in 2008 [3]. Generally, the highest incidence rates are found in Switzerland, U.S. whites, Italy, and many other European countries, whereas low rates are found in Africa, Asia, and South America. The rates in U.S. Hispanics and Asians are substantially higher compared with the rates in most cancer registries in Asia and Latin America. The high breast cancer incidence rates in white women in the United States and in most European countries reflect the long-standing high prevalence of reproductive factors associated with increased risk of breast cancer, including early menarche, late child bearing, fewer pregnancies, use of menopausal hormone therapy, as well as increased detection through mammography [11,12].

Prostate cancer is the second most frequently diagnosed cancer and the sixth leading cause of cancer death among men worldwide, with 914,000 new cases and 258,000 deaths projected to occur in 2008. Incidence rates (per 100,000) vary nearly 50-fold worldwide, ranging from 3.9 in India to 178.8 in U.S. blacks. Generally, the highest rates are recorded in North America, Oceania, and Northern and Western Europe, whereas the lowest rates are found in Asia and North Africa [3].

With respect to stomach cancer, incidence rates (per 100,000) vary from 3.3 in men and 2.0 in women in Egypt to 65.9 in men and 25.9 in women in Korea and it's the fourth most commonly diagnosed cancer and the second leading cause of cancer death worldwide, with an estimated 990,000 new cases cancer in 2008. Large regional variations may reflect differences in prevalence of *Helicobacter pylori* infection, which accounts for more than 60% of gastric cancer worldwide [13]. Incidence rates for stomach cancer have declined steadily in several western countries [14], with rates decreasing by more than 80% since 1950 in the United States [15]. In contrast to this scenario, incidence rates have increased for cancer of the gastric cardia (the proximal part of the stomach) in the United States and many European countries, including Denmark and the United Kingdom [16]. This increase is thought to reflect a rise in the gastroesophageal reflux disease associated with the obesity epidemic [17].

Liver cancer is the sixth most commonly diagnosed cancer and the third leading cause of cancer death worldwide, with an estimated 748,000 new liver cancer cases during 2008. Nearly 85% of these cases occur in less developed countries, with China alone accounting for more than 50% of the total [3]. There is a 20- to 40-fold difference in international variations in liver cancer rates. The highest rates are found in Asia and West and Central Africa, and the lowest in Europe, Oceania, and North America [18,19,20]. U.S. Hispanics and Asians have higher rates than U.S. whites, but they have lower rates than their counterparts in Asia and Latin America. The international variation in liver cancer rates is largely explained by the distribution of chronic hepatitis B virus (HBV) and hepatitis C virus (HCV) infections [18], with HBV infection generally dominating in high-risk areas, including Asia and Sub-Saharan Africa, and HCV infection dominating in low-risk areas, including most parts of Europe and North America. These two viruses account for 78% (HBV, 53%; HCV, 25%) of the total liver cancer deaths globally, with the estimates by region varying from about 64% in the Americas to about 90% in Japan and Singapore [21].

While incidence and mortality rates for most cancers (including lung, colorectum, female breast, and prostate) are decreasing in the United States and many other western countries, they are increasing in several less developed and economically transitioning countries, including Brazil, because of adoption of unhealthy western lifestyles such as smoking and physical inactivity and consumption of calorie-dense food. While smoking prevalence is declining in economically developed countries, it is increasing in some developing countries in South America, Asia, and Africa [22]. Most developing countries also continue to be disproportionately affected by cancers related to infectious agents, such as cervix, liver, and stomach cancers. The proportion of new cancer cases diagnosed in less developed countries is projected to increase from about 56% of the world total in 2008 to more than 60% in 2030 because of the increasing trends in cancer rates and expected increases in life expectancy and growth of the population. In general, smoking, dietary patterns, and reproductive behaviors have been known to be the major risk factors for cancer in western (host) countries, and infectious agents in economically developing countries. However, these patterns are changing rapidly.

There are several reasons why nutrition (conceived broadly to include diet, body size, and physical activity) should be causally linked to cancer at one or more anatomic sites [23]. Nevertheless, the nutrition and cancer field has been problematic, particularly with respect to the etiologic roles of dietary factors and physical activity. For a number of important foods, macronutrients, and micronutrients (total dietary fat and fat subtypes, dietary fiber and whole grains, fruits and vegetables, folate, lycopene, selenium, calcium, and vitamin D, to name just a few), the causal links to cancers remain unclear [23].

Oxidative stress (OS), a disturbance between oxidants/antioxidants balance in favor of the former, has been the subject of intensive research in recent years and has been linked to the pathogenesis of several chronic diseases including cancer, osteoporosis, type 2 diabetes, neurodegenerative diseases and cardiovascular disease [24].

Carcinogenesis is a multistep process involving mutation and the subsequent selective clonal expansion of the mutated cell. Chemical and physical agents including those that induce reactive oxygen species (ROS) can induce and/or modulate this multistep process. Several modes of action by which carcinogens induce cancer have been identified, including through production of ROS. Some studies have shown an important role for ROS in tumor development [25,26].

Reactive Oxygen/nitrogen Species (ROS/RNS)

Oxygen is an important element that plays a significant role in many processes of the human body including cellular metabolism, intercellular and intracellular signaling and acts as a key component for an effective immune system and response [27]. Under physiological conditions, there is a constant endogenous production of ROS and reactive nitrogen species (RNS), produced from mitochondria, peroxisomes, and inflammatory cell activation [28]. ROS can also be produced by exogenous sources, including environmental agents, pharmaceuticals, and industrial chemicals. To counterbalance ROS-mediated injury, an endogenous antioxidant defense system exists; however, when oxidation exceeds the defense mechanisms, OS arises. The defense mechanisms include enzymatic endogenous antioxidants such as superoxide dismutase (SOD), catalase (CAT), glutathione peroxidase (GPx) and glutathione-S-transferase, and non-enzymatic endogenous antioxidants (vitamins E and C, coenzyme Q, b-carotene, and glutathione (GSH)) [29].

In aerobic healthy organisms the production of reactive ROS is approximately balanced with antioxidant defense systems [30]. The balance is not perfect, however, so that some ROS-mediated damage occurs continuously. ROS can be generated in response to both endogenous and exogenous stimuli [28,31,32].

Under physiological concentrations, ROS act as signaling molecules mediating cell growth, migration and differentiation whereas at higher concentrations, they induce cell death, apoptosis and senescence. In the process of aerobic metabolism, electron leakage along the electron transport chain in the mitochondria results in the production of the superoxide anion ($O_2^{\bullet-}$). Other biological reactions, including oxidative bursts produced by phagocytes and enzyme systems such as cytochrome P450 and xanthine oxidase, also contribute to the production of these highly reactive species [33].

Among the various types of ROS, hydrogen peroxide (H_2O_2) is generated from almost all sources of OS and can diffuse freely in and out of cells and tissues. This indicates that H_2O_2 is a key oxygen metabolite involved in OS. However, H_2O_2 itself is not a reactive radical, rather the agent is a precursor to the most highly toxic hydroxyl radical ($^{\bullet}OH$) radical. Intracellular biomolecules, such as protein kinases, lipids (LH), and DNA, are potential targets of $^{\bullet}OH$. In particular, DNA is sensitive to damage from exposure to H_2O_2, which induces cell death by apoptosis, pyknosis and/or necrosis. Thus, oxidative DNA damage induced by $^{\bullet}OH$ is a key factor influencing the mutagenic and carcinogenic load in living organisms [34].

Excessive production or accumulation of ROS can have detrimental effects by participating in reduction-oxidation (redox) reactions causing damage to macromolecules, cell membranes and DNA [24]. This can alter biological properties of membranes, enzymes and receptors, impair cell functioning, and lead to cell death [35]. For this reason, a complex network of defense systems has developed in humans to protect against excessive production of and damage by reactive species in an effort to maintain 'redox homeostasis' [24]. ROS can be viewed as critical determinants of intracellular redox states and thus serve as important cellular regulatory mechanisms in both health and disease.

Antioxidants

In a broad definition, an antioxidant is any substance that, when present at low concentrations compared with those of an oxidizable substrate, significantly delays or prevents oxidation of that substrate [36]. Antioxidants may react directly with the reactive radicals to destroy them by accepting or donating electron(s) to eliminate the unpaired condition of the radical, or they may indirectly decrease the formation of free radicals by inhibiting the activities or expressions of free radical generating enzymes or by enhancing the activities and expressions of other antioxidant enzymes [37].

Antioxidant supplementation has been shown to decrease OS, but there is still controversy with respect to cancer treatment. Much debate has arisen about whether antioxidant supplementation alters the efficacy of cancer chemotherapy. The use of antioxidant supplements by patients with cancer is estimated to be between 13% and 87% [38,39,40,41]. This wide range of percentages might be attributed to the variability of definitions of complementary and alternative medicine used in the different studies, and to differences in the cancer types, age, education, economic status, and ethnicity of the groups assessed [42].

There is a controversy with respect to antioxidant supplementation in cancer, based on some evidence. Firstly, there is a widespread concern that the use of antioxidant supplements during cancer treatment may protect tumor cells from the oxidative damage induced by cancer therapies, thereby reducing the effectiveness of treatment and increasing the risk of mortality [43]. Second, antioxidants may protect normal cells from the oxidative damage that occurs during radiotherapy and certain chemotherapy regimens; however, the same mechanism could protect tumor cells and potentially reduce effectiveness of cancer treatments.

In a recent meta-analysis of randomized controlled trials no overall association was found between the consumption of antioxidant supplements and cancer risk [44]. However, previous experimental and epidemiological studies have indicated that persons with a low intake of fruits and vegetables that are rich in antioxidant substances are more susceptible to cancer [45,46,47]. Much debate has focused on the use of antioxidant supplements by patients undergoing chemotherapy due to concerns that the antioxidants may interfere with the mechanism of action of the therapeutic agent and subsequently decrease its efficacy [48].

Others argue that antioxidant supplements are beneficial to patients by enhancing the efficacy of the chemotherapy, as well as alleviating the side effects [49]. Block et al. [50] conducted a systematic review and found no evidence to support the view that antioxidant supplementation given concurrently with ROS-generating chemotherapy diminished the efficacy of the chemotherapy in patients with advanced cancers or relapsed patients. Antioxidant supplementation actually helped reduce some adverse reactions including neurotoxicity, thrombocytopenia, and diarrhea, thus enabling increased or uninterrupted dosing in patients who may otherwise discontinue treatment due to side effects.

Defense mechanisms against free radical-induced OS involve: (i) preventative mechanisms, (ii) repair mechanisms, (iii) physical defenses, and (iv) antioxidant defenses. Enzymatic antioxidant defenses include SOD, GPx, and CAT. Non-enzymatic antioxidants are represented by ascorbic acid (Vitamin C), α-tocopherol (a form of vitamin E), GSH, carotenoids, flavonoids (FOH), and other antioxidants. Under normal conditions, there is a balance between both the activities and the intracellular levels of these antioxidants. This balance is essential for the survival of organisms and their health [24]. Now, we'll try to understand the main defense mechanisms against free radical-induced OS.

Mechanisms of Antioxidant Actions

Free Radical Scavengers that Act as Reducers or Break Lipid Chains

The efficacy of antioxidants is dependent on the type of the oxidants. For example, α-tocopherol is a potent radical-scavenging antioxidant but it is a poor antioxidant against lipid peroxidation (LPO) by lipoxygenase. Carotenoids may be weak radical-scavenging antioxidants but can be potent inhibitors of the oxidation induced by singlet oxygen. Oxidative damage can be attenuated not only by scavenging radicals but also by sequestering metal ions, decomposing H_2O_2 and/or hydroperoxides (ROOH), quenching active pro-oxidants, and repairing damage. However, this subject is more complicated than it superficially appears. In other words: does enough antioxidant reach the target *in vivo*? Biological systems are inherently quite heterogeneous. There are both hydrophilic and hydrophobic domains. The effective antioxidant concentration, that is, bioavailability, is one of the important factors influencing the antioxidant capacity. Furthermore, localization and mobility at the microenvironment are also important, especially for lipophilic antioxidants. It is well known that water-soluble antioxidants such as vitamin C and uric acid are aqueous phase antioxidants but are not effective for radicals generated in a lipophilic domain. Lipophilic antioxidants such as α-tocopherol, β-carotene, and ubiquinol are incorporated into membranes and lipoproteins. They can be localized at the protein-lipid surface or interior. The long side chains of tocopherols, tocotrienols, and ubiquinols, which are essential for their incorporation and retention in membranes and lipoproteins, reduce the mobility within and between the membranes and lipoproteins. Therefore, the antioxidant activity may vary dramatically in the membranes and lipoproteins. These data suggest that antioxidant capacity depends on the environment and that the results evaluated in the homogeneous solution may not be directly extrapolated to a heterogeneous system [51].

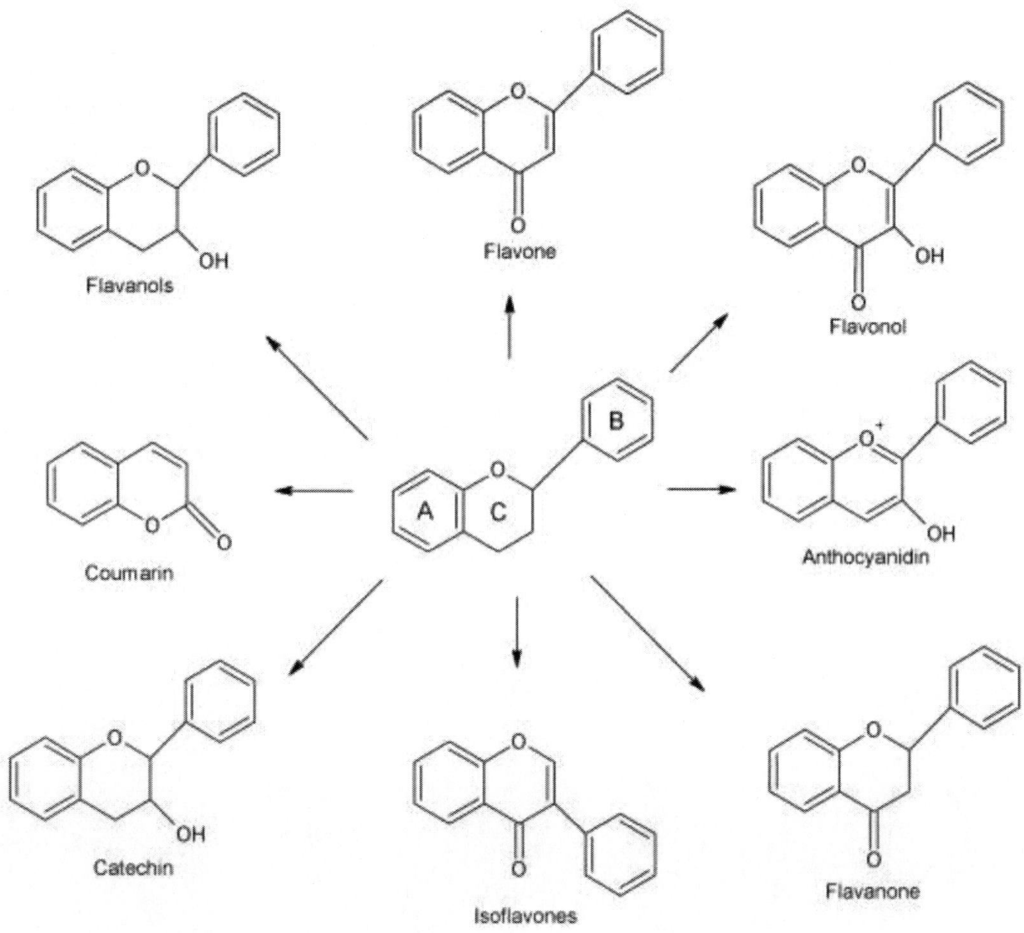

Figure 1. The basic structure of a polyphenol and its related compounds.

Polyphenols

Polyphenols are secondary metabolites of plants and include a myriad of chemical structures, from simple molecules such as phenolic acids, to highly polymerized compounds, such as condensed tannins. The most abundant family of polyphenols present in human diets is the FOH. FOH is a chemically defined family of polyphenols that have a basic structure of two aromatic rings (ring A and ring B) linked through three carbons that frequently form an oxygenated heterocycle (ring C). Different arrangements of hydroxyl and/or carbonyl groups, and carbon–carbon double bonds in the basic structure define the different subgroups of FOH as shown in Figure 1 [52]. Many mechanisms have been proposed for polyphenol prevention of OS and ROS/RNS generation both *in vitro* and *in vivo*. In the radical scavenging mechanism, polyphenols sacrificially reduce ROS/RNS, such as $^{\bullet}OH$, $O_2^{\bullet -}$, nitric oxide, or peroxynitrite ($OONO^-$) after generation, preventing damage to biomolecules or the formation of more reactive ROS [53].

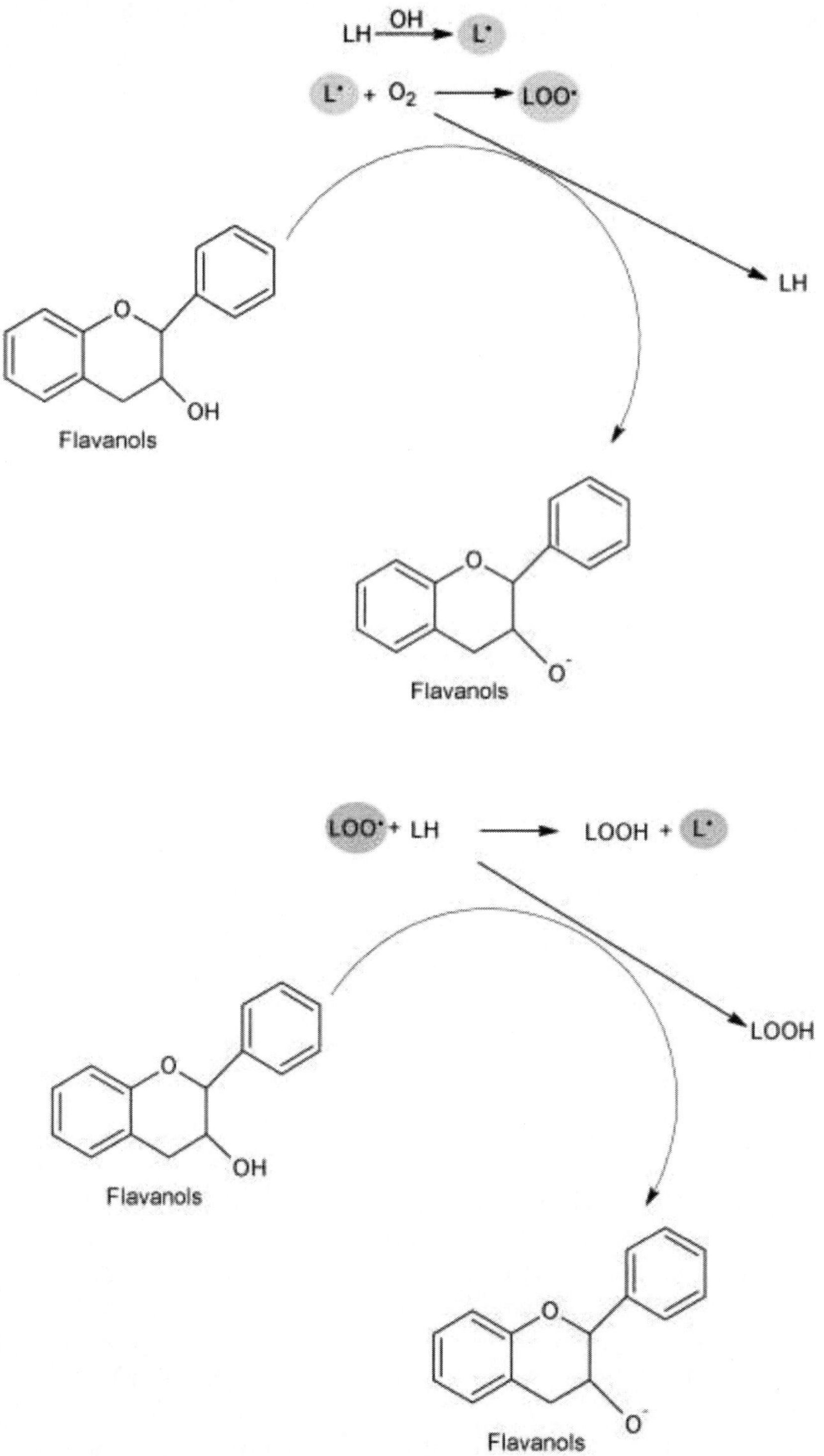

Figure 2. Chain reaction of lipid peroxidation, neutralization of radical formation by flavonoids.

LH oxidation, which is a major event in the oxidation of biological systems, occurs as a chain reaction involving LH and molecular oxygen as substrates, and metals as catalysts (see

Figure 2). The inhibition of the lipid oxidation chain reaction may be considered one of the most important mechanisms explaining the antioxidant actions of FOH. Generally, chain-breaking antioxidants inhibit or retard lipid oxidation by interfering with chain propagating reactions. As shown in Figure 5, FOH can donate hydrogen atoms to lipid ($L^•$) or lipid peroxyl ($LOO^•$) radicals to hamper lipid oxidation propagation. The products of these reactions are non radical species, i.e., the original LH, or the corresponding lipid hydroperoxide (LOOH), and the radical derived from the antioxidant or FOH [52].

However, a major limitation for the 'antioxidant action' of polyphenols associated with free radical chain reactions breaking and metals sequestration (described forward), is the relatively low polyphenol bioavailability observed even after the consumption of foods rich in these compounds. Thus, a potential action of polyphenols as free radical scavengers is unlikely to be physiologically relevant in most organs, except for those exposed to a high polyphenol concentration such as the gastrointestinal tract and perhaps, the blood [54].

Vitamins

Vitamins are organic compounds the body requires for the growth and maintenance of normal cell and organ functions. Because they cannot be made in sufficient quantities, they are required in small amounts in the diet.

α-Tocopherol, shown in Figure 3, has been defined as a radical-chain breaker, which, due to its hydrophobic nature, operates in a LH environment. The effects of α-tocopherol as an antioxidant are thus restricted to its direct effects in membranes and lipoprotein domains. Consequently, other definitions such as "secondary antioxidants" as an inhibitor of "enzymes that produce radicals," or activation of genes coding for "antioxidant enzymes," are confusing. Tocopherols react with free radicals, notably peroxide radicals, and with singlet molecular oxygen, which is the basis of its function as an antioxidant. RRR-α-tocopherol is the major peroxyl radical scavenger in biological lipid phases such as membranes or low-density lipoproteins. In membranes, such high reactivity is important because tocopherols react with $LOO^•$ radicals to yield a relatively stable LOOH, and the tocopheroxyl radical interrupts the radical chain reaction, thereby affording protection against LPO. Vitamin E is the major lipid-soluble antioxidant protecting LH against peroxidative damage. Studies indicate that oxidative cleavage of the phytyl side chain is a major metabolic pathway in humans, operative at saturated vitamin E plasma concentrations. In a study by Chitra et al., aimed to evaluate early and late effects of radiation and α-tocopherol on the secretion of saliva and on the selected saliva salivary parameters in oral cavity cancer patients, the conclusion was that supplementation with α-tocopherol improved the salivary flow rate, thereby maintaining the salivary parameters [54].

Vitamin C or L-ascorbic acid (Figure 4) is water soluble and is present in its deprotonated state under most physiological conditions. It is considered to be the most important vitamin in extracellular fluids and has many cellular activities of an antioxidant nature as well. Vitamin C has been shown to scavenge superoxide, hydrogen, peroxide, $^•OH$ and peroxyl radicals efficiently. Ascorbic acid can also protect membranes against peroxidation by enhancing the activity of tocopherol, the chief lipid-soluble vitamin [54].

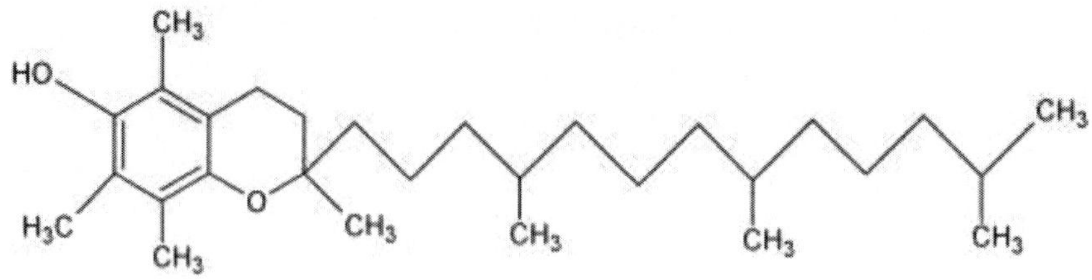

Figure 3. Alpha-tocopherol - just one form of vitamin E.

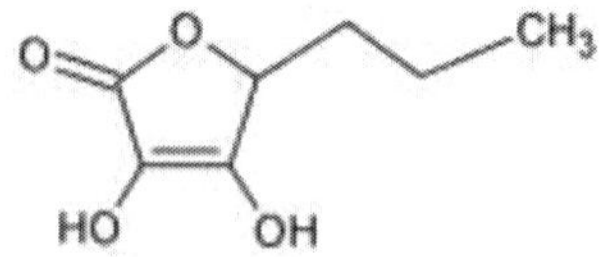

Figure 4. Vitamin C.

Carotenoids are natural compounds with lipophilic properties; β-carotene is the most prominent (Figure 5).

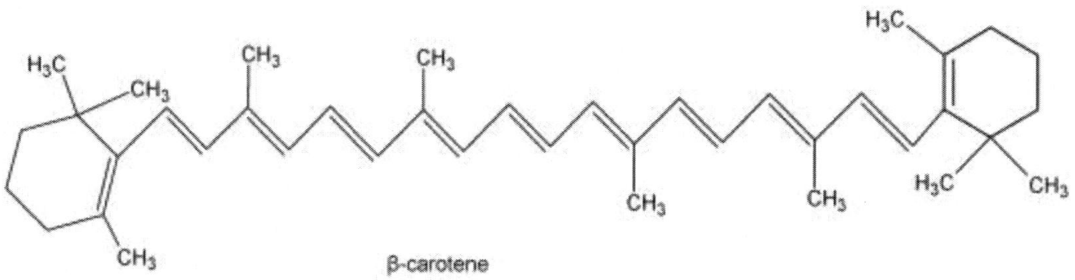

Figure 5. β-carotene.

Most carotenoids contain an extended system of conjugated double bonds, which is responsible for their antioxidant activity; β-carotene deactivates $^{\bullet}O_2$, depending largely on their physical quenching. Carotenoids have also been shown to be capable of inhibiting free-radical reactions (Figure 6). β-carotene very efficiently reduces trichloromethylperoxyl radicals, inhibiting the oxidation of model compounds by peroxyl radicals [54].

Antioxidants that Act as Metal Chelators

Because iron is a primary cause of ROS generation *in vivo* and because it plays such a pivotal role in contributing to OS, DNA damage, and cell death, iron has been the target of many antioxidant therapies. Due to their ability to coordinate iron, polyphenols are one large class of antioxidants that have been extensively examined for treatment and prevention of conditions associated with iron-generated ROS and OS [53]. Several studies have demonstrated that antioxidants and metal chelators may be of beneficial use in the treatment of neurodegenerative diseases, such as Alzheimer's disease. Transition metals such as copper (Cu^{+}) and iron are known to aggravate OS. These metals (Ferrous (Fe^{2+}) and Cu^{+}) react with

H_2O_2, which is a product formed by the dismutation of the $O_2^{\bullet-}$ by SOD, to produce the highly reactive •OH. Unlike iron, copper generates more singlet oxygen than •OH upon its reaction with H_2O_2. Fe^{2+} and Cu^{+} are oxidized to Fe^{3+} and Cu^{2+}, respectively. Oxidized metal ions Fe^{3+} and Cu^{2+} are reduced in the presence of reducing agents such as ascorbic acid ($AscH^{-}$) and a cellular reductant such as NADH thereby allowing the recycling with the formation of another molecule of H_2O_2, which generates another •OH radical. The •OH is highly reactive and can react directly with proteins and other macromolecules to produce carbonyls (aldehydes and ketones), cross-linking and LPO. Chelating metal ions can decrease their activity thereby reducing the formation of ROS [55]. It is important to consider that chelation of transition metals will not always result in an antioxidant action. As the redox properties of a metal change by chelation, it will be the reduction potentials of each polyphenol-metal complex that determine the subsequent behavior.

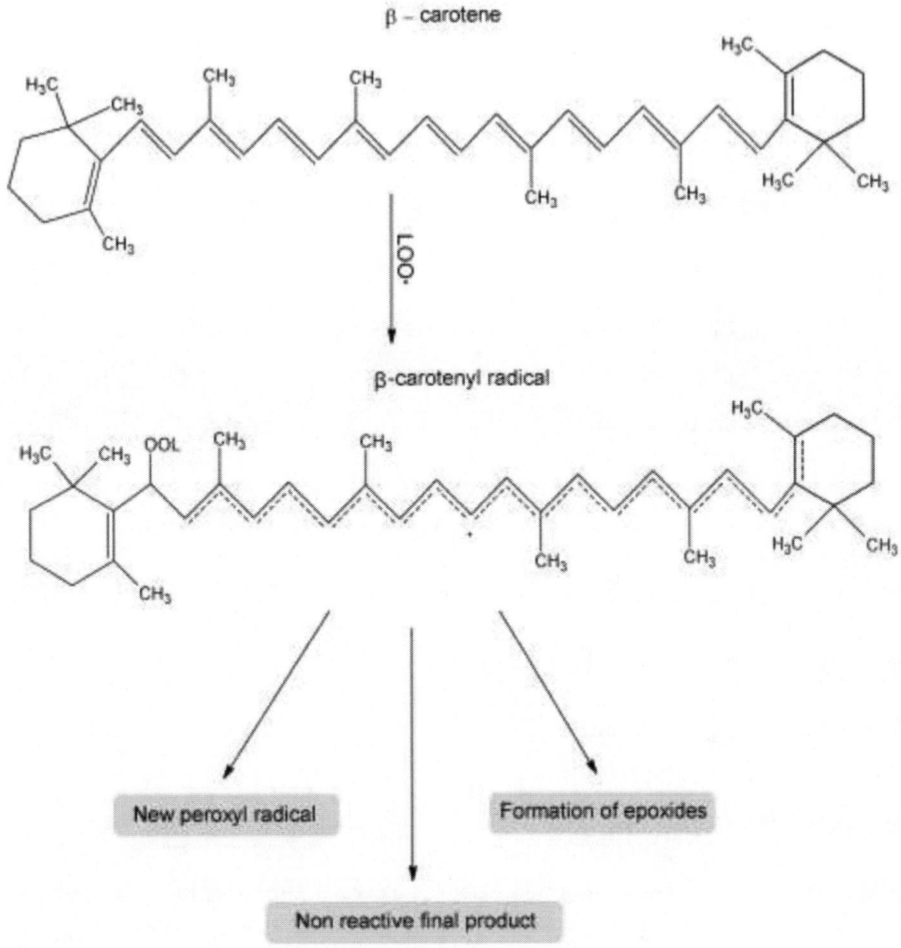

Figure 6. Stabilization of the peroxyl **radical by** β-carotene.

In the intracellular milieu, Fe^{2+} is complexed with a variety of compounds, e.g., phosphates, citrate, etc., with different abilities to promote radical formation. To operate as an antioxidant, the polyphenol-metal complex has to be less efficient in promoting radical formation than the physiological metal-complexes. Finally it is important to indicate that polyphenol-metal complexes have also shown other antioxidant actions, such as mimicking the effects of SOD as was reported for the quercetin–Fe^{2+} complex. Because iron-mediated damage to biomolecules such as LH and DNA is implicated in disease development, the iron-chelating mechanism of polyphenol antioxidant activity must be fully explored in addition to radical scavenging to understand polyphenol antioxidant behavior (Figure 7). Polyphenols with gallol or catechol groups are generally the most potent antioxidants, primarily because of the large iron-binding stability constants for these groups. Also, compounds with the hydroxy-keto moiety can chelate iron, giving rise to antioxidant activity. As compared to radical scavenging, however, the iron-binding mechanism for polyphenol antioxidant activity is relatively underdeveloped.

Therefore, additional research is needed in several areas, including stability constant measurements for iron binding, pKa measurements of polyphenols, and additional cell studies and DNA damage prevention experiments to correlate *invitro* and *in vivo* antioxidant activity of these compounds [53].

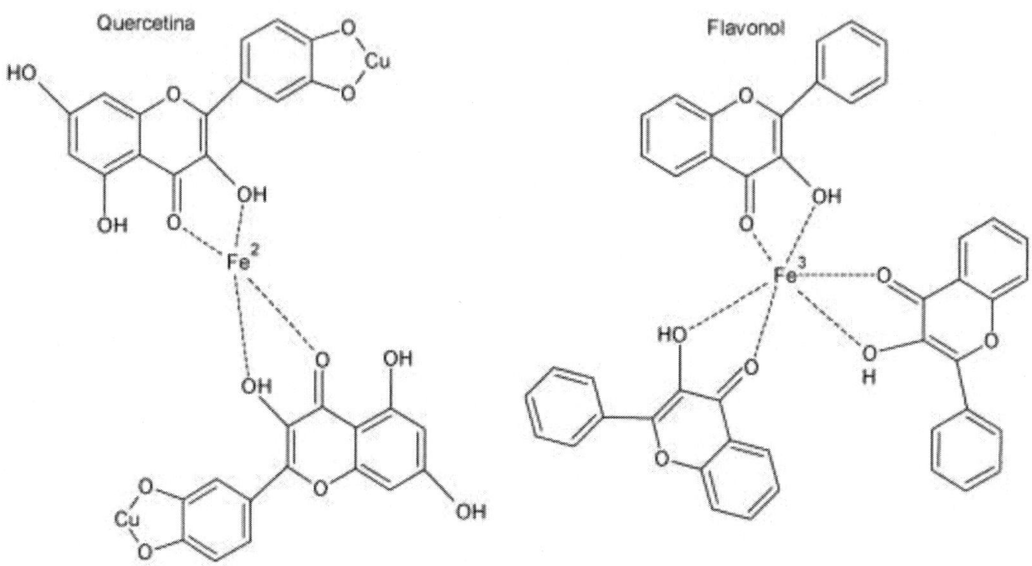

Figure 7. Iron chelation by polyphenols.

Antioxidants and DNA Damage

Cellular DNA may be protected against oxidation by antioxidants, and oxidized DNA lesions are removed by several repair systems such as base excision repair (BER), nucleotide excision repair (NER) and mismatch repair that have overlapping specificity and may interact or function as back-up systems [56]. Polymorphisms in several of these DNA repair-related genes have been found to be associated with the risk of developing different tumor types, although results are not always unequivocal [57]. Individual variation in BER/NER and OS genes is one of the host factors that may influence UV radiation-related cancer risk, such as melanoma [57]. A low activity of DNA repair towards oxidized DNA may increase the risk of cancer by increasing the accumulation of errors in the genome. It has been reported that low repair activity towards oxidized DNA is associated with an increased risk of cancer in case–control studies, although this could be due to reverse causality [56]. Although oxidative DNA damage is believed to stand for an early event, mitochondrial DNA (mtDNA) has, by its turn, been reported to be even more susceptible to oxidation than nuclear DNA. The greater accumulation of damage in mtDNA may be related to mitochondria being the main producers of ROS in the cells as well as the limited repair capacity of mtDNA since the proteins responsible for DNA repair are expressed at lower levels in mitochondria. Moreover, mtDNA is not protected by histones [58].

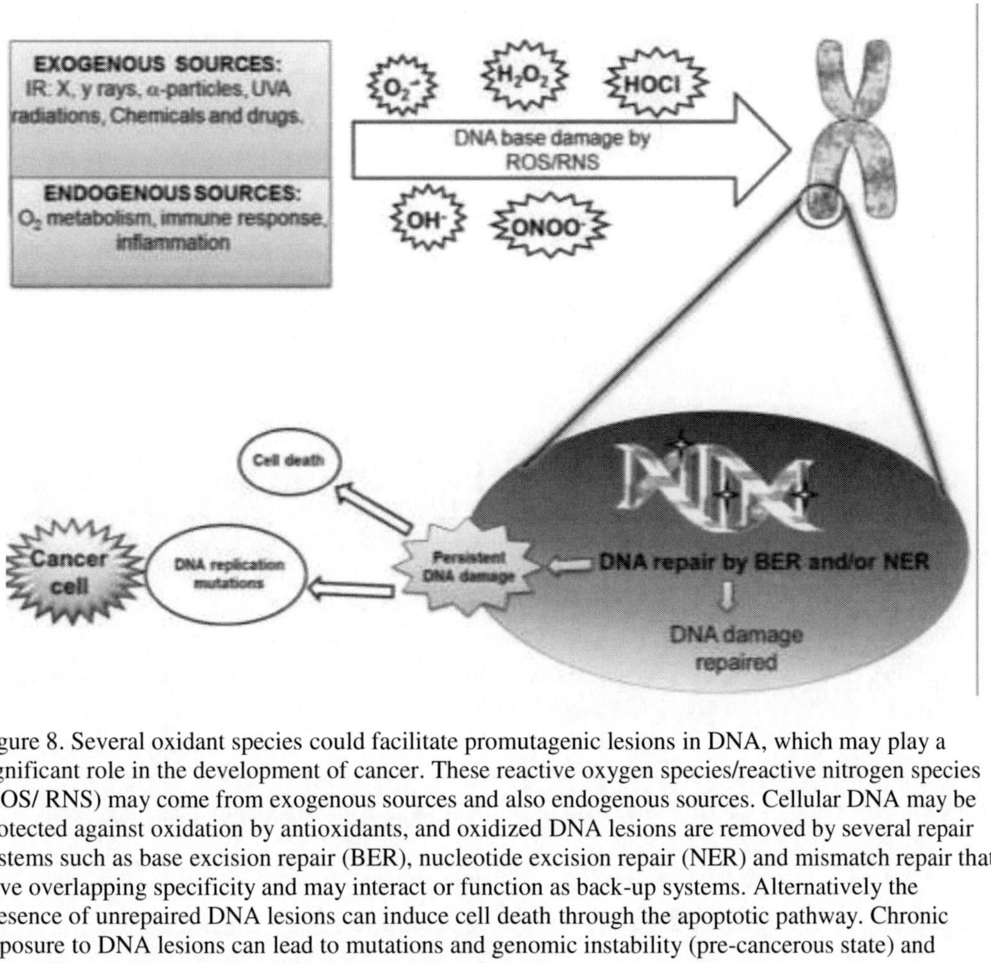

Figure 8. Several oxidant species could facilitate promutagenic lesions in DNA, which may play a significant role in the development of cancer. These reactive oxygen species/reactive nitrogen species (ROS/ RNS) may come from exogenous sources and also endogenous sources. Cellular DNA may be protected against oxidation by antioxidants, and oxidized DNA lesions are removed by several repair systems such as base excision repair (BER), nucleotide excision repair (NER) and mismatch repair that have overlapping specificity and may interact or function as back-up systems. Alternatively the presence of unrepaired DNA lesions can induce cell death through the apoptotic pathway. Chronic exposure to DNA lesions can lead to mutations and genomic instability (pre-cancerous state) and eventually to malignant transformations (cancerous state).

ROS produced in cells, largely as by-products of metabolic processes, constantly threaten the integrity and correct functioning of cellular DNA. Several oxidant species have the capacity to produce promutagenic lesions in DNA, which may play a significant role in the development of cancer [59]. These attacks can be divided into two broad categories: exogenous and endogenous (Figure 8). Exogenous and environmental sources of oxidation relate to specific exposures of the organism to ionizing radiations like X-, γ- or cosmic rays and α-particles from radon decay, oxidizing chemicals and UVA solar light. Endogenous (intracellular) attacks correspond to natural origin such as through cellular signaling and metabolic processes or during inflammation. The oxidatively induced DNA damage associated with ROS typically are apurinic/apyrimidinic (abasic) DNA sites, oxidized purines and pyrimidines, single strand and double strand DNA breaks. Two of the most common endogenous DNA base modifications are 8-oxo-7,8-dihydroguanine (8-oxoGua) and 2,6-diamino-4-hydroxy-5-formamidopyrimidine [60].

Table 1. Antioxidants and their possibles mechanisms in cancer

ANTIOXIDANT	EFFECT ON CANCER
Quercetin	- Inhibited NF-kB and and AP-1 - dose dependent [66] - Induces the tumor suppressor p53 [66] - Modification of signal transduction pathways [144,149] - Induction of apoptosis [144,149] - Inhibition of Phase I enzymes and induction of Phase II enzymes [144,149]
Selenium	- Destroys peroxides [67] - Induces apoptosis [67]
Vitamin E	- Oxidative cleavage of the phytyl side chain [59] - Increase the efficacy of several chemotherapeutic drugs [154]
Vitamin C	- Stimulate immune function [152] - Inhibit nitrosamine formation [152] - Block the metabolic activation of carcinogens [152] - Protection against oxidative DNA damage [152]
Polyphenol	- Inhibition of growth factor signaling [122] - Inhibition of key cellular enzymes [122] - Inhibition of gene transcription [122] - Induction of tumor suppressor genes [122]
Resveratrol	- Regulating cell proliferation and apoptosis [123]
Curcumin	- Inhibit free radicals from mediating peroxidation of membrane lipids or oxidative DNA damage [120,132,133] - Inhibiting intracellular transcription factors and secondary messengers [120,132,133]
Carotenoids	- Interrupt the chain reaction of lipid oxidation and to quench peroxyl radicals [159] - Inhibition of cell growth and malignant transformation and the promotion of apoptosis [161]

Activation of transcription factors activator protein 1 (AP-1) and nuclear factor kappa β (NF-kβ), play a pivotal role in neoplastic transformation [61]. These transcription factors are regulated by upstream kinases, such as mitogen activated protein kinase signaling pathways [62]. Fruits and vegetables contain relatively high amounts of components with inherent antioxidant properties, such as vitamin C, carotenoids and FOH, which has led to the suggestion that dietary antioxidants may augment cellular antioxidant defenses and help protect cellular components from oxidative damage [59]. It was shown that quercetin inhibited NF-kβ and AP-1 in a dose dependent manner. In addition, quercetin also induces the tumor suppressor p53, which promotes DNA repair and has proven to be chemopreventative [62].

The micronutrient selenium has antioxidant action by virtue of its being an integral part of GPx, which destroys peroxides. While its activity in normal cells results in the inhibition of transformation by radiation, in part by increasing inherent levels of antioxidants and doubling the breakdown of peroxide and in stimulating DNA repair in cells with functional p53 (normal cells). The apoptotic effects of selenium on cancer cells have been seen largely in cell cultures. Selenium induces apoptosis in prostate cancer cells and protected normal human fibroblasts [63]. However, until now, there are many doubts about this subject. For example, in an *in vitro* experiment, the presence of vitamins A, C and E in incubation solutions acted synergistically, increasing the level of DNA lesions in cells caused by the exposure of the material on tested irinotecan (a common chemotherapeutic agent) concentrations. Analysis of the efficacy of DNA repair, performed after 2 hours of post incubation, showed the decrease of DNA percentage. Knowledge about the interrelationships of antioxidants, other nutrients, and xenobiotics in model systems and in animal models, is very necessary for providing a rational basis for any potential therapeutic use [64].

In Table 1, some antioxidants and their effects on cancer are listed.

Endogenous Enzymatic Antioxidants

There are three main types of antioxidant defense enzymes: the SODs, including manganese superoxide dismutase (MnSOD) and cytosolic copper/zinc superoxide dismutase (CuZnSOD) (SOD1), CAT, and the GPx (Figure 9). All of them function to protect the cell from damage due to ROS. In addition, several other enzymes are implicated in oxidative damage repair. The reduction of oxidized GSH produced by action of GPxs is catalyzed by glutathione reductase. Accumulating evidence suggests that, in addition to their ''antioxidant'' functions, these enzymes participate in cell signaling processes [58]. Transforming growth factor β1 has been shown to suppress the expression of antioxidant enzymes in some cells leading to increased cellular OS [65]. Recently, it has also been shown that some of these enzymes are associated with modification of histone acetylation and histone acetyltransferase activity, both of which have critical roles in eukaryotic gene transcription, and others are associated with decreased cell proliferation in vascular endothelial cells and increased proliferation of fibroblasts [65]. Mitochondria from several malignant animal tumors, and from many tumor cells in culture, show low MnSOD activity [36]. Low activities of CuZnSOD, CAT and GPx are frequently reported in transformed cell lines and sometimes in biopsies of animal tumors [36]. Studies on human tissues have given variable results, but in general there is no clear evidence for marked decreases in MnSOD or other antioxidant enzymes in freshly-analyzed human cancerous tissue [36].

The thioredoxin (Trx) and thioredoxin reductases (TrxR) are also involved in antioxidant defense through the Trx redox cycle. These proteins are responsible for mediating numerous cytoplasmic functions and are implicated in the control of cell growth in which the redox functions are essential for growth stimulation and apoptosis. Trx is also a key enzyme for DNA synthesis by directly serving as an electron donor to ribonucleotide reductase. In addition, the level of TrxR in tumor cells is often 10-fold or even greater than in normal tissues and tumor proliferation seems to be crucially dependent on an active Trx system [65].

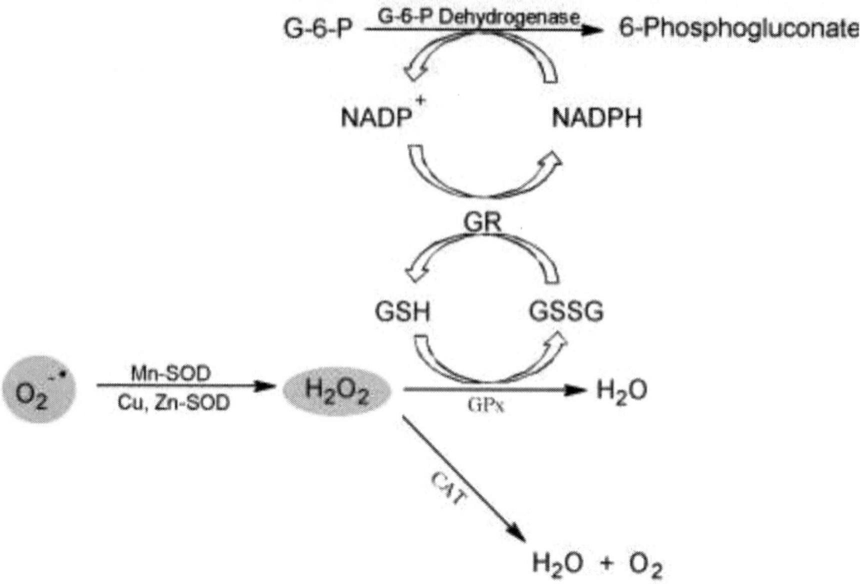

Figure 9. Superoxide dismutase (SOD), glutathione peroxidase (GPx), and catalase (CAT) are the main endogenous enzymatic defense systems of all aerobic cells. They give protection by directly scavenging superoxide radicals and hydrogen peroxide, converting them to less reactive species. SOD catalyzes the **dismutation of superoxide radical (O2•) to hydrogen peroxide** (H_2O_2). CAT the important part of enzymatic defense, neutralizes H_2O_2 into H2O. GPx neutralizes H_2O_2 by taking hydrogens from GSH molecules resulting in two H_2O and one glutathione disulfide (GSSG). Glutathione reductase (GR) then regenerates GSH from GSSG.

SOD

One of the most effective intracellular enzymatic antioxidants is SOD (EC 1.15.1.1). This enzyme, whose activity was first demonstrated in 1969, catalyzes the dismutation of the $O_2^{\bullet-}$ to molecular oxygen and H_2O_2. The H_2O_2 formed in this reaction is then destroyed by the action of CAT and GPx. It should be noted that SOD is the only enzyme family with activity against superoxide radicals (Figure 10) [66]. In humans, there are three forms of SOD: the cytosolic CuZnSOD, which contains copper and zinc in its active center, the mitochondrial MnSOD (that contains manganese in the active site), and the extracellular SOD [58]. Another function of SOD is to protect dehydratases (dihydroxy acid dehydratase, aconitase, 6-phosphogluconate dehydratase and fumarases A and B) against inactivation by superoxide radicals [67]. However, it is still unknown whether SOD1 or other key antioxidant enzymes are hyperactivated in cancer cells and whether they have important roles in tumorgenesis [68].

$$2O_2^{-\bullet} + 2H^+ \xrightarrow{SOD} H_2O_2 + O_2$$

Figure 10. Reaction of superoxide dismutase (SOD). SOD converts superoxide radicals to hydrogen peroxide and oxygen.

CAT

CAT is a tetrameric haeminenzyme consisting of four identical tetrahedrally arranged subunits of 60 kDa. Therefore, it contains four ferriprotoporphyrin groups per molecule, and its molecular mass is about 240 kDa [67]. Mainly localized in the peroxisomes of mammalian cells, which decomposes H_2O_2 to water and molecular oxygen (Figure 11) Thus, it lowers the risk of •OH formation from H_2O_2 *via* the Fenton reaction. In addition, CAT is involved in the detoxification of other substrates that work as H^+ donors, such as phenols and alcohols [58]. CAT is one of the most efficient enzymes known. It is so efficient that it cannot be saturated by H_2O_2 at any concentration [67]. Even though CAT is not essential for some cell types under normal conditions, it plays an important role in the acquisition of tolerance to OS in the adaptive response of cells [67].

$$2H_2O_2 \xrightarrow{\text{Catalase}} 2H_2O + O_2$$

Figure 11. Reaction of catalase. Catalase converts hydrogen peroxide to water and oxygen.

In animals, CAT is present in all major body organs, being especially concentrated in the liver. Since H_2O_2 diffuses readily, this enzyme in erythrocytes can also protect other tissues against oxidative damage. The brain, heart and skeletal muscle contain lower levels of CAT than the liver [36].

GPx

GPx, for which at least four different mammalian forms are known, oxidizes two molecules of GSH to glutathione disulfide (GSSG) (the oxidized form of GSH), which can subsequently be reduced to GSH again by glutathione reductase (Figure 12) [58]. Although their expression is ubiquitous, the levels of each isoform vary depending on the tissue type [69]. The ratios of reduced to oxidized GSH/GSSG in normal cells are high. So, there must be a mechanism for reducing GSSG back to GSH. This is achieved by glutathione reductase enzymes, which catalyze the reaction.

The selenium-containing peroxidases (EC 1.11.1.19), of which GPx may be considered the most important example, catalyze the reduction of a variety of hydroperoxides (ROOH or H_2O_2) in the presence of the reduced form of GSH. Selenium is a trace element essential for the normal function of the body and can be present in inorganic form, metallic form (Se^0) or oxyanions, such as selenite ($SeO(OH)_2$) and selenate ($SeO_2(OH)_2$), and also in organic forms, such as selenocysteine (SeCys) and selenomethionine (SeMet), analogs of sulfur-containing amino acids cysteine and methionine, respectively. Once selenium compounds are recognized as selenium species, they are transformed into selenide, a common intermediate metabolite, and then used for the synthesis of selenoproteins (selenoenzymes) or excreted after being methylated stepwise [70]. Most selenoproteins exhibit oxidoreductase activities. For example, five selenoprotein GPx, three TrxR and all three function on the basis of amino acid selenocysteine contributing to their oxidoreductase activity. Selenoproteins are thought to be closely linked with cancer and carcinogenesis because there are numerous epidemiological reports on an inverse correlation between selenium intake and occurrence of cancer risk [71]. However, the exact mechanism of how selenium intake protects against cancer is unknown. On the other hand, when a normal cell turns into a tumor cell, selenoproteins in the tumor switch their role to protect the malignant phenotype [55,72]. It is, therefore, not surprising that TrxR and Trx have been found to be overexpressed in many aggressive tumors [73]. Moreover, the tumor cell may require enough electrons from the Trx system for ribonucleotide reductase to keep up a constant DNA synthesis. Thus, the Se-containing mammalian TrxRs have emerged as new targets for anti-cancer drug development [55]. The anticarcinogenic role of GPx-1, GPx-4 and Selenoproteins appears to rely mostly on their function as ROOH degradation enzymes. In contrast, GPx-2 and TrxR-1 certainly act as a "double-edged sword" exhibiting anti- and pro-carcinogenic properties. This dual role of GPx-2 has been recently highlighted by an approach using small interfering RNA (siRNA) to knock down GPx-2 expression, which inhibited migration and invasion of human adenocarcinoma cells, but supported tumor cell growth in mice [74]. Further studies are necessary to elucidate the effect of selenoproteins on various types of cancer, focusing not only on prostate and colorectal tumors, which are the most cited in the literature [70].

$$2GSH + H_2O_2 \xrightarrow{\text{Glutathione peroxidase}} GSSG + 2H_2O$$

$$GSSG + NADPH + H^+ \xrightarrow{\text{Glutathione reductase}} 2GSH + NADP^+$$

$$H_2O_2 + NADPH + H^+ \xrightarrow{\text{GSH}} 2H_2O + NADP^+$$

Figure 12. Reactions of glutathione peroxidase and reductase.

Oxidative Stress and Carcinogenesis

Evidence from both *in vitro* and *in vivo* studies has linked environmental agents like radiation, xenobiotics and chlorinated compounds, to the induction of significant cellular damage via ROS-mediated toxicity. In addition, cigarette smoking (known to contain approximately 60 carcinogenic agents) has been considered as one of the most established environmental sources of ROS-mediated carcinogenesis. For example, after chronic exposure, these carcinogenic agents can promote irreversible DNA lesions that can impose an increased risk for developing lung cancer. On the other hand, alcohol consumption is the second leading risk factor associated with neck, oral, and head cancers. Alcohol has been shown to facilitate ROS production, release cytokines and also promote an *in vivo* oxidative microenvironment. Furthermore, exposure to ionizing and ultraviolet radiations also induces ROS-mediated alterations in major pathways associated with the control of cellular growth and survival. For instance, ultraviolet B rays can damage DNA directly and also increase ROS concentrations in epidermal cells [31].

Genetic alterations, chronic inflammation, and malignant transformation are the main events leading to cancer and all of these conditions are associated with excessive ROS generation, resulting in OS. In addition, chronic and accumulative OS induces deleterious modifications to a variety of macromolecular components, such as LH, protein and DNA (Figure 13) [31].

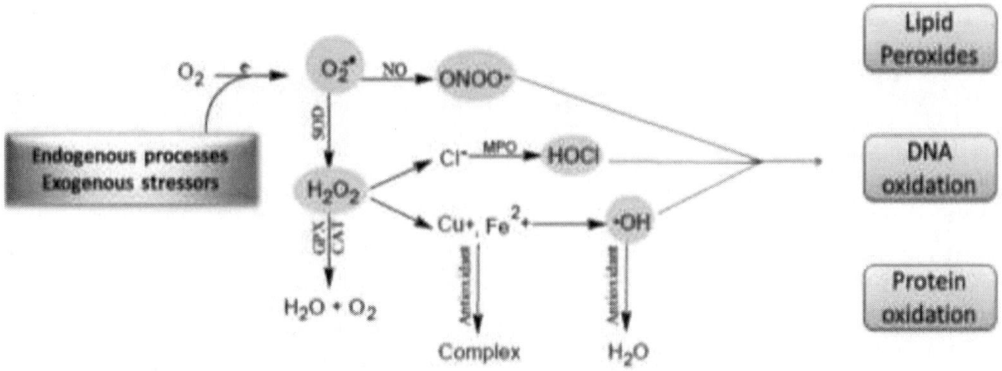

Figure 13. Reactive species of oxygen (ROS) and nitrogen (RNS) are generated by endogenous as well as exogenous sources, causing damage and accumulation of proteins, lipids and DNA, when defensive (repair) mechanisms of body become weak. ROS are either free radicals, reactive anions containing oxygen atoms, or molecules containing oxygen atoms that can either produce free radicals or are chemically activated by them. Summary of ROS and RNS types and sources, and action point of antioxidants: superoxide anion (O2-•), **hydroxyl radical** (•OH) and other species such as hydrogen peroxide (H2O2), hypochlorous acid and peroxynitrite (ONOO-). Antioxidant defense, superoxide dismutase (SOD), catalase (CAT), or glutathione peroxidase (GPx).

Lipid Peroxidation

Polyunsaturated fatty acids, containing two or more double bonds, are readily oxidized by ROS to produce $LOO^{\bullet}$ radicals and LOOH, a process called lipid peroxidation or LPO [75]. Once the process of LPO is initiated, it proceeds as a free radical-mediated chain reaction involving initiation, propagation, and termination [76]. Initiation of LPO is started by the abstraction of a hydrogen atom from polyunsaturated fatty acid moiety of membrane phospholipids by the attack of reactive species [76]. The fatty acid radicals formed in the initiation step will react with the neighboring lipid molecules and generate new free radicals. The propagation phase can repeat many times until it is stopped by chain breaking antioxidants [75,77,78] (Figure 14).

The breakdown of LPO products results in the formation of many reactive aldehydes, such as malondialdehyde (MDA) and 4-hydroxy-2-nonenal [79]. These aldehydes have shown reactivity with protein and DNA and form adducts with these macromolecules [80,81,82,83]. MDA and MDA-MDA dimers are mutagenic [28,84]. Isoprostanes, prostaglandin like compounds, are generated from the free radical-initiated peroxidation of arachidonic acid [85,86,87]. They are formed *in vivo* and can be detected in plasma, tissue and urine, and are elevated by OS inducers such as chloroform, carbon tetrachloride, and cigarette smoking [88,89].

LPO has been implicated in the pathogenesis of various diseases such as cardiovascular disease, cancer, neurological disorders, and aging. LPO also induces disturbances in the fine structure, integrity, fluidity, permeability, and functions of biomembranes, modifies low density lipoprotein and high density lipoprotein to pro-atherogenic and pro-inflammatory forms, and generates potentially toxic products. The reactive carbonyl compounds, the secondary products of LPO, modify proteins and DNA bases.

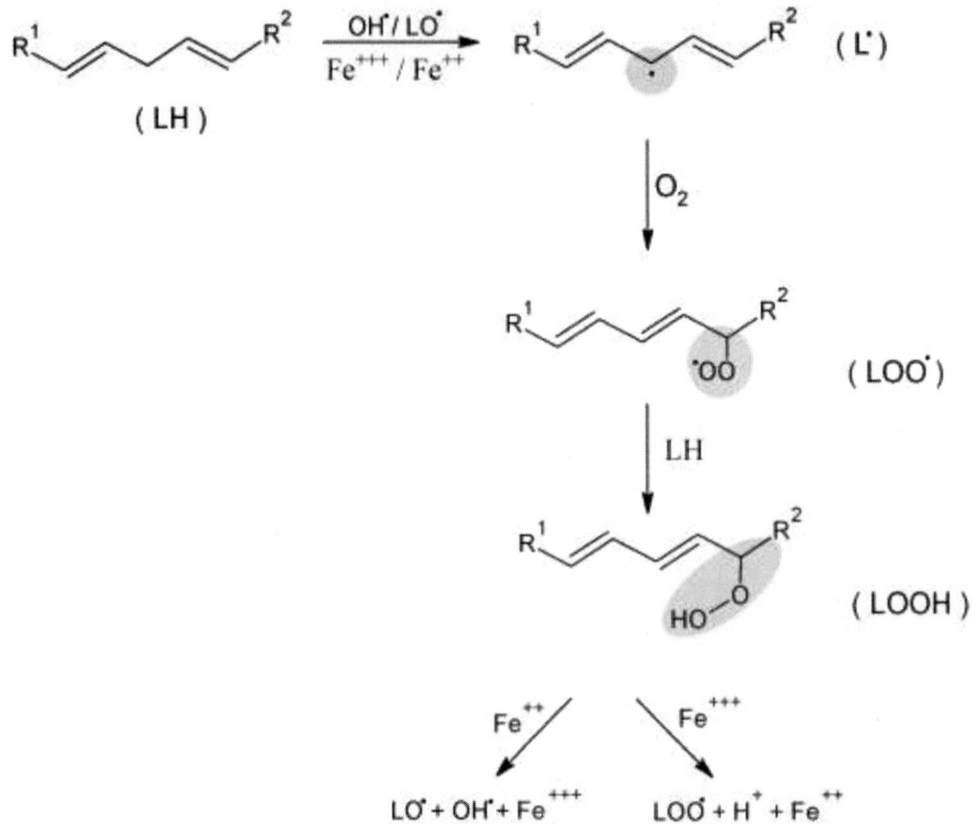

Figure 14. Sequence of reactions involved in the lipid oxidation, LH- lipid molecule; L. -lipid radical; LOO●- lipid peroxyl radical; LOOH- lipid hydroperoxyl.

Consistent with this notion, numerous studies show increased levels of LPO products in the biological fluids and tissues from the cancer patients compared with healthy subjects.

Protein Oxidation

ROS inducing protein damage, oxidative damage to protein-coding or noncoding RNA, may potentially cause errors in protein synthesis or dysregulation of genes expression that could induce to cancer [89]. Reactive species can react directly with protein or they can react with sugars and LH, generating products that in turn react with the protein [90,91]. Within the protein, either the peptide bond or the side chain may be targeted. Basic mechanisms involved in the oxidation of proteins by ROS were elucidated by studies in which amino acids, peptides, and proteins were exposed to ionizing radiations under conditions where •OH or a mixture of •OH and $O_2^{\bullet-}$ are formed [92]. It has been demonstrated that the attack by •OH leads to an abstraction of a hydrogen atom from the protein polypeptide backbone and form a carbon-centered radical [92]. Oxidative damage to proteins ROS-mediated may have significant biological consequences. It can result in modification of enzyme activity (stimulation or inhibition) [93,94]. Damage to membrane transport proteins may produce cellular ionic homeostasis and lead to alterations in intercellular calcium and potassium that will trigger a series of changes in cells [83,95]. Cellular OS can modify intercellular communication, protein kinase activity, membrane structure and function, and gene expression, and result in modulation of cell growth [83]. Changes to receptor proteins and gap junction proteins may also modify signal transfer in cells. In selective cases alteration of protein structure may allow the target protein to be further attacked by proteinases [83].

LPO-induced formation of DNA-protein cross-links is one of the many mechanisms in which protein oxidative damage is generated. *In vitro* models have implicated constituent protein residues and amino acid components as significant targets in long-term exposure to ROS-induced OS.

Evidence suggests that in the presence of exogenous metals, proteins are highly susceptible to damage by a variety of oxidants like H_2O_2 by participating in Fenton reaction, as shown in Figure 15 [31].

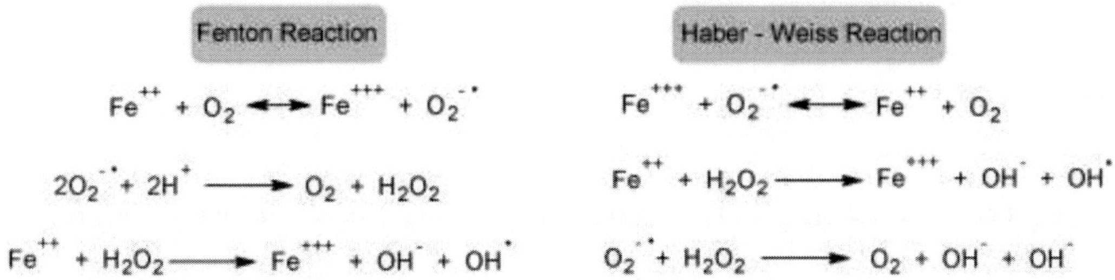

Figure 15. Fenton and Haber-Weiss Reactions.

Protein oxidation products such as bityrosine, a secondary by-product of the mutagenic photoreactive effect of ultraviolet radiation, and carbonyl group formation have both been proposed as important biomarkers of ROS-mediated environmental toxicity [31].

Advanced oxidation protein products, another biomarker of protein oxidation, are formed during OS by the action of chloraminated oxidants, mainly hypochlorous acid and chloramines, produced by myeloperoxidase in activated neutrophils. They are defined as dityrosine containing cross-linked protein products and are considered as reliable markers to estimate the degree of oxidative modifications of proteins [96,97]. However, while protein oxidation has been implicated in a number of aging processes and diseases, most notably Alzheimer's disease, a clear link between protein oxidation and carcinogenesis has not been established [98].

DNA Damage

The most important oxygen-free radical causing damage to basic biomolecules (proteins, membrane LH, and DNA) is the $^{\bullet}OH$. The $^{\bullet}OH$ can be produced by various mechanisms, especially by the Fenton reaction of H_2O_2 (which diffuses into the nucleus) and metals and other endogenous and exogenous ROS. The $^{\bullet}OH$ attacks DNA strands when it is produced adjacent to cellular and mtDNA causing the addition of DNA based new radicals, which lead to the generation of a variety of oxidation products [99]. Being highly reactive, the $^{\bullet}OH$ is the predominant ROS that targets DNA. H_2O_2, a precursor to $^{\bullet}OH$, is less reactive and more readily diffusible and more likely to be involved in the formation of oxidized bases through

Fenton and Haber-Weiss reactions [90]. The interaction of $^{\bullet}OH$ with the nucleobases of the DNA strand, such as guanine, leads to the formation of 8-hydroxyguanine or its nucleoside form deoxyguanosine (8-hydroxy-2-deoxyguanosine). Initially, the reaction of the $^{\bullet}OH$ addition leads to the generation of radical adducts, and then by one electron abstraction, the 8-hydroxy-2-deoxyguanosine (8-OH-dG) is formed [100].

Considerable evidence shows the increase of 8-OH-dG levels in various human cancers and in animal tumor models [101,102,103]. An 8-OH-dG-mediated transversion of guanine:cytosine to thymine:adenine is the most well-known event found in mutated oncogenes and tumor suppressor genes. During DNA replication, the formation of 8-OH-dG by the reaction of ROS with deoxyguanosine triphosphate mediates transversion adenine: thymine to cytosine: guanine. Thus, 8-OH-dG is considered a biomarker of ROS-induced DNA damage and is also widely used to examine the mutagenic and carcinogenic loads derived from OS [34]. In addition, RNS, produced during the process of chronic inflammation, can cause nitrative DNA damage to form 8-nitroguanine and its formation has been observed in various human samples. Experimental evidence suggested that 8-nitroguanine is a mutagenic DNA lesion, which preferentially leads to guanine:thymine transversions [104]. Therefore, 8-nitroguanine could also be used as a potential biomarker to evaluate the risk of inflammation, during which high levels of ROS are usually produced.

ROS can also mediate an indirect attack to DNA primarily by reacting with other cellular components, such phospholipids, resulting in a generation of secondary reactive intermediates that irreversibly couple with DNA bases forming DNA adducts, which is central in the carcinogenesis process [31].

mtDNA is more susceptible to oxidation than nuclear DNA [105], and evidences suggest that oxidative mtDNA is involved in the development of many human cancers including colon [106], liver [107], breast [108], lung [109], bladder [110], prostate [111], esophageal cancer [112], ovarian [113], head and neck [114], and nasopharyngeal [115]. Mutant mtDNA has been reported to be 220 times more abundant than a mutated nuclear DNA biomarker of cancer cells.

Role of Antioxidants in Cancer

Nutrition has long been suspected to play an important role in cancer etiology. Accumulating evidence suggests that diet, in addition to cancer causing substances, also contains many cancer preventive agents [116]. Carcinogenesis is a multi-step process which begins with initiation followed by promotion and progression [117]. It is becoming increasingly clear that many dietary agents can retard or prevent the process of carcinogenesis with reduced cancer outcomes by multiple mechanisms supported by laboratory experiments, including antioxidation, induction of detoxification enzymes and inhibition of bioactivation enzymes, estrogenic and antiestrogenic activity, antiproliferation, cell cycle arrest and apoptosis, promotion of differentiation, regulation of host-immune function, and inhibition of angiogenesis [118]. The cancer protective effect of food constituents is also supported by epidemiological data [116]. In recent years, many studies have demonstrated strong chemopreventive qualities, in other words, the use of agents to inhibit the development or progression of malignant changes in cells, and possibly of the cancer´s treatment effect with one or more cytotoxic antineoplastic drugs of whole food and bioactive food components against cancers of the skin, lung, breast, colon, liver, stomach, prostate and other sites [116]. This implies that many cancers could be prevented by changes in dietary habits [116]. The promising dietary chemopreventive compounds, which have demonstrated anticancer effects, include vitamins and carotenoids, FOH, and the phenolic compounds that they contain [119].

Green Tea Compounds

Green tea is widely acclaimed for its potent antioxidant activity. The predominant green tea polyphenol is catechin, consisting of epigallocatechin-3-gallate (EGCG), epigallocatechin, epicatechin-3-gallate and epicatechin [120]. Green tea polyphenols have been reported to possess antimutagenic, anticarcinogenic, hypolipidemic, and neuroprotective effects attributable to their antioxidant effects, free radical scavenging, and chelation of metal ions [121]. Numerous mechanisms have been proposed to account for the cancer preventive effects of green tea and EGCG in laboratory animal models [122]. These mechanisms include the inhibition of growth factor signaling, inhibition of key cellular enzymes, inhibition of gene transcription, and induction of tumor suppressor genes [122]. Under conditions of high OS, tea polyphenols may be able to directly react with and scavenge free radicals, thus blocking tissue damage. There is considerable and increasing evidence that green tea and EGCG can enhance the expression of endogenous antioxidant systems in both animal models and humans, important to chemoprevention [122].

Certain FOH compounds, including epicatechin and catechin, were found to be inversely associated with lung cancer among tobacco smokers [118]. However, EGCG has been shown to be the most potent FOH for the inhibition of carcinogenesis and the reduction of OS among these catechins [120]. The inhibitory effects of EGCG on Wnt and Hedgehog signaling have been reported in various cancers like breast, prostate, lung and colon cancer, antler progenitor cells, intestinal tumorigenesis and adenomas [120,123]. Moreover, the effect of EGCG in inhibition of metastasis was demonstrated recently [117]. Hepatocyte growth factor was shown to promote the autophosphorylation and enhance the activity of matrix metalloproteinase and urokinase-type plasminogen activator, these effects can eventually lead to cancer cell proliferation, colony dispersion, migration, and invasion of tumors [117]. EGCG blocks hepatocyte growth factor induced invasion and metastasis of hypopharyngeal carcinoma cells and suppressed the molecular tumor motility and the molecular changes induced by hepatocyte growth factor suggesting that EGCG may serve as a therapeutic agent to inhibit hepatocyte growth factor-induced invasion in hypopharyngeal carcinoma patients [117]. EGCG also possibly plays a role in chemoprevention and chemotherapy of various types of cancers, mainly prostate cancer, and colon cancer [124]. *In vitro* studies show that EGCG at high concentrations (10 to 1,000 μM) inhibits a wide range of biomedically-relevant molecular targets and disease related cellular processes, including anticancer molecular targets [124].

Tea polyphenols can also act as pro-oxidants depending on the cell type, dose and/or time of treatment, as they can enhance ROS production and therefore induce apoptosis [125,126]. The mechanism by which polyphenol can act as a pro-oxidant is unclear. Metal ions appear to be involved and most of the cell culture medium is rich in iron ions. Polyphenols can oxidize readily in cell culture medium. Oxidation generates H_2O_2, resulting in the production of ROS

[127]. The observations that inclusion of CAT in the cell culture system prevented EGCG-induced apoptosis of human lung cancer cell line H661 and H-ras-transformed human bronchial epithelial cell line, suggest that H_2O_2 generated from EGCG plays a role in apoptosis induction [126]. The pro-oxidant effects of these compounds have also been suggested as potential mechanisms for cancer prevention [122]. Under typical cell culture conditions, green tea polyphenols are unstable and undergo auto-oxidative reactions resulting in the production of ROS [122]. Pro-oxidant effects of EGCG have been reported in large xenograft tumors, but it has not been established if such effects occur in normal or hyperplastic tissue at low doses [122]. One particularly interesting possibility is that tea polyphenols, at dietary levels, induce low levels of OS which "prime" endogenous antioxidant systems to deal with larger oxidative insults arising from ultraviolet light and other carcinogens [122].

Curcumin

Curcumin is a lipophilic molecule developed from the plant *Curcuma Longa Linn*, commonly called turmeric [128]. Research has shown curcumin to be a potent antioxidant, anti-inflammatory, antiproliferative, antimetastatic, antiangiogenic, antidiabetic, hepatoprotective in cell culture and animal studies [129]. Various *in vitro* as well as *in vivo* studies demonstrated that curcumin can inhibit the growth of various cancer cells from different organs including blood, brain, breast, gastrointestinal system, head and neck, liver, pancreas, colon, prostate, ovary and skin cancers [129,130]. The potent anticancer property of curcumin is attributed to its antioxidant effects that inhibit free radicals from mediating peroxidation of membrane LH or oxidative DNA damage which are both important initiators of cancer development [131]. Despite this, the mechanism by which curcumin exerts its anti-neoplastic activity is not fully understood, but there are over 20 different potential molecular pathways that are currently being studied [128]. Moreover, studies have shown that it induces apoptosis in oncogenic cells by inhibiting various intracellular transcription factors and secondary messengers such as (NF-kβ), AP-1, c-Jun, the janus kinase/signal transducers and activators of transcription (JAK-STAT) pathway, and various others and exhibits potent anti-inflammatory activity, due to the inhibition of IkB kinase required for the activation of NF-kβ, an important transcriptional regulator of inflammatory pathways involved in carcinogenesis and various other pathologic conditions [120,132,133].

Curcumin is also well known for its potential to inhibit carcinogenesis induced by chemical carcinogens, at both initiation and progression stages in various preclinical studies [133]. Curcumin specifically inhibits the expression of cyclooxygenase-2 (COX-2), which plays an important role in colon carcinogenesis [120]. In addition, cancer cells are known to have alterations in multiple cellular signaling pathways among which Wnt and Hedgehog signaling pathways appear to play prominent roles especially because these two developmental pathways are also important in the biology of cancer stem cells and epithelial mesenchymal transition phenotypic cells [123]. Moreover, the molecules in both Wnt and Hedgehog signaling pathways appear to be critical for the processes of cancer cell invasion and metastasis [123]. Therefore, curcumin and others products that target Wnt and Hedgehog signaling could be useful for the prevention of tumor progression and/or could also be useful for the treatment of human malignancies [123]. Curcumin is of special interest for the treatment of leukemia because of its ability to prevent resistance to chemotherapy [131]. On the other hand, it also acts as an immunopotentiator and further protects lymphocytes from genotoxic effects, which are known inducers of secondary cancers [131]. On the other hand, it also acts as an immunopotentiator and further protects lymphocytes from genotoxic effects, which are known inducers of secondary cancers [131].

Curcumin seems to play a role in both chemoprevention and chemotherapy for colon carcinogenesis [128]. The chemopreventive effect of curcumin is mainly due to the inhibition of COX-2, which leads to inhibition of prostaglandin E that normally causes subsequent colon cancer growth [128]. These chemopreventive effects of curcumin resemble those of nonsteroidal anti-inflammatory drugs and COX-2 inhibitors and thus seem to act strongly via inhibition of arachidonate metabolism, reducing cell proliferation, and inducing apoptosis [128]. Curcumin also has been shown to inhibit the growth of transformed cells and colon carcinogenesis at the initiation, promotion and progression stages in carcinogen-induced rodent models, which can potentially be a superior therapeutic strategy for these cancers [134]. Inclusion of curcumin, which effectively inhibits EGFRs and IGF-1R in chemo-surviving cells, into colon cancer chemotherapeutics is likely to inhibit the growth of the chemo-surviving cells and reduce the likelihood of subsequent relapse following chemotherapy at no additional toxicity [135].

Although the antioxidant properties appear to be critical for the chemopreventive effects of curcumin, curcumin also acts as a pro-oxidant by producing ROS [136]. Dance-Barnes et al. suggest that, in the lung, curcumin exerts a tumor-promoting activity causing a statistically significant increase in tumor multiplicity and a clear shift from the predominantly hyperplasia development [137]. In this study, the results demonstrated that after 1 week of curcumin exposure in the diet, mice exhibited an increased level of proteins modified by oxidative damage [137]. Thus, the curcumin-mediated increase in ROS probably predisposes lung tissue to increased genomic instability and tumor progression [138]. In another study, curcumin was shown to cause hyperplasia of the mucosal epithelium in the cecum and colon of male and female rats, an increased incidence of hepatocellular adenoma in male and female mice, a significant increase in thyroid gland follicular cell hyperplasia in female mice and a small but significant increase in sister chromatid exchanges and chromosomal aberrations in cultured Chinese hamster ovary cells [138].

Resveratrol

For decades, several studies have focused on the potential anticancer activity of resveratrol in various kinds of cancers by interfering in different cellular events associated with initiation, promotion, and progression of multistage carcinogenesis [139,140]. These studies suggest that resveratrol has the ability to suppress the proliferation of a wide variety of tumor cells, including lymphoid and myeloid cancers, multiple myeloma, cancers of the breast, prostate, stomach, colon, pancreas, and thyroid, melanoma, head and neck squamous cell carcinoma, ovarian carcinoma, and cervical carcinoma [141]. Resveratrol suppresses many types of cancers by regulating cell proliferation and apoptosis through a variety of mechanisms [123]. The mechanisms of anti-cancer action of resveratrol depend on its ability to induce apoptosis in cancer cells through multiple, related signaling pathways, as for example, inducing loss of mitochondrial membrane potentials, triggering the release of cytochrome C and Smac/Diablo, and subsequently activating caspase-9 (CASP9) and caspase-3 (CASP3) or inducing apoptosis by down-regulating lysosomal cathepsin D and its post-transcriptional factors [140]. The growth-inhibitory effects of resveratrol are mediated through cell-cycle arrest; a decreased cell viability through induction of apoptosis by increasing proapoptotic factors; a down-regulation of survivin, cyclin D1, cyclin E, Bcl-2, Bcl-xL and cIAPs; and an activation of caspases; a suppression of the activation of several transcription factors; and a down-regulation genes products such as COX-2, *5-lipoxygenase*, *vascular endothelial growth factor*, and interleukines (IL) IL-1, IL-6 and IL-8 [131,140,141]. Resveratrol protects the genome at the DNA damage stage by acting as an antioxidant via its inhibition of inflammation, suppression of metabolic carcinogen activation, de novo expression of genes that encode detoxifying proteins and possibly even via radical scavenging properties [139].

Resveratrol also has been shown to potentiate the apoptotic effects of cytokines, chemotherapeutic agents and γ-radiation [140,141]. In addition, cancer cells are known to have alterations in multiple cellular signaling pathways among which Wnt and Hedgehog signaling pathways appear to play prominent roles [123]. Moreover, the molecules in both the Wnt and Hedgehog signaling pathways appear to be critical for the processes of cancer cell invasion and metastasis [123]. It was found that resveratrol suppresses Wnt and Hedgehog signaling pathways [123]. Studies also suggest that the resveratrol inhibits tumorigenesis through the regulation of phosphatidylinositol-3-kinase and Akt proteins, which have been implicated in the development and progression of skin cancer and inhibited tumor-induced neovascularization in the lung metastasis model [117]. In addition, resveratrol also modulates DNA double-strand break repair pathways in p53-dependent manner, suggesting the regulatory effect of resveratrol on p53 signaling [120].

Because tumors develop resistance to chemotherapeutic agents, the cancer research community continues to search for effective chemosensitizers [142]. One promising possibility is to use dietary agents that sensitize tumors to the chemotherapeutics [142]. The tumors shown to be sensitized by resveratrol include lung carcinoma, acute myeloid leukemia, promyelocytic leukemia, multiple myeloma, prostate cancer, oral epidermoid carcinoma, and pancreatic cancer [142]. The chemosensitization of tumor cells by resveratrol appears to be mediated through its ability to modulate multiple cell-signaling molecules, including drug transporters, cell survival proteins, cell proliferative proteins, and members of the NF-kβ and STAT3 signaling pathways [142].

Despite its potential, the use of resveratrol as an anticancer drug is severely constrained because of its tendency to prolong gastric ulceration [143]. In addition to delaying ulcer healing, resveratrol also aggravates acute gastric ulceration induced by the non-steroidal anti-inflammatory drugs by reducing the synthesis of prostaglandin via a specific inhibition of cyclooxygenase that also hampered angiogenesis [143]. Resveratrol has also been found to suppress the phorbol ester-induced COX-2 mRNA expression [143]. It has been suggested that trans-resveratrol, the stereoisomeric form of resveratrol, acts as an angiogenesis inhibitor that may cause the delay of ulcer healing [143]. In addition, at low concentrations, a pro-oxidant effect was also demonstrated for resveratrol in HL-60 leukemia cells, *in vitro* conditions, and was characterized by NADPH oxidase-dependent elevation of intracellular superoxide [139]. Depending on treatment conditions and the intracellular milieu, resveratrol might, therefore, be able to act as pro-oxidant and to differentially influence transcription factors and cellular signaling cascades, which are extremely sensitive to even subtle changes in the redox setting [139].

Quercetin

Quercetin, in certain fruits (apples and grapes) and vegetables (onions and broccoli), is the most abundant naturally occurring FOH [144]. Several previous studies reported that quercetin possesses various beneficial biological activities including antioxidant, anti-inflammatory, anti-atherosclerotic and antitumor properties [144]. Quercetin has also been reported to have anti-tumor effects against a variety of cancer cells *in vitro*, including melanoma, leukemia, human head and neck squamous cell carcinoma, prostate, lung, hepatoma, oral, and colon cancer cell lines [144,145,146,147,148]. Anticarcinogenic and chemopreventive properties may be due to various mechanisms including free radical scavenging, modification of signal transduction pathways, induction of apoptosis, inhibition of Phase I enzymes responsible for activation of carcinogens and induction of Phase II enzymes responsible for the detoxification of carcinogens [144,149]. Quercetin's ability to interact with electrons at higher concentrations plays a central role in its mechanism of action, mainly by the activation of proteins and DNA damage leading to the induction of many downstream pathways [150]. The anticancer mechanisms of quercetin include: (1) inhibiting cell proliferation; (2) antioxidant properties; modulating a number of key targets in cellular signal transduction pathways related to the apoptosis and cell proliferation such as down-regulating anti-apoptosis proteins of the Bcl-2 family; (3) up-regulating pro-apoptotic members; (4) inducing apoptosis through a CASP3 and CASP9 dependent mechanism by releasing cytochrome c and *poly polymerase* cleavage; (5) inhibiting the proteasome activity through modulation of signaling components such as serine/theonine kinase, Akt/protein kinase B, phosphatidylinositol-3 kinase and extracellular-regulated kinase [148,150,151]. Some studies also demonstrated that quercetin can induce apoptosis through suppressing COX-2 in *in vivo* and *in vitro* models [146,151]. Another study suggests that quercetin can restrain neoplastic cell growth by inhibiting various tyrosine kinases [149]. In addition, recent studies have shown that quercetin has antitumor effects on several malignant cell lines such as HL-60, K562, NB4 and Jurkat [151]. Quercetin is also capable of detoxifying free radicals or inactivating radicals intermediates generated by anti-neoplastic drugs and enhancing the cytotoxic action of the chemotherapeutic drugs without damaging normal cells and synergistically potentiates the anti-proliferative effect of anti-neoplastic drugs in these cells [147].

Vitamins C and E

Numerous epidemiological studies have shown an inverse association between vitamin C intake and the risk from different types of cancers. Foods rich in vitamin C include citrus fruit, cabbage, dark green vegetables, cantaloupe, strawberries, and potatoes [124]. Although vitamin C has been known to stimulate immune function, inhibit nitrosamine formation, and block the metabolic activation of carcinogens, its cancer-preventive effects may be associated mainly with its protective effects against OS [152]. OS that leads to oxidative damage, by generating moderate amounts of ROS, could be responsible for causing cancer through multiple mechanisms [152]. The carcinogenic effect of OS has been primarily focused on the genotoxicity of ROS. These can alter signal transduction cascades as well as induce changes in transcription factors that mediate immediate cellular stress responses [153]. Vitamin C can protect against oxidative DNA damage, which is implicated in tumor initiation [152]. In addition, *in vivo* studies have shown that vitamin C is also known to exert anti-cancer activity selectively on cancer cells by generating pro-oxidant activity, depending on blood concentrations, without affecting normal cells [154]. At normal physiologic concentrations, vitamin C acts as an antioxidant that inactivates ROS [155]. However, at high pharmacologic concentrations, vitamin C can act as pro-oxidant by generating oxidative species such extracellular H_2O_2 [155]. Interestingly, the OS promoted by ascorbate seems to preferentially target cancer cells, which exhibit a greater sensitivity towards ascorbate compared to their normal counterparts [155]. Several *in vitro* studies have shown that the extracellular vitamin C that generates H_2O_2, kills cancer cells selectively but does not harm the normal cells [155,156]. Extracellular H_2O_2 from high doses of vitamin C diffuses into the cancer cells and causes toxicity in these cells by *adenosine triphosphate* depletion which eventually leads to cell death [155,156]. Additionally, H_2O_2 toxicity compromises the DNA integrity in the cancer cells [156].

In normal cells H_2O_2 is readily neutralized by antioxidant enzymes such as CAT, GPx and SOD. The level of these enzymes in cancer cells is low which causes the toxicity and cancer cell death [155,156]. The mechanism by which vitamin C can act as a pro-oxidant may be possibly due to its ability to regenerate vitamin E, which in excess can cause displacement of other important antioxidants, interference with essential defense mechanisms, such as apoptosis, damage to essential LH and competition for absorption of other essential compounds [124].

Some studies suggest that vitamin E decreases the risk for the development of esophageal, colon, prostate, mammary, and lung tumorigenesis in animal studies, suggesting that this vitamin may have a strong potential for applications in the prevention of human cancers [124]. On the other hand, the Selenium and Vitamin E Cancer Preventions Trial (SELECT), showed that dietary supplementation with 400 IU/d of all-racemic alpha-tocopheryl acetate significantly increased the risk of prostate cancer among healthy men. Vitamin C and E have been reported to increase the efficacy of several chemotherapeutic drugs either *in vitro* or *in vivo*, and similar data have been obtained with radiotherapy [154]. These vitamins may be used as a radioprotector that effectively scavenges the free radicals formed during radiation exposure [157].

However, some studies show increased mortality with high vitamin E supplementation [158]. Pro-oxidant effects at high doses, displacement of other important antioxidants, vitamin E interference with essential defense mechanisms, such as apoptosis, damage to essential LH, and competition for absorption of other essential compounds are possible explanations for a lack of benefit of vitamin [158].

Carotenoids Compounds

Carotenoids, a group of fat-soluble pigments present in many foods, particularly fruits and vegetables, have abundant conjugated double bonds to interrupt the chain reaction of lipid oxidation and to quench peroxyl radicals [155]. They have been postulated to reduce the risk of cancer through their antioxidant properties by reducing oxidative DNA damage [160]. They can also influence cell growth regulation, including the inhibition of growth and malignant transformation and the promotion of apoptosis in transformed cells and may thereby protect against carcinogenesis [160]. Carotenoids exhibit antioxidant activity *in vitro* [161].

Epidemiological data have shown that diets rich in β-carotene are associated with a decreased incidence of cancer compared with those with normal diets [158]. Evidence suggests that foods containing these carotenoids are associated with a decreased risk for cancers of the mouth, pharynx, larynx, esophagus, and lung [124]. Thus, based on these data, it has been suggested that β-carotene should be helpful in preventing cancer [158].

One study found that β-carotene given for 21 days before methotrexate application, a cytotoxic agent in the treatment of leukemia and other malignancies, provided significant protection from the hepatotoxicity of methotrexate [119]. The pretreatment with β-carotene probably protected the hepatocyte membrane integrity by preventing the peroxidation of fatty acids by free radicals and inhibiting an important mechanism that causes liver damage and by probably protecting cells from DNA changes and apoptosis with the ability of connecting singlet oxygen radicals and scavenging peroxide radicals [119]. The inhibition of lung metastasis by β-carotene has been shown in mice and these carotenoids have been shown to inhibit o estrogen signalling of 17β-estradiol, and attenuate the adverse effect in hormone-dependent breast cancer [117,156].

Moreover, an inverse association between β-carotene and risk of overall breast cancer has been observed in several case-control and prospective studies [160]. β-carotene has been shown to inhibit both estrogen receptor–positive and estrogen receptor–positive breast tumor cell growth *in vitro* and also to inhibit estrogen signaling of 17β-estradiol and thus inhibit estrogen-induced cell proliferation [161]. Estrogenic stimulation is believed to play a causal role in the pathogenesis of breast cancer, and higher serum estrogen concentration has been observed to contribute to the risk of recurrence in women who have been diagnosed and treated for early-stage breast cancer [161]. These data suggest that longer-term exposure to carotenoids is associated with a greater likelihood of breast cancer–free survival in women who have been diagnosed and treated for early-stage breast cancer [161].

Some carotenoids, such as β-carotene, have a provitamin A activity [160]. Vitamin A derivatives play an essential role in cell proliferation, differentiation, and apoptosis in normal and neoplastic ovarian tissue [162]. Retinoic acid, the primary active metabolite of vitamin A, mediates numerous gene transcriptions through retinoid nuclear receptors, and hence, is considered to be one of the most promising chemopreventive and chemotherapeutic agents against ovarian cancer [161]. Based on this hypothesis high intake of β-carotene may be protective among women against risk of ovarian cancer [160,162].

Lycopene is a carotenoid without provitamin A activity and is found in foods such as tomato, watermelon, and pink grapefruit [163]. Epidemiological evidence and a small number of animal studies indicate that lycopene rich diets may have a protective effect against chronic diseases, including cancer [163]. Lycopene also has antitumor and anti-inflammatory properties [163]. Among the more than 600 naturally occurring carotenoids, lycopene is the most efficient antioxidant [164]. Some properties of lycopene are attributed to its ability to scavenge free radicals and physically quench singlet molecular oxygen [123,163,164]. Palozza et al. suggest that lycopene products could be potent anticancer compounds in chemopreventive and therapeutic applications and provide a novel mechanistic insight into the inhibitory effects of lycopene on the growth of human cancer cells [165].

Lycopene has a protective effect against prostate cancer [124]. An *in vivo* and *in vitro* study has been reported, which indicates that short-term intake of tomatoes induces changes in the concentrations of serum components that modulate potential genes of prostatic cancer cells *in vivo* [166]. Experimental studies *in vitro* also showed that lycopene inhibited cell growth in breast, prostate and endometrial cancer cells with regulation of cell-cycle related genes [123]. Sarkar et al. have shown that lycopene supplements reduced tumor size and PSA level, *in vivo,* in localized prostate cancer suggesting its promising effects on prostate cancer prevention and/or treatment [123]. Experimental studies have shown that lycopene reduced inflammatory signals, prevented oxidative DNA damage, and regulated the expression or activity of IGF/Akt, Wnt/β-catenin, and AR signaling [167]. It is believed that the effects of lycopene on these pathways contribute to the observed cell growth inhibition and apoptosis induction [167]. An *in vivo* study showed that the application of lycopene before abdominopelvic radiotherapy has the potential to reduce oxidative damage caused by radiotherapy in rats by decreasing LPO and stimulating antioxidant enzyme activities [167]. Moreover, lycopene has been shown to inhibit estrogen signalling of 17β-estradiol, and attenuate the adverse effect of hormone-dependent breast cancer [160].

Epidemiologic studies of dietary or blood levels of carotenoids in relation to cancer risk have yielded inconsistent results with both inverse and null findings [160,162]. Results from two clinical trials, the α-Tocopherol, β-Carotene Cancer Prevention Study and the Carotene [168] and Retinol Efficacy Trial [169], indicate an adverse effect of h-carotene supplements on lung cancer risk among smokers and drinkers. These findings not only raise health concerns about potential pro-oxidant effects of β-carotene but also add further complexity to our understanding of the underlying antiproliferative mechanisms of antioxidants [162].

Primary prevention lung cancer clinical trials demonstrate a potential risk of increased lung cancer and overall mortality associated with β-carotene supplementation for smokers [158]. The paradox lies in the fact that many dietary intake studies have shown an association of increased intake of β-carotene with decreased risk of lung cancer whereas intervention studies with high-dose β-carotene supplementation have shown an increased risk of lung cancer in smokers [158]. Most recently, reports were published highlighting supplements as a cause for a higher incidence of cancer [170]. Bjelakovic et al. conducted a meta-analysis of 67 randomized controlled trials which showed that vitamin E, vitamin A, and β-carotene supplements may be associated with an increased incidence of mortality [170].

ATBC Cancer Prevention Study was a randomized placebo control study of approximately 30,000 male subjects of age 50–69 years who were heavy smokers. There were four treatment groups: 50 mg α-tocopheryl acetate alone, 20 mg of β-carotene alone, a combination of the two, and a placebo group. Subjects received their respective treatment for 5–8 years. The results were that those who were treated with β-carotene had an increased incidence of lung cancer (16–18%) and an 8% increased rate of mortality [180]. Further research is needed to define the biologically plausible explanation for the possible association between β-carotene supplementation and an increase in lung cancer rates in individuals at high risk for lung cancer [181]. Burton and Ingold noted that β-carotene action depends on whether it exists in low oxygen concentrations or high concentrations of oxygen or whether other oxidants in the microenvironment can govern pro-oxidant versus antioxidant effects

[171]. β-Carotene has enhanced antioxidant activity at a lower oxygen tension [158]. At even higher oxygen tension, any antioxidant activity of β-carotene is offset by its pro-oxidant activity [158]. Thus, β-carotene would be contraindicated in situations of high oxygen tension, such as hyperoxia, oxygen therapy, reperfusion injury, and likely exposure to other oxidants (smoking) [158].

Oncology Therapy and Antioxidants

The use of antioxidant supplementation in patients with cancer is controversial, because it may interfere with the mechanism of action of the chemotherapy and subsequently decrease its efficacy. Others argue that antioxidant supplementation is beneficial when associated with chemotherapy by enhancing its efficacy, as well as alleviating toxic side effects [50].

A few publications support the view that antioxidant supplementation can help reduce some adverse effects of chemotherapeutic agents including neurotoxicity, thrombocytopenia, and diarrhea, thereby enabling increased or uninterrupted dosing in patients who otherwise may discontinue treatment due to side effects [50].

Radiotherapy

The principal therapeutic effect of radiation occurs indirectly via the ionization of water molecules in the cytoplasm to ROS, for example, $O_2^{\bullet-}$ and $^{\bullet}OH$s. In addition, radiotherapy is based on the fact that ionizing radiation destroys tumor cells and induces direct lesions in the DNA or biological molecules via ROS formation. Some of this radiation damage can be repaired, leaving a cell that remains viable with the ability to proliferate. On the other hand, antioxidants are compounds that can counteract free radicals and prevent them from causing tissue and organ damage. Bairati et al. reported that among 540 head and neck cancer patients who were randomly assigned to receive either α-tocopherol with or without β-carotene versus placebo concurrent with their radiation therapy, those who received both antioxidants had a statistically significant 38% reduction in severe, acute side effects [172]. Nevertheless, these results suggest that caution should be advised regarding the use of high-dose α - tocopherol supplements for cancer prevention [172, 173].

Several others studies have provided evidence that antioxidants can decrease the effectiveness of radiation therapy [174]. Ferreira et al. randomly assigned 54 head and neck cancer patients, who were undergoing radiation therapy, to receive an oil-based oral rinse that contained either α-tocopherol or placebo before and after each daily dose of radiation. Vitamin E was associated with a 36% reduction in symptomatic mucositis, however, a decrease in 2-year overall survival was observed (32%) with supplemental vitamin E versus 63% with placebo; $p=0.13$) but this was not statistically significant. In another cohort study 90 patients were evaluated with non metastatic breast cancer who received conventional therapy either alone or in association with high doses of β-carotene, vitamin C, niacin, selenium, coenzyme Q10, and/or zinc. Breast cancer-specific survival and disease-free survival were shorter in the nutrient-supplemented group than in the non-supplement group, but the differences were not statistically significant [175].

The Food and Drug Administration has approved the use of some antioxidants during oncological treatments, such as amifostine, a thiol-containing antioxidants, which act to increase the radio-resistance of normal salivary gland tissues. However, neither the prospective, randomized phase III trial or randomized comparative trial with amifostine [176, 177] nor meta-analyses [178, 179] have provided conclusive evidence of increased radio resistance of tumors with this therapy.

Chemotherapy Drugs

One of the main mechanisms of chemotherapy drugs against cancer cells is the formation of ROS and RNS. Drugs with free radical mechanisms include alkylating agents (e.g., melphalan, cyclosphosphamide), anthracyclines (e.g., doxorubicin, epirubicin), podophillin derivates (e.g., etoposide), platinum coordination complexes (e.g., cisplatin, carboplatin) and camptothecins (e.g., topotecan, irinotecan). Other chemotherapy drugs generate lower levels of OS, and free radical damage is thought to be of less importance in their mechanisms of action, such as the taxanes (e.g., paclitaxel, docetaxel), vinca alkaloids (e.g., vincristine, vinblastine), and antimetabolites (e.g., methotrexate, fluorouracil, cytarabine). In addition, antioxidants have multiple mechanisms of action, and depending on their use, have been noted to have the potential to serve as oxidant molecules themselves. This represents a dilemma for patients with cancer in trying to understand whether antioxidant therapy will increase their quality of life through protection of normal tissues or interfere with the eventual clinical outcome of their disease [50].

Pathak et al. examined whether the concurrent administration of a high-dose antioxidant mixture containing vitamins C and E, and β-carotene with paclitaxel and cisplatin improved tumor response and survival in 136 patients with advanced non–small cell lung cancer and observed no survival or tumor response benefits with the antioxidants [180]. However, the authors' conclusion that the antioxidant supplementation was safe is not warranted because the study was not sufficiently powered to evaluate a reduction in survival or tumor response [180]. In a systematic review of the randomized trials of antioxidants and chemotherapy, Ladas et al. found such a wide range of cancer diagnoses, chemotherapy regimens, and antioxidant supplementation that they could not draw definitive conclusions about the safety and efficacy of the antioxidant interventions [181]. Although several studies [reviewed by Mills et al. [182]] have suggested that melatonin supplementation may improve the survival of chemotherapy-treated patients with some solid tumors, it is not clear whether this effect was mediated exclusively by the antioxidant action of this hormone [182]. For example, in a randomized clinical trial of cisplatin plus etoposide and melatonin, Lissoni et al. observed improved tumor response rates in 100 patients with metastatic non–small-cell lung cancer [183]. The same group of investigators also observed similar results with melatonin in a study of 250 patients with various metastatic solid tumors who received several different chemotherapy regimens [184]. These intriguing results should now be independently confirmed in larger trials [185].

Conclusion and Perspectives

In conclusion, molecular epidemiological studies have identified a causal relationship between chronic exposure to OS and the development of environmental carcinogenesis. In particular, it has been estimated that exposure to environmental carcinogens can contribute significantly in the development of human cancers through OS-mediated macromolecular damage. In addition, OS has also been implicated in inducing mutations that debilitate the normal functioning of a variety of repair mechanisms and thus allow for the loss-of-function of cell cycle control genes. Exposure to many environmental and occupational carcinogens have shown positive correlations with biomarkers of ROS-mediated macromolecular damage, thus providing supporting evidence between environmental toxicity and the development of carcinogenesis. With respect to antioxidant therapy, there are several controversial publications regarding cancer treatment. Some studies suggest that antioxidant supplementation may affect cancer treatment outcome, but they are still limited in the quality and number of patients used. On the other hand, there are papers showing that antioxidant supplementation provided during chemotherapy administration reduced the toxic effects of ROS/RNS produced by the chemotherapuetic agents. The effects of antioxidant supplements on human health, particularly in relation to cancer, should not be overemphasized because their use might be harmful for some cancers. Therefore, research into the potential therapeutic effects of novel antioxidant molecules (or existing antioxidants but in different doses) remains a high priority but questions about safety and utility in cancer must be clarified.

References

[1] Howlader N, Noone AM, Krapcho M, Garshell J, Neyman N, Altekruse SF, et al. National Cancer Institute. SEER Cancer Statistics Review, 1975-2009 (Vintage 2009 Populations). [Internet]. Bethesda, Maryland. [Updated on: 2012 August ; accessed on 2013 Jun 16] Available from: http://seer.cancer.gov/csr/1975_2009_pops09.

[2] Antonsson A, Nancarrow DJ, Brown IS, Green AC, Drew PA, Watson DI, et al. (2010). High-risk human papillomavirus in esophageal squamous cell carcinoma. *Cancer Epidemiol Biomarkers Prev.*19(8):2080-7.

[3] Ferlay J, Shin HR, Bray F, Forman D, Mathers C, Parkin DM. *International Agency for Research on Cancer.* GLOBOCAN 2008, Cancer Incidence and Mortality Worldwide: IARC CancerBase [Internet]. Lyon, France. [Updated on: 2011 December; accessed on 2013 Jun 20], Available from: http://globocan.iarc.fr.

[4] Jemal A, Center MM, DeSantis C, Ward EM (2010) Global patterns of cancer incidence and mortality rates and trends. *Cancer Epidemiol Biomarkers Prev.* 19(8):1893-907.

[5] Youlden DR, Cramb SM, Baade PD (2008). The international epidemiology of lung cancer: Geographical distribution and secular trends. *J Thorac Oncol.* 3(8):819–31.

[6] Bray FI, Weiderpass E (2010). Lung cancer mortality trends in 36 European countries: secular trends and birth cohort patterns by sex and region 1970-2007. *Int J Cancer.* 126(6):1454-66.

[7] Ezzati M, Henley SJ, Lopez AD, Thun MJ (2005). Role of smoking in global and regional cancer epidemiology: current patterns and data needs. *Int J Cancer.* 116(6):963-71.

[8] Ezzati M, Lopez AD (2003). Estimates of global mortality attributable to smoking in 2000. *Lancet.* 362(9387):847-52.

[9] Center MM, Jemal A, Smith RA, Ward E (2009). World wide variations in colorectal cancer. *CA Cancer J Clin.* 59(6):366-78.

[10] Edwards BK, Ward E, Kohler BA, Eheman C, Zauber AG, Anderson RN, et al. (2010). Annual report to the nation on the status of cancer, 1975-2006, featuring colorectal cancer trends and impact of interventions (risk factors, screening, and treatment) to reduce future rates. *Cancer.* 116(3):544-73.

[11] Parkin DM, Fernández LM (2006). Use of statistics to assess the global burden of breast cancer. *Breast J.* 2 Suppl 1:S70-80.

[12] Zahl PH, Maehlen J, Welch HG (2008). The natural history of invasive breast cancers detected by screening mammography. *Arch Intern Med.* 168(21):2311-6.

[13] Parkin DM (2002). The global health burden of infection-associated cancers in the year. *Int J Cancer.* 118(12):3030-44.

[14] Bertuccio P, Chatenoud L, Levi F, Praud D, Ferlay J, Negri E, et al. (2009) Recent patterns in gastric cancer: a global overview. *Int J Cancer.* 125(3):666-73.

[15] Jemal A, Siegel R, Ward E, Hao Y, Xu J, Thun MJ (2009). Cancer statistics, 2009. *CA Cancer J Clin.* 59(4):225-49.

[16] Botterweck AA, Schouten LJ, Volovics A, Dorant E, van Den Brandt PA (2000). Trends in incidence of adenocarcinoma of the esophagus and gastric cardia in ten European countries. *Int J Epidemiol.* 29(4):645-54.

[17] El-Serag HB (2007). Time trends of gastro esophageal reflux disease: a systematic review. *Clin Gastroenterol Hepatol.* 5(1):17-26.

[18] Bosch FX, Ribes J, Díaz M, Cléries R (2004). Primary liver cancer: worldwide incidence and trends. *Gastroenterology.* 127(5 Suppl 1):S5-S16.

[19] Raza SA, Clifford GM, Franceschi S (2007). Worldwide variation in the relative importance of hepatitis B and hepatitis C viruses in hepatocellular carcinoma: a systematic review. *Br J Cancer.* 96(7):1127-34.

[20] Seeff LB, Hoofnagle JH (2006). Epidemiology of hepatocellular carcinoma in areas of low hepatitis B and hepatitis C endemicity. *Oncogene.* 25(27):3771-7.

[21] Perz JF, Armstrong GL, Farrington LA, Hutin YJ, Bell BP (2006). The contributions of hepatitis B virus and hepatitis C virus infections to cirrhosis and primary liver cancer worldwide. *J Hepatol.* 45(4):529-38.

[22] Shafey O, Dolwick S, Guindon GE. *Tobacco Control Country Profiles* [Internet]. 2 ed. Atlanta (GA): American Cancer Society, WHO, International Union against Cancer; 2003. [accessed on 2013 Jun 21] Available from http://www.who.int/tobacco/global_data/country_profiles/en/

[23] Schatzkin A, Subar AF, Moore S, Park Y, Potischman N, Thompson FE, et al. (2009). Observational epidemiologic studies of nutrition and cancer: the next generation (with better observation). *Cancer Epidemiol Biomarkers Prev.* 18(4):1026-32.

[24] Valko M, Leibfritz D, Moncol J, Cronin MT, Mazur M, Telser J (2007). Free radicals and antioxidants in normal physiological functions and human disease. *Int J Biochem Cell Biol.* 39(1):44-84.

[25] Kumar B, Koul S, Khandrika L, Meacham RB, Koul HK (2008). Oxidative stress is inherent in prostate cancer cells and is required for aggressive phenotype. *Cancer Res.* 68(6):1777-85.

[26] Ishikawa K, Takenaga K, Akimoto M, Koshikawa N, Yamaguchi A, Imanishi H, et al. (2008). ROS-generating mitochondrial DNA mutations can regulate tumor cell metastasis. *Science.* 320(5876):661-4.

[27] Sitkovsky M, Lukashev D (2005). Regulation of immune cells by local-tissue oxygen tension: HIF1 alpha and adenosine receptors. *Nat Rev Immunol.* 5(9):712-21.

[28] Klaunig JE, Kamendulis LM (2004). The role of oxidative stress in carcinogenesis. *Annu Rev Pharmacol Toxicol.* 44:239-67.

[29] Federico A, Morgillo F, Tuccillo C, Ciardiello F, Loguercio C (2007). Chronic inflammation and oxidative stress in human carcinogenesis. *Int J Cancer.* 121(11):2381-6.

[30] Kadiiska MB, Gladen BC, Baird DD, Germolec D, Graham LB, Parker CE, et al (2005). Biomarkers of oxidative stress study II: are oxidation products of lipids, proteins, and DNA markers of CCl4 poisoning? *Free Radic Biol Med.* 38(6):698-710.

[31] Ziech D, Franco R, Georgakilas AG, Georgakila S, Malamou-Mitsi V, Schoneveld O, et al. (2010). The role of reactive oxygen species and oxidative stress in environmental carcinogenesis and biomarker development. *Chem Biol Interact.* 188(2):334-9.

[32] Ushio-Fukai M and Nakamura Y (2008). Reactive Oxygen Species and Angiogenesis: NADPH Oxidase as Target for Cancer Therapy. *Cancer Lett.* 266(1):37–52.

[33] Serafini, Mauro (2006). The role of antioxidants in disease prevention. *Medicine.* 34(12):533-35.

[34] Lee JC, Son YO, Pratheeshkumar P, Shi X (2012). Oxidative stress and metal carcinogenesis. *Free Radic Biol Med.* 53(4):742-57.

[35] Dalle-Donne I, Rossi R, Colombo R, Giustarini D, Milzani A (2006). Biomarkers of oxidative damage in human disease. *Clin Chem.* 52(4):601-23.

[36] Halliweell B, Gutteridge JMC (1999). Antioxidant defenses. In: Halliweell B, Gutteridge JMC. Free Radicals in Biology and Medicine. 3th edition. City: New York, Oxford Science Publications; 105-245.

[37] Lü JM, Lin PH, Yao Q, Chen C (2010). Chemical and molecular mechanisms of antioxidants:experimental approaches and model systems. *J. Cell. Mol. Med.* Aug; 14(4):840-860.

[38] Boon H, Stewart M, Kennard MA, Gray R, Sawka C, Brown JB, et al. (2000) Use of complementary/alternative medicine by breast cancer survivors in Ontario: prevalence and perceptions. *J Clin Oncol.* 18(13):2515-21.

[39] Burstein HJ, Gelber S, Guadagnoli E, Weeks JC (1999). Use of alternative medicine by women with early-stage breast cancer. *N Engl J Med.* 340(22):1733-9.

[40] Gupta D, Lis CG, Birdsall TC, Grutsch JF (2005). The use of dietary supplements in a community hospital comprehensive cancer center: implications for conventional cancer care. *Support Care Cancer.* 13(11):912-9.

[41] Kumar NB, Hopkins K, Allen K, Riccardi D, Besterman-Dahan K, Moyers S (2002). Use of complementary/integrative nutritional therapies during cancer treatment: implications in clinical practice. *Cancer Control.* 9(3):236-43.

[42] Verhoef MJ, Balneaves LG, Boon HS, Vroegindewey A (2005). Reasons for and characteristics associated with complementary and alternative medicine use among adult cancer patients: a systematic review. *Integr Cancer Ther.* 4(4):274-86
[43] Nechuta S, Lu W, Chen Z, Zheng Y, Gu K, Cai H, et al. (2011). Vitamin supplement use during breast cancer treatment and survival: a prospective cohort study. *Cancer Epidemiol Biomarkers Prev.* 20(2):262-71.
[44] Myung SK, Kim Y, Ju W, Choi HJ, Bae WK (2011). Effects of antioxidant supplements on cancer prevention: meta-analysis of randomized controlled trials. *Annals of Oncology* 21(1):166-179.
[45] Sandhu JK, Haggani AS, Birnboim HC (2000). Effect of dietary E on spontaneous or nitric oxide donor-induced mutations in a mouse tumor model. *J Natl Cancer Inst* 92:1429-1433.
[46] Wright GL, Wang S, Fultz ME, Arif I, Matthews K, Chertow BS (2002). Effect of vitamin A deficiency on cardiovascular function in the rat. *Can J Physiol Pharmacol* 80:1-7.
[47] Hercberg S, Galan P, Preziosi P et al. (1998). The potential role of antioxidants vitamins in preventing cardiovascular diseases and cancers. *Nutrition* 14:513-20.
[48] D'Andrea GM (2005). Use of antioxidants during chemotherapy and radiotherapy should be avoided. *CA Cancer J Clin* 55:319-21).
[49] Conklin KA (2004). Chemotherapy-associated oxidative stress: impact on chemotherapeutic effectiveness. *Integr Cancer Ther* 3:294-300.
[50] Block KI, Koch AC, Mead MN, Tothy PK, Newman RA, Gyllenhaal C (2008). Impact of antioxidant supplementation on chemotherapeutic toxicity: a systematic review of the evidence from randomized controlled trials. *Int J Cancer.* 123(6):1227-39.
[51] Niki E, Noguchi N. Evaluation of antioxidant capacity (2000). What capacity is being measured by which method? *IUBMB Life.* 50(4-5):323-9.
[52] Galleano M, Verstraeten SV, Oteiza PI, Fraga CG (2010). Antioxidant actions of flavonoids: Thermodynamic and kinetic analysis. *Arch Biochem Biophys.* 501(1):23-30.
[53] Perron NR, Brumaghim JL (2009). A Review of the Antioxidant Mechanisms of Polyphenol Compounds Related to Iron Binding. *Cell Biochem Biophys.* 53(2):75–100.
[54] Fuchs-Tarlovsky V (2013). Role of antioxidants in cancer therapy. *Nutrition.* 29(1):15-21.
[55] Lu J, Holmgren A (2009). Selenoproteins. *J. Biol. Chem.* 284(2):723-727.
[56] Guarnieri S, Loft S, Riso P, Porrini M, Risom L, Poulsen HE, et al. (2008). DNA repair phenotype and dietary antioxidant supplementation. *Br J Nutr.* 99(5):1018-1024.
[57] Ibarrola-Villava M, Peña-Chilet M, Fernandez LP, Aviles JA, Mayor M, Martin-Gonzalez M, et al. (2011). Genetic polymorphisms in DNA repair and oxidative stress pathways associated with malignant melanoma susceptibility. *Euro. J. Cancer.* 47(17):2618-2625.
[58] Silva JP, Coutinho OP (2010). Free radicals in the regulation of damage and cell death - basic mechanisms and prevention. *Drug Discov Ther.* 4(3):144-67.
[59] Lorenzo Y, Azqueta A, Luna L, Bonilla F, Domínguez G, Collins AR (2009). The carotenoid beta-cryptoxanthin stimulates the repair of DNA oxidation damage in addition to acting as an antioxidant in human cells. *Carcinogenesis.* 30(2):308-14.
[60] Kryston TB, Georgiev AB, Pissis P, Georgakilas AG (2011). Role of oxidative stress and DNA damage in human carcinogenesis. *Mutat Res.* 711(1-2):193-201.

[61] Lee KW, Kang NJ, Heo YS, Rogozin EA, Pugliese A, Hwang MK, et al. (2008). Raf and MEK protein kinases are direct molecular targets for the chemopreventive effect of quercetin, a major flavonol in red wine. *Cancer Res.* 68(3):946-55.
[62] Mendoza EE, Burd R (2011). Quercetin as a systemic chemopreventative agent: structural and functional mechanisms. *Mini Rev Med Chem.* 11(14):1216-21.
[63] Borek C (2004). Dietary Antioxidants and Human Cancer. *Integr Cancer Ther.* 3(4):333-41.
[64] Kontek R, Drozda R, Sliwiński M, Grzegorczyk K. et al. (2010). Genotoxicity of irinotecan and its modulation by vitamins A, C and E in human lymphocytes from healthy individuals and cancer patients. *Toxicol In Vitro.* 24(2):417-424.
[65] Cebrian A, Pharoah PD, Ahmed S, Smith PL, Luccarini C, Luben R, et al. (2006) Tagging single-nucleotide polymorphisms in antioxidant defense enzymes and susceptibility to breast cancer. *Cancer Res.* 66(2):1225-33.
[66] Kinnula VL (2005). Focus on antioxidant enzymes and antioxidant strategies in smoking related airway diseases. *Thorax.* 60(8):693-700.
[67] Matés JM (2000). Effects of antioxidant enzymes in the molecular control of reactive oxygen species toxicology. *Toxicology.* 153(1-3):83-104.
[68] Cairns RA, Harris IS, Mak TW (2011). Regulation of cancer cell metabolism. *Nature Reviews Cancer.* 11:85-95.
[69] Matés JM, Sánchez-Jiménez F (1999). Antioxidant enzymes and their implications in pathophysiologic processes. *Front Biosci.* 15(4):339-45.
[70] Almondes KG, Leal GV, Cozzolino SM, Philippi ST, Rondó PH (2010). The role of selenoproteins in cancer. *Rev Assoc Med Bras.* 56(4):484-8.
[71] Papp LV, Lu J, Holmgren A, Khanna KK (2007). From selenium to selenoproteins: synthesis, identity, and their role in human health. *Antioxid Redox Signal.* 9:775–806.
[72] Kim HJ, Chae HZ, Kim YJ, Kim YH, Hwangs TS, Park EM, Park YM (2003). Preferential elevation of Prx I and Trx expression in lung cancer cells following hypoxia and in human lung cancer tissues. *Cell Biol Toxicol.* 19:285–98.
[73] Berggren M, Gallegos A, Gasdaska JR, Gasdaska PY, Warneke J, Powis G. (1996) Thioredoxin and thioredoxin reductase gene expression in human tumors and cell lines, and the effects of serum stimulation and hypoxia. *Anticancer Res.* 16:3459–66.
[74] Banning A, Kipp A, Schmitmeier S, Löwinger M, Florian S, Krehl S, et al. (2008). Glutathione peroxidase 2 inhibits cyclooxygenase-2-mediated migration and invasion of HT-29 adenocarcinoma cells but supports their growth as tumors in nude mice. *Cancer Res.* 68:9746-53.
[75] Rice-Evans C, Burdon R (1993). Free radical-lipid interactions and their pathological consequences. *Prog Lipid Res.* 32(1):71-110.
[76] Gago-Dominguez M, Castelao JE (2005). Role of lipid peroxidation in the epidemiology and prevention of breast cancer. *Cancer Epidemiol Biomarkers Prev.* 14(12):2829-39.
[77] Foy HM (1999). Mycoplasma pneumoniae pneumonia: current perspectives. *Clin Infect Dis.* 28(2):237.
[78] Niki E, Yoshida Y, Saito Y, Noguchi N (2005). Lipid peroxidation: mechanisms, inhibition, and biological effects. *Biochem Biophys Res Commun.* 338(1):668-76.
[79] Tuma DJ (2002). Role of malondialdehyde-acetaldehyde adducts in liver injury. *Free Radic Biol Med.* 32(4):303-8.

[80] Kikugawa K, Taguchi K, Maruyama T (1987). Reinvestigation of the modification of nucleic acids with malonaldehyde. *Chem Pharm Bull (Tokyo).* 35(8):3364-9.

[81] Nicholls R, de Jersey J, Worrall S, Wilce P (1992). Modification of proteins and other biological molecules by acetaldehyde: adduct structure and functional significance. *Int J Biochem.* 24(12):1899-906.

[82] Uchida K, Stadtman ER (1993). Covalent attachment of 4-hydroxynonenal to glyceraldehyde-3-phosphate dehydrogenase. A possible involvement of intra- and intermolecular cross-linking reaction. *J Biol Chem.* 268(9):6388-93.

[83] Klaunig JE, Xu Y, Isenberg JS, Bachowski S, Kolaja KL, Jiang J, et al (1998). The role of oxidative stress in chemical carcinogenesis. *Environ Health Perspect.* 106 Suppl 1:289-95.

[84] Spalding JW (1988). NTP Toxicology and carcinogenesis studies of malondialdehyde sodium salt (3-hydroxy-2-propenal, sodium salt) in F344/N rats and B6C3F1 mice. *Natl Toxicol Program Tech Rep Ser.* 331:1-182.

[85] Morrow JD, Hill KE, Burk RF, Nammour TM, Badr KF, Roberts LJ (1990) A series of prostaglandin F2-like compounds are produced in vivo in humans by a non-cyclooxygenase, free radical-catalyzed mechanism. *Proc Natl Acad Sci U S A.* 87(23):9383-7.

[86] Liu T, Stern A, Roberts LJ, Morrow JD (1999). The isoprostanes: novel prostaglandin-like products of the free radical-catalyzed peroxidation of arachidonic acid. *J Biomed Sci.* 6(4):226-35.

[87] Morrow JD, Roberts LJ (2002). The isoprostanes: their role as an index of oxidant stress status in human pulmonary disease. *Am J Respir Crit Care Med.* 166(12 Pt 2):S25-30.

[88] Delannoy E, Courtois A, Freund-Michel V, Leblais V, Marthan R, Muller B (2010). Hypoxia-induced hyper reactivity of pulmonary arteries: role of cyclooxygenase-2, isoprostanes, and thromboxane receptors. *Cardiovasc Res.* 85(3):582-92.

[89] Klaunig JE, Wang Z, Pu X, Zhou S (2011). Oxidative stress and oxidative damage in chemical carcinogenesis. *Toxicol Appl Pharmacol.* 254(2):86-99.

[90] Klaunig JE, Xu Y, Bachowski S, Jiang J (1997). Free-radical oxygen-induced changes in chemical carcinogenesis. In: Wallace KB. *Free Radic Toxicol.* 375–400.

[91] Freeman TA, Parvizi J, Della Valle CJ, Steinbeck MJ (2009). Reactive oxygen and nitrogen species induce protein and DNA modifications driving arthrofibrosis following total knee arthroplasty. *Fibrogenesis Tissue Repair.*13;2(1):5.

[92] Stadtman ER (2004). Role of oxidant species in aging. *Curr Med Chem.* 11(9):1105-12.

[93] White AA, Crawford KM, Patt CS, Lad PJ (1976). Activation of soluble guanylate cyclase from rat lung by incubation or by hydrogen peroxide. *J Biol Chem.* 251(23):7304-12.

[94] Bellomo G, Mirabelli F, Richelmi P, Orrenius S (1983). Critical role of sulfhydryl group(s) in ATP-dependent Ca2+ sequestration by the plasma membrane fraction from rat liver. *FEBS Lett.* 163(1):136-9.

[95] Kerr LD, Inoue J, Verma IM (1992). Signal transduction: the nuclear target. *Curr Opin Cell Biol.* 4(3):496-501.

[96] Witko-Sarsat V, Friedlander M, Capeillère-Blandin C, Nguyen-Khoa T, Nguyen AT, Zingraff J, et al. (1996). Advanced oxidation protein products as a novel marker of oxidative stress in uremia. *Kidney Int.* 49(5):1304-13.

[97] Cakatay U (2005). Protein oxidation parameters in type 2 diabetic patients with good and poor glycaemic control. *Diabetes Metab.* 31(6):551-7.

[98] Klaunig JE, Kamendulis LM, Hocevar BA (2010). Oxidative stress and oxidative damage in carcinogenesis. *Toxicol Pathol.* 38(1):96-109.

[99] Valko M, Izakovic M, Mazur M, Rhodes CJ, Telser J (2004). Role of oxygen radicals in DNA damage and cancer incidence. *Mol Cell Biochem.* 266(1-2):37-56.

[100] Kasai H (1997). Analysis of a form of oxidative DNA damage, 8-hydroxy-2'-deoxyguanosine, as a marker of cellular oxidative stress during carcinogenesis. *Mutat Res.* 387(3):147-63.

[101] Diakowska D, Lewandowski A, Kopeć W, Diakowski W, Chrzanowska T (2007). Oxidative DNA damage and total antioxidant status in serum of patients with esophageal squamous cell carcinoma. *Hepatogastroenterology.* 54(78):1701-4.

[102] Valavanidis A, Vlachogianni T, Fiotakis C (2009). 8-hydroxy-2' -deoxyguanosine (8-OHdG): A critical biomarker of oxidative stress and carcinogenesis. *J Environ Sci Health C Environ Carcinog Ecotoxicol Rev.* 27(2):120-39.

[103] Muguruma M, Unami A, Kanki M, Kuroiwa Y, Nishimura J, Dewa Y, et al. (2007). Possible involvement of oxidative stress in piperonyl butoxide induced hepatocarcinogenesis in rats. *Toxicology.* 236(1-2):61-75.

[104] Kawanishi S, Hiraku Y (2006). Oxidative and nitrative DNA damage as biomarker for carcinogenesis with special reference to inflammation. *Antioxid Redox Signal.* 8(5-6):1047-58.

[105] Brandon M, Baldi P, Wallace DC (2006). Mitochondrial mutations in cancer. *Oncogene.* 25(34):4647-62.

[106] Polyak K, Li Y, Zhu H, Lengauer C, Willson JK, Markowitz SD, et al. (1998) Somatic mutations of the mitochondrial genome in human colorectal tumours. *Nat Genet.* 20(3):291-3.

[107] Nishikawa M, Nishiguchi S, Shiomi S, Tamori A, Koh N, Takeda T, et al. (2001). Somatic mutation of mitochondrial DNA in cancerous and noncancerous liver tissue in individuals with hepatocellular carcinoma. *Cancer Res.* 61(5):1843-5.

[108] Tan DJ, Bai RK, Wong LJ (2002). Comprehensive scanning of somatic mitochondrial DNA mutations in breast cancer. *Cancer Res.* 62(4):972-6.

[109] Suzuki M, Toyooka S, Miyajima K, Iizasa T, Fujisawa T, Bekele NB, et al. (2003). Alterations in the mitochondrial displacement loop in lung cancers. *Clin Cancer Res.* 9(15):5636-41.

[110] Chen GF, Chan FL, Hong BF, Chan LW, Chan PS (2004). Mitochondrial DNA mutations in chemical carcinogen-induced rat bladder and human bladder cancer. *Oncol Rep.* 12(2):463-72.

[111] Petros JA, Baumann AK, Ruiz-Pesini E, Amin MB, Sun CQ, Hall J, et al. (2005) mtDNA mutations increase tumorigenicity in prostate cancer. *Proc Natl Acad Sci USA.* 18;102(3):719-24.

[112] Tan DJ, Chang J, Liu LL, Bai RK, Wang YF, Yeh KT, et al. (2006). Significance of somatic mutations and content alteration of mitochondrial DNA in esophageal cancer. *BMC Cancer.* 18;6:93.

[113] Van Trappen PO, Cullup T, Troke R, Swann D, Shepherd JH, Jacobs IJ, et al. (2007). Somatic mitochondrial DNA mutations in primary and metastatic ovarian cancer. *Gynecol Oncol.* 104(1):129-33.

[114] Zhou S, Kachhap S, Sun W, Wu G, Chuang A, Poeta L, et al. (2007). Frequency and phenotypic implications of mitochondrial DNA mutations in human squamous cell cancers of the head and neck. *Proc Natl Acad Sci USA*. 104(18):7540-5.
[115] Pang LJ, Shao JY, Liang XM, Xia YF, Zeng YX (2008). Mitochondrial DNA somatic mutations are frequent in nasopharyngeal carcinoma. *Cancer Biol Ther.* 7(2):198-207.
[116] Lawenda BD, Kelly KM, Ladas EJ, Sagar SM, Vickers A, Blumberg JB (2008). Should supplemental antioxidant administration be avoided during chemotherapy and radiation therapy? *J Natl Cancer Inst*. 100:773-83.
[117] Shu L, Cheung K, Khor TO, Chen C, Kong A (2010). Phytochemicals: cancer chemoprevention and suppression of tumor onset and metastasis. *Cancer Metastasis Rev*. 29:483-502.
[118] Cui Y, Morgenstern H, Greenland S, Tashkin DP, Mao JT, Cai L, et al. (2008). Dietary flavonoid intake and lung cancer-a population-based case-control study. *Cancer.*112(10):2241-8.
[119] Vardi N, Parlakpinar H, Cetin A, Erdogan A, Ozturk IC (2010). Protective effect of β-carotene on methotrexate-induced oxidative liver damage. *Toxicol Pathol*. 38:592-7.
[120] Tarapore RS, Siddiquiy IA, Mukhtar H. Modulation of Wnt/b-catenin signaling pathway by bioactive food components (2012). *Carcinogenesis.* 33(3):483–91.
[121] Shin J, Kim G, Jang H (2007). Antioxidant and pro-oxidant effects of green tea extracts in oxygen radical absorbance capacity assay. *J Med Food*. 10(1):32–40.
[122] Lambert JD, Elias RJ (2010). The antioxidant and pro-oxidant activities of green tea polyphenols: a role in cancer prevention. *Arch Biochem Biophys*. 501(1):65-72.
[123] Sarkar FH, Li Y, Wang Z, Kong D (2010). The role of nutraceuticals in the regulation of wnt and hedgehog signaling in cancer. *Cancer Metastasis Rev*. 29:383-94.
[124] Mosby TT, Cosgrove M, Sarkardei S, Platt KL, Kaina B (2012). Nutrition in adult and childhood cancer: role of carcinogens and anti-carcinogens. *Anticancer Res.* 32: 4171-4192.
[125] Hou Z, Lambert JD, Chin K, Yan CS (2004). Effects of tea polyphenols on signal transduction pathways related to cancer chemoprevention. *Mutat Res.* 555:3–19.
[126] Lambert JD, Yang CS (2013). Mechanisms of cancer prevention by tea constituents. *J Nutr.* 133(10):3262S-7S.
[127] Halliwell B (2007). Dietary polyphenols: good, bad, or indifferent for your health? *Cardiov Res* 73:341–7.
[128] Markle B, May EJ, Majumdar APN (2010). Do nutraceutics play a role in the prevention and treatment of colorectal cancer? *Cancer Metastasis Rev*. 29:395–404.
[129] Anand P, Thomas SG, Kunnumakkara AB, Sundaram C, Harikumar KB, Sung B, et al. (2008). Biological activities of curcumin and its analogues (congeners) made by man and mother nature. *Biochem Pharmacol*. 76:1590–611.
[130] Aggarwal BB, Harikumar KB (2009). Potential therapeutic effects of curcumin, the anti-inflammatory agent, against neurodegenerative, cardiovascular, pulmonary, metabolic, autoimmune and neoplastic diseases. *Int J Biochem Cell Biol.* 41:40–59.
[131] Kelkel M, Jacob C, Dicato M, Diederich M (2010). Potential of the dietary antioxidants resveratrol and curcumin in prevention and treatment of hematologic malignancies. *Molecules.* 15:7035-74.
[132] Kunnumakkara AB, Diagaradjane P, Anand P, Kuzhuvelil HB, Deorukhkar A, Gelovani J, et al. (2009). Curcumin sensitizes human colorectal cancer to capecitabine

by modulation of cyclin D1, COX-2, MMP-9, VEGF and CXCR4 expression in an orthotopic mouse model. *Int J Cancer.* 125:2187–97.
[133] Bansal SS, Goel M, Aqil F, Vadhanam MV, Gupta RC (2011). Advanced drug delivery systems of curcumin for cancer chemoprevention. *Cancer Prev Res.* 4(8);1158–71.
[134] Patel BB, Sengupta R, Qazi S, Vachhani H, Yu Y, Arun K, et al (2008). Curcumin enhances the effects of 5-fluorouracil and oxaliplatin in mediating growth inhibition of colon cancer cells by modulating EGFR and IGF-1R. *Int. J. Cancer.* 122:267–73.
[135] Patel BB, Gupta D, Elliott AA, Sengupta V, Yu Y, Majumdar AP (2010). Curcumin Targets FOLFOX-surviving colon cancer cells via inhibition of EGFRs and IGF-1R. *Anticancer Res.* 30:319-25.
[136] Basnet P, Skalko-Basnet N (2011). Curcumin: an anti-inflammatory molecule from acurry spice on the path to cancer treatment. *Molecules.* 16:4567-98.
[137] Dance-Barnes ST, Kock ND, Moore JE, Lin EY, Mosley LJ, D'Agostino Jr RB, et al. (2009). Lung tumor promotion by curcumin. *Carcinogenesis.* 30(6):1016-23.
[138] National Institute of Environmental Health Sciences. Toxicology and carcinogenesis Studies of Turmeric Oleoresin (CAS No. 8024-37-1) (Major Component 79-85% Curcumin, CAS No. 458-37-7) in F344/N Rats and B6C3F1 Mice (Feed Studies). 1993.
[139] Gatz SA, Wiesmüller L (2008). Take a break-resveratrol in action on DNA. *Carcinogenesis.* 29(2):321–32.
[140] Chun-Fu W, Jing-Yu Y, Fang W, Xiao-Xiao W (2011). Resveratrol: botanical origin, pharmacological activity and applications. *Chin J Nat Med.* 11(1):1-15.
[141] Aggarwal BB, Bhardwaj A, Aggarwal RS, Seeram NP, Shishodia S, Takada Y (2004). Role of resveratrol in prevention and therapy of cancer: preclinical and clinical studies. *Anticancer Res.* 24:2783-840.
[142] Gupta Subash C, Kannappan R, Reuter S, Kim JH, Aggarwal BB (2011). Chemosensitization of tumors by resveratrol. *Ann NY Acad Sci.* 1215:150-60.
[143] Guha P, Dey A, Sarkar B, Dhyani MV, Chattopadhyay S, Bandyopadhyay SK (2008) Improved antiulcer and anticancer properties of a trans-resveratrol analog in mice. *J Pharmacol Exp Ther.* 328(3):829-38.
[144] Lam TK, Rotunno M, Lubin JH, Wacholder S, Consonni D, Pesatori AC, et al. (2010). Dietary quercetin, quercetin-gene interaction, metabolic gene expression in lung tissue and lung cancer risk. *Carcinogenesis.* 31(4):634-42.
[145] Lin C, Hou W, Shen SC, Juan SH, Ko CH, Wang LM, et al. (2008). Quercetin inhibition of tumor invasion via suppressing PKCd/ERK/AP-1-dependent matrix metalloproteinase-9 activation in breast carcinoma cells. *Carcinogenesis.* 29(9):1807-15.
[146] Siegelin MD, Reuss DE, Habel A, Rami A, von Deimling A (2009). Quercetin promotes degradation of surviving and thereby enhances death-receptor–mediated apoptosis in glioma cells. *Neuro Oncol.* 11(2):122-31.
[147] Attia SM (2010). The impact of quercetin on cisplatin-induced clastogenesis and apoptosis in murine marrow cells. *Mutagenesis.* 25(3):281-8.
[148] Cheng S, Gao N, Zhang Z, Chen G, Budhraja A, Ke Z, et al. (2010). Quercetin induces tumor selective apoptosis through downregulation of Mcl-1 and activation of Bax. *Clin Cancer Res.* 16(23):5679-91.

[149] Linsalata M, Orlando A, Messa M, Refolo MG, Russo F (2010). Quercetin inhibits human DLD-1 colon cancer cell growth and polyamine biosynthesis. *Anticancer Res.* 30:3501-08.

[150] Vargas AJ, Burd R (2010). Hormesis and synergy: pathways and mechanisms of quercetin in cancer prevention and management. *Nutr Rev.* 68(7):418-28.

[151] Niu G, Yin S, Xie S, Li Y, Nie D, Ma L, et al. (2011) Quercetin induces apoptosis by activating caspase-3 and regulating Bcl-2 and cyclooxygenase-2 pathways in human HL-60 cells. *Acta Biochim Biophys Sin.* 43:30-7.

[152] Lee KW, Lee HJ, Surh YJ, Lee CY (2003). Vitamin C and cancer chemoprevention: reappraisal. *Am J Clin Nutr.*78:1074–8.

[153] Reuter S, Gupta V, Chaturvedi MM, Aggarwal BB (2010). Oxidative stress, inflammation, and cancer: How are they linked? *Free Radic Biol Med.* 49(11):1603–16.

[154] Takahashi H, Mizuno H, Yanagisawa A (2012). High-dose intravenous vitamin C improves quality of life in cancer patients. *Personalized Medicine Universe.* 1:49-53.

[155] Verrax J, Calderon PB (2008). The controversial place of vitamin C in cancer treatment. *Biochem Pharmacol.* 76:1644-52.

[156] Salerno JP (2013). High dose IV vitamin C for treatment of prostate adenocarcinoma. *Personalized Medicine Universe.* 1-3.

[157] Chandrasekharan DK, Kagiya TV, Nair CKK (2009). Radiation Protection by 6-palmitoyl ascorbic acid-2-glucoside: studies on DNA damage in vitro, ex vivo, in vivo and oxidative stress in vivo. *J. Radiat. Res.* 50(3):203-12.

[158] Soni MG, Thurmond TS, Miller ER, Spriggs T, Bendich A, Omaye ST (2010). Safety of vitamins and minerals: controversies and perspective. *Toxicol Sci.* 118(2):348–55.

[159] Akinnuga AM, Bamidele O, Ebunlomo OA, Adeniyi OS, Adeleyea GS, Ebomuche LC (2010). Hypoglycaemic effects of dietary intake of ripe and unripe lycopersiconesculentum (tomatoes) on streptozotocin-induced diabetes mellitus in rats. *OJBS.*10(2):50-3.

[160] Larsson SC, Bergkvist L, Wolk A (2010). Dietary carotenoids and risk of hormone receptor-defined breast cancer in a prospective cohort of Swedish women. *Eur J Cancer.* 46: 1079-85.

[161] Rock CL, Natarajan L, Pu M, Thomson CA, Flatt SW, Caan BJ, et al. (2009) Longitudinal biological exposure to carotenoids is associated with breast cancer-free survival in the Women's Healthy Eating and Living Study. *Cancer Epidemiol Biomarkers Prev.* 18: 486-94.

[162] Tung K, Wilkens LR, Wu AH, McDuffie K, Hankin JH, Nomura AMY, et al. (2005). Association of dietary vitamin A, carotenoids, and other antioxidants with the risk of ovarian cancer. *Cancer Epidemiol Biomarkers Prev.* 14:669-76.

[163] Meydan D, Gursel B, Bilgici B, Can B, Ozbek N (2011). Protective effect of lycopene against radiation-induced hepatic toxicity in rats. *J Int Med Res.* 39:1239-52.

[164] Van Breemen RB, Sharifi R, Viana M, Pajkovic N, Zhu d, Yuan L, et al. (2001). Antioxidant effects of lycopene in African American men with prostate cancer or benign prostate hyperplasia: a randomized, controlled trial. *Cancer Prev Res.* 4:711-8.

[165] Palozza P, Colangelo M, Simone R, Catalano A, Boninsegna A, Lanza P, et al. (2010). Lycopene induces cell growth inhibition by altering mevalonate pathway and Ras signaling in cancer cell lines. *Carcinogenesis.* 31:1813-21.

[166] Talvas J, Caris-Veyrat C, Guy L, Rambeau M, Lyan B, Minet-Quinard R, et al. (2010). Differential effects of lycopene consumed in tomato paste and lycopene in the form of a purified extract on target genes of cancer prostatic cells. *Am J Clin Nutr.* 91:1716-24.
[167] Wertz K (2009). Lycopene effects contributing to prostate health. *Nutr Cancer.* 61:775-783.
[168] ATBC Cancer Prevention Study Group (1994). The alpha-tocopherol, beta carotene cancer prevention study group: the effect of vitamin E and beta carotene on the incidence of lung cancer and other cancers in male smokers. *N Engl J Med.* 330:1029-5.
[169] Omenn GS, Goodman GE, Thornquist MD, Balmes J, Cullen MR, Glass A, et al. (1996). Risk factors for lung cancer and for intervention effects in CARET, the β-carotene and retinol efficacy trial. *J Natl Cancer Inst* 88:1550-9.
[170] Bjelakovic G, Nikolova D, Gluud LL, Simonetti RG, Gluud C (2010). Antioxidant supplements for prevention of mortality in healthy participants and patients with various diseases. In: *The Cochrane Library prepared by The Cochrane Collaboration,* Hoboken, NJ, U.S.A., John Wiley & Sons, 1-235.
[171] Burton, GW, Ingold KU (1984). Beta-carotene: an unusual type of lipid antioxidant. *Science.* 224:569–73.
[172] Bairati I, Meyer F, Gélinas M, Fortin A, Nabid A, Brochet F, et al. (2005). Randomized trial of antioxidant vitamins to prevent acute adverse effects of radiation therapy in head and neck cancer patients. *J Clin Oncol.* 20;23(24):5805-13.
[173] Bairati I, Meyer F, Gélinas M, Fortin A, Nabid A, Brochet F (2005). A randomized trial of antioxidant vitamins to prevent second primary cancers in head and neck cancer patients. *J Natl Cancer Inst.* 97(7):481-8.
[174] Ferreira PR, Fleck JF, Diehl A, et al. (2004). Protective effect of alpha-tocoferol in head and neck cancer radiation-induced mucositis: a double-blind randomized trial. *Head* Neck. 26(4):313-21.
[175] Lesperance ML, Olivotto IA, Forde N, Zhao Y, Speers C, Foster H, et al. (2002) Mega-dose vitamins and minerals in the treatment of non-metastatic breast cancer: an historical cohort study. *Breast Cancer Res Treat.* 76(2):137-43.
[176] Wasserman TH, Brizel DM, Henke M, Monnier A, Eschwege F, Sauer R, et al. (2005). Influence of intravenous amifostine on xerostomia, tumor control, and survival after radiotherapy for head-and- neck cancer: 2-year follow-up of a prospective, randomized, phase III trial. *Int J Radiat Oncol Biol Phys.* 63(4):985-90.
[177] Komaki R, Lee JS, Milas L, Lee HK, Fossella FV, Herbst RS, et al. (2004). Effects of amifostine on acute toxicity from concurrent chemotherapy and radiotherapy for inoperable non-small-cell lung cancer: report of a randomized comparative trial. *Int J Radiat Oncol Biol Phys.* 58(5):1369-77.
[178] Mell LK, Malik R, Komaki R, Movsas B, Swann RS, Langer C, et al. (2007) Effect of amifostine on response rates in locally advanced non-small-cell lung cancer patients treated on randomized controlled trials: a meta-analysis. *Int J Radiat Oncol Biol Phys.* 68(1):111-8.
[179] Buentzel J, Micke O, Adamietz IA, Monnier A, Glatzel M, de Vries A (2006). Intravenous amifostine during chemoradiotherapy for head-and-neck cancer: a randomized placebo-controlled phase III study. *Int J Radiat Oncol Biol Phys.* 64(3):684-91.

[180] Pathak AK, Bhutani M, Guleria R, Bal S, Mohan A, Mohanti BK, et al. (2005). Chemotherapy alone vs. Chemotherapy plus high dose multiple antioxidants in patients with advanced non small cell lung cancer. *J Am Coll Nutr.* 24(1):16-21.
[181] Ladas EJ, Jacobson JS, Kennedy DD, Teel K, Fleischauer A, Kelly KM (2004). Antioxidants and cancer therapy: a systematic review. *J Clin Oncol.* 22(3):517-28.
[182] Mills E, Wu P, Seely D, Guyatt G (2005). Melatonin in the treatment of cancer: a systematic review of randomized controlled trials and meta-analysis. *J Pineal Res.* 39(4):360-6.
[183] Lissoni P, Chilelli M, Villa S, Cerizza L, Tancini G (2003). Five years survival in metastatic non-small cell lung cancer patients treated with chemotherapy alone or chemotherapy and melatonin: a randomized trial. *J Pineal Res.* 35(1):12-5.
[184] Lissoni P, Barni S, Mandalà M, Ardizzoia A, Paolorossi F, Vaghi M, et al. (1999). Decreased toxicity and increased efficacy of cancer chemotherapy using the pineal hormone melatonin in metastatic solid tumour patients with poor clinical status. *Eur J Cancer.* 35(12):1688-92.
[185] Lawenda BD, Kelly KM, Ladas EJ, Sagar SM, Vickers A, Blumberg JB (2008). Should supplemental antioxidant administration be avoided during chemotherapy and radiation therapy? *J Natl Cancer Inst.* 100(11):773-83.

In: Free Radicals
Editor: Bill Stone

ISBN: 978-1-63117-177-2

Chapter III

Vitamin E Isoforms: Multiple Mechanisms of Action against Carcinogenesis

Sharon E. Campbell[1]*, Aashish S. Morani[1], William L. Stone[2], Koyamangalath Krishnan[3] and Victoria E. Palau[4]
[1]Departments of Biomedical Sciences
[2]Pediatrics
[3]Internal Medicine
[4]James H. Quillen College of Medicine, East Tennessee State University, Johnson City, US and Bill Gatton College of Pharmacy

Abstract

Cancer is the second leading cause of death in the United States and is expected to become the primary cause of disease-related death within the next decade. There are significant country-to-country variations in cancer incidence, which suggests that nutrition and dietary factors are important to the carcinogenesis process. An increased risk of cancer is associated with obesity and a high body mass index demonstrating that nutrition has a central role in the promotion of cancer. Healthy eating habits protect against cancer, while unhealthy eating habits increase the risk of cancer. Mediterranean societies have a lower risk for many cancers than those of northern Europe and the Americas. Mediterranean diets consist of a high consumption of fruits, vegetables, grains, beans, nuts, and seeds, with olive oil as an important source of monounsaturated fat. These foods are rich in lipid soluble antioxidants such as vitamin E. Vitamin E may prevent cancer by decreasing the formation of mutagens arising from the oxidation of lipids, decreasing oxidative stress in the epithelial cells as well as modulating molecular mechanisms that influence cell death, cell cycle, and transcriptional events. Vitamin E is a major fat-soluble antioxidant and it occurs naturally as eight compounds (alpha-, beta-,

* Corresponding author: Department of Biomedical Sciences, James H. Quillen College of Medicine, East Tennessee State University, Johnson City, TN 37614, USA, Email: CAMPBESE@mail.etsu.edu

gamma-, and delta-tocopherol or alpha-, beta-, gamma-, and delta-tocotrienol). Since the recognition of vitamin E in 1922 as an essential nutrient for reproduction, alpha-tocopherol has been considered the major form of vitamin E. It has the highest concentration in the plasma and has been studied more in epidemiological and clinical studies than any other form of vitamin E. Recent data suggests that other isoforms of vitamin E may be important in the control of cancer. These isoforms of vitamin E have varying anti-carcinogenic potencies. Data indicate that gamma-tocopherol may be a more effective anti-cancer agent than alpha-tocopherol. Our laboratories and others have demonstrated that tocotrienols are even more effective than tocopherols at inhibiting cell proliferation in cancer cells. Differences in apoptotic induction among the various vitamin E isoforms are reflective of different avenues of apoptotic signaling and may be tissue specific. Dietary fat has been linked to an increase in a number of cancers including colon, prostate, and breast cancer. Vitamin E modulates a number of molecular mechanisms involved in fat metabolism. These include: the peroxisome proliferator activator receptor (PPAR), arachidonic acid metabolism, *de novo* sphingolipid metabolism, and cholesterol metabolism. Vitamin E family members have demonstrated the potential to activate pathways involved in cell proliferation, differentiation, apoptosis, and cell cycle. This chapter reviews data that identify the molecular targets of vitamin E action against the development of cancer.

Keywords: tocopherols, tocotrienols, vitamin E, signal transduction, peroxisome proliferator activator receptor, sphingolipids

Abbreviations

AA	arachidonic acid
ACF	aberrant crypt foci
AOM	azoxymethane
a-T3E	6-O-carboxypropyl-alpha-tocotrienol
ATBC	Alpha Tocopherol Beta Carotene
a-TEA	alpha-tocopheryloxyacetic acid
ATF3	activating transcription factor 3
a-TOB	alpha-tocopheryloxybutyrate
a-TTP	alpha-tocopherol transfer protein
a-VEA	alpha-tocopheryl acetate
a-VES	alpha-tocopheryl succinate
B[a]P	benzo[a]pyrene
BFGF	basic fibroblast growth factor
cdks	cyclin dependent kinases
CE	cholesteryl ester
CEHC	carboxyethyl-hydroxychroman
COX-2	cyclooxygenase-2
CTGF	connective tissue growth factor
ECM	extracellular matrix
EGFR	epidermal growth factor receptor

ERK	extracellular signal-regulated kinase
FGF1	fibroblast growth factor 1
g-H2AX	gamma histone 2A, family member X
HASMC	human aortic smooth muscle cell
HBP	highly basic protein
HCC	hepatocellular carcinoma
HDL	high density lipoprotein
HEL	human erythroleukemia cell
HNSCC	head and neck squamous cell carcinoma
HUVEC	human umbilical vein endothelial cells
IFITM-1	interferon inducible protein 9-27
LDL-R	low-density lipoprotein receptor
MDR	multidrug resistant 1
MMP	matrix metalloproteinase
NBP2	neuroblastoma cells
NNK	4-(methylnitrosamino)-1-(3-pyridyl)-1-butanone
NO	nitric oxide
PG	prostaglandin
PI3K	phosphatidylinositol-3-kinase-dependent kinase
PIN	intraepithelial neoplasia
PKB	protein kinase B
PKC	protein kinase C
PP2A	phosphatase 2A
PPAR	peroxisome proliferator activator receptor
Rac	racemic
Rb	retinoblastoma protein
ROS	reactive oxygen species
SELECT	Selenium and Vitamin E Cancer Prevention Trial
SR-BI	scavenger receptor class B type I
TAK-1	TNF associated factor 1
TGFβ2	transforming growth factor beta 2
TRAMP	transgenic adenocarcinoma mouse prostate
VEGF	vascular endothelial growth factor
VEGFR	vascular endothelial growth factor receptor

Introduction

Diet Plays a Role in Cancer Risk

Cancer occurs by successive mutations to DNA that allows the cancer cell to develop a selective growth advantage. These DNA mutations can occur through reactions with reactive oxygen species (ROS) and free radicals or radiation. Ames suggests that deficiencies in micronutrients such as folic acid, vitamin B12, vitamin B6, niacin, vitamin C, vitamin E, iron, or zinc mimics the damaging effects of radiation on DNA [1]. DNA damage that occurs as a result of micronutrient deficiencies could result in DNA damage that leads to cancer. Differences in the incidence of many cancers throughout the world suggest that diet has a role in the process of carcinogenesis. Diets rich in antioxidants (such as vitamin E) may prevent cancer by decreasing the formation of mutagens arising from the oxidation of lipids, by decreasing oxidative stress in the epithelial cells and by molecular mechanisms that influence cell death, cell cycle, and transcriptional events.

Vitamin E Compounds Other than Alpha Tocopherol are Physiologically Relevant

Vitamin E consists of eight naturally-occurring, structurally-related lipid soluble compounds classified into two distinct families: tocopherols and tocotrienols as seen in Figure 1. Each family has four members (alpha, gamma, delta, and beta). It was discovered in 1922 that alpha-tocopherol deficiency impairs mammalian fertility [2]. This discovery and the predominance of alpha-tocopherol over other tocopherols in the plasma have resulted in the concept that alpha-tocopherol is the more relevant form of Vitamin E. This convention came into question when it was discovered that gamma-tocopherol, but not alpha-tocopherol plasma concentrations are reduced with age [3].

In 1985, Handelman, *et al.* discovered that supplementation with alpha-tocopherol, reduces the plasma concentration of gamma-tocopherol [4]. Gamma-tocopherol was brought to center stage in 1993 when Cooney *et al.* demonstrated that it has superiority over alpha-tocopherol when detoxifying nitrogen dioxide [5].

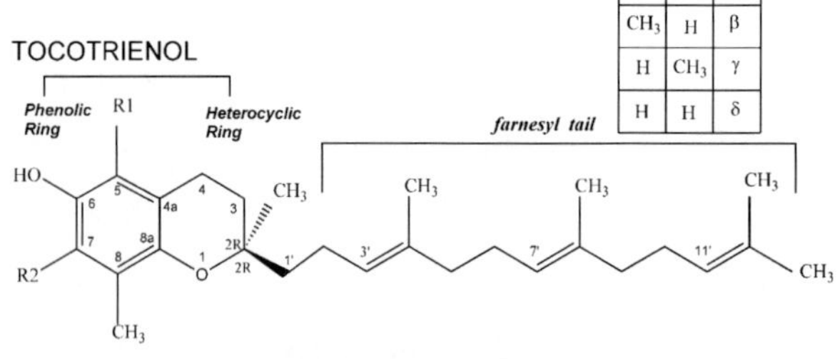

R1	R2	E
CH_3	CH_3	α
CH_3	H	β
H	CH_3	γ
H	H	δ

Figure 1. The naturally occurring compounds of vitamin E have two families, the tocopherols (top) and the tocotrienols (bottom). Both families have a chroman head group consisting of a phenolic ring and a heterocyclic ring. The tocopherols have a phytyl tail, where the tocotrienols have an unsaturated, farnesyl tail. There are four family members per lineage and include alpha, beta, gamma, and delta-tocopherol and the corresponding tocotrienols. These isoforms vary based upon the placement of methyl groups around the phenolic ring. The dash-bordered table in the center of the figure lists the location of the methyl group placement for each vitamin E isoform. The hydroxyl group on the phenolic ring is the site of antioxidant activity for all vitamin E isoforms (—¨—¨—).

Peroxynitrite is a powerful mutagen that is formed during the activation of phagocytes and may lead to the initiation of cancer through chronic inflammation. Christen *et al.* determined that this reaction was quenched solely by gamma-tocopherol and remained unaffected in the presence of alpha-tocopherol. Further, gamma-tocopherol, but not alpha-tocopherol can inhibit the activity of cyclooxygenase-2 (COX-2) [6], the up regulation of which is a known prognostic factor in a number of epithelial cancers and is associated with reduced survival [7-10]. Later alpha-tocopherol was found to reduce the anti-cancer activity of other isoforms [11]. These seminal research findings changed the landscape of vitamin E research, leading to more than three decades of research demonstrating that vitamin E isoforms other than alpha-tocopherol have implications in the prevention of cancer.

Vitamin E has Antioxidant Properites BUT Also Plays a Role in Signal Transduction Modulation

Since the early 1980's, vitamin E's primary mode of action was thought to be as lipid-soluble antioxidant, but not all of alpha-tocopherol's published actions could be explained by the antioxidant hypothesis. In 1994, Stauble and Azzi found that alpha-tocopherol could activate the AP-1 transcription factor and inhibit the activation of protein kinase C [12]. This study demonstrated that alpha-tocopherol, but not beta-tocopherol could modulate two independent signal transduction pathways. Since beta-tocopherol could not modulate these pathways, it was concluded that these effects of alpha-tocopherol were independent of antioxidant activity. Increasing evidence is validating the hypothesis that vitamin E functions as a modulator of signal transduction. These data have led to the testing of vitamin E isoforms, analogues and metabolites as anti-cancer agents. This chapter reviews the signal transduction pathways that are modulated by vitamin E isoforms and the implications for vitamin E as an anti-cancer agent.

The Biology of Vitamin E

Vitamin E is at Least Eight Structurally Related Compounds

As shown in Figure 1, both families of vitamin E (tocopherols and tocotrienols) have a chroman head group consisting of a phenolic ring fused to a heterocyclic ring and hydrocarbon tail. The tocopherols have a saturated phytyl side chain (tail) attached to the 2-position of the chromanol ring whereas tocotrienols have an unsaturated farnesyl tail attached at this position with three double bonds. All of the natural forms of vitamin E exist as the R-stereoisomer where chiral carbons exist. The tocopherols have three chiral carbons, existing at the 2, 4', and 8' positions. The tocotrienols have one chiral carbon at the number 2 position. For tocopherols, the RRR-tocopherol is most bioavailable. Likewise, the R-tocotrienols are most actively absorbed by humans compared to the S-isomers.

Alpha-, gamma-, beta-, and delta-tocopherols (or tocotrienols) are distinguished by the number and positions of methyl groups attached to the chromanol ring. The position of antioxidant activity occurs on the phenolic ring at carbon number 6, where the attached hydroxyl group may release its hydrogen in order to quench free radicals. This hydrolyzed form of vitamin E is recycled through a reaction with ascorbic acid [13-18].

Synthetic Vitamin E is Not Identical to Natural Vitamin E

In addition to the natural forms of vitamin E, a number of synthetic forms of vitamin E exist as shown in Figure 2. The most common synthetic form of vitamin E is all-racemic (rac)-alpha-tocopherol, which contains a mixture of (R) and (S) stereoisomers for each chiral carbon. The rule for obtaining the number of possible steroisomers for a diasteromer is 2^n, where n is the number of chiral carbons the molecule contains. Since alpha-tocopherol contains 3 chiral carbons, the number of different diasteromers in all-rac-alpha-tocopherol is 8; meaning the all-racemic mixture is one-eighth RRR-alpha-tocopherol (the most actively absorbed diasteromer of alpha-tocopherol). This means that only one-eighth of all-rac-alpha-tocopherol is the natural RRR-isoform. Unfortunately, this distinction has been ignored by investigators in the past and the term all-rac-alpha-tocopherol has been used interchangeably with RRR-alpha-tocopherol, vitamin E, or alpha-tocopheryl-acetate (discussed below). The lack of diligence to discern the difference between these alpha-tocopherol forms has resulted in some confusion as to how to interpret the results from these studies. This chapter will use due diligence to discern the difference between these forms of alpha-tocopherol when possible. When not possible, a parenthetical notation will be made.

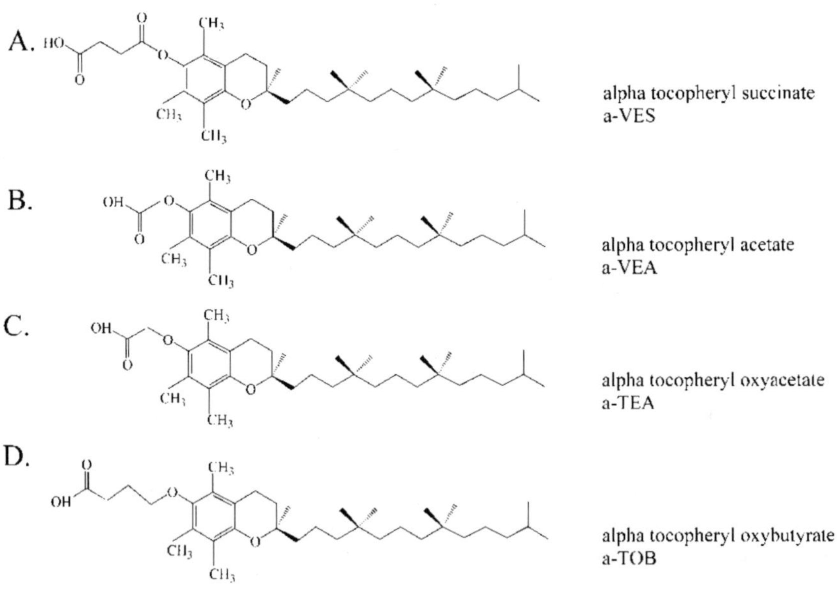

Figure 2. Synthetic isoforms of alpha-tocopherol mask the site of antioxidant activity making them redox silent and more potent anti-cancer agents. Some redox silent synthetic forms of vitamin E are esters such as alpha tocopheryl succinate (A) and alpha-tocopheryl acetate (B). Other redox silent vitamin E isoforms are ethers such as alpha tocopheryloxyacetate (C) or alpha tocopheryloxybutyrate (D).

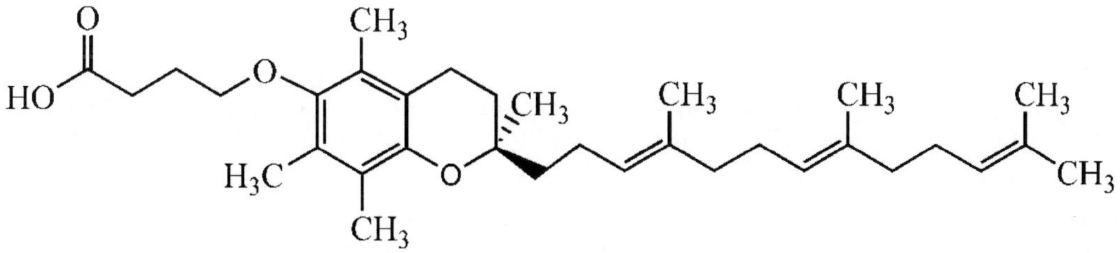

6-O-carboxypropyl-alpha-tocotrienol
a-T3E

Figure 3. Synthetic isoform of alpha-tocotrienol, 6-O-carboxypropyl-alpha-tocotrienol (a-T3E) is a redox silent ether analogue and an efficient anti-cancer agent.

Numerous redox inactive forms of vitamin E have been synthesized whereby the hydroxyl group at carbon number 6 is converted to an ester or ether analog. Examples of these tocopherol analogs can be seen in Figure 2 and include: alpha-tocopheryl-acetate (a-VEA), alpha-tocopheryl succinate (a-VES), alpha-tocopheryloxyacetic acid (a-TEA), and alpha-tocopheryloxybutyrate (a-TOB). Similarly, modifications to the tocotrienol family of vitamin E to prepare redox inactive (silent) ester and ether analogs are currently being investigated [19-21]. As shown in Figure 3, one ether analog of tocotrienol (6-O-carboxypropyl-alpha-tocotrienol (a-T3E)) has been tested in several different cancer cell lines [22-24]. Both the methyl groups and the type of hydrocarbon tail (phytyl vs. farnesyl) have a considerable influence on the biochemistry and potential chemopreventive properties of the different forms of vitamin E [25].

Vitamin E Transport and Metabolism Occur in the Liver with Different Reaction Kinetics Depending Upon Various Conditions

In the intestine all forms of vitamin E are absorbed without discrimination. In the liver, the alpha-tocopherol transfer protein (a-TTP) is preferential for RRR-alpha-tocopherol incorporation into VLDL and subsequent distribution to peripheral tissues [26]. While the selectivity of the a-TTP is for RRR-alpha-tocopherol, the SRR-alpha-tocopherol and gamma-tocopherol have identical plasma uptakes (micromoles per liter of plasma) over time following a single oral dose, suggesting that in the absence of RRR-alpha-tocopherol, other tocopherols can be transported from the liver to the tissues [26]. Further, in tissue culture cell lines, gamma-tocopherol up-take into cells is much higher than alpha-tocopherol, suggesting that once gamma-tocopherol is transported to the plasma, greater concentrations can be achieved in tissues [27, 28].

The bioavailability, absorption, and homeostasis of vitamin E are determined by a wide variety of factors, all of which may not be known. For example, there appears to be a threshold at which the a-TTP becomes saturated and diminishes tocopherol turnover [29]. Smokers have decreased RRR alpha tocopherol levels in lymphocytes and platelets even though their plasma levels were similar to nonsmokers [30]. Following administration, RRR-alpha-tocopherol is eliminated significantly faster in smokers compared with non-smokers. Smokers also take up less newly absorbed RRR-alpha-tocopherol [30]. Further, the plasma uptake of a-VEA consumed with meals varies depending upon the fat content and food matrix given with the vitamin E [31]. There are differences in the biokinetics among subjects with varying lipid status [32]. For example, there is a decreased uptake of alpha-tocopherol into plasma, lipoproteins, erythrocytes, platelets, and lymphocytes in hyperlipidemics [32].

All forms of vitamin E are metabolized by an initial ω-hydroxylation followed by beta-oxidation rendering a carboxyethyl-hydroxychroman (CEHC) metabolic product as shown in Figure 4. These reactions are catalyzed by cytochrome p450 enzymes and CEHC metabolites are excreted in the urine [33-36]. Structural features of the tocopherols and tocotrienols play a role in the ω-hydroxylation/beta-oxidation reaction kinetics. For example, the methylation at the C5 (as seen with the alpha- and beta- isoforms) of the chromanol ring was associated with markedly low activity, while tocotrienols had much higher V_{max} values [37]. Remarkably, side-chain stereochemistry had no effect on ω-hydroxylation [37]. Finally, microsomal activity of CYP4F2 revealed Michaelis-Menten kinetics for alpha-tocopherol, but reflected allosteric cooperativity for other vitamers, especially tocotrienols [37]. Furthermore, the variation in the CYP4F2, CYP4F14, and ω-hydroxylase proteins has an effect on the metabolism of vitamin E [38-40].

Vitamin E Interactions

Few investigations have examined the influence of combining vitamin E isoforms or other dietary compounds upon the metabolism and accumulation of tocopherols or tocotrienols. For example, rats fed alpha-tocopherol diets had higher levels of vitamin E in feces, colonocytes, plasma and liver than rats fed the gamma-tocopherol diets [41]. Dietary iron does not influence tocopherol levels in plasma, liver, or feces; however, higher dietary iron intake decreases tocopherol levels in colonocytes [41]. Sesamin, a sesame lignin, causes elevation of tissue tocopherols, by strongly inhibiting tocopherol metabolism through inhibition of CYP3A [36]. Dietary flavonoids result in an increase in alpha-tocopherol concentrations in plasma and liver in rats [42]. These flavonoids also result in reduced alpha-tocopherol oxidation in a human LDL *ex vivo* model, but do not affect the vitamin E metabolism in hepatocyte cultures [42].

The Role of Vitamin E Isoforms on Apoptosis

Apoptosis is often referred to as "programmed cell death." It was initially described by morphological characteristics including: cell shrinkage, membrane blebbing, chromatin condensation, and nuclear fragmentation. The apoptotic pathway regulates the homeostasis between cell death and cell life and is the most common pathway by which the body rids itself of damaged or nonproductive cells. Defects or gene mutations in the apoptosis pathway can lead to genetic instability, allowing propagation of damaged cells, giving them a selective growth advantage, which subsequently may lead to carcinogenesis. Thus, finding compounds that can alter the defects in the apoptotic pathway in cancer cells is important to cancer prevention and treatment. These apoptotic pathways and vitamin E action are summarized in Figure 5.

2, 5, 7, 8-tetramethyl-2-(β-carboxyethyl)-6-hydrochroman (CEHC)

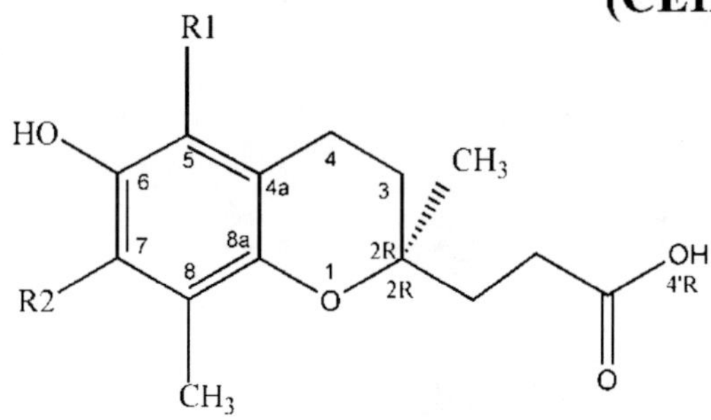

R1	R2	E
CH_3	CH_3	α
CH_3	H	β
H	CH_3	γ
H	H	δ

Figure 4. The major metabolic product of vitamin E isoforms metabolism by w-hydroxylation and subsequent beta-oxidation carboxyethyl-hydrochroman (CEHC). As with vitamin E the substituted methyl groups around the phenolic ring designate alpha-, beta-, gamma- and delta -CEHC.

Natural Vitamin E Isoforms are Effective Apoptotic Modulators in Cancer Cell Lines

Natural vitamin E isoforms have been shown to be effective apoptotic modulators in cancer cell lines from various tissue types and differing genetic abnormalities. For example, delta-tocotrienol induces concentration-dependent apoptosis in cancer cell lines of various tissue types; MDA-MB-435 (melanoma/metastatic ductal carcinoma), HCT-8 (colon cancer), HL-60 (leukemia), and SF-295 (glioblastoma) cell lines demonstrating effectiveness regardless of tissue type [43]. Delta-tocotrienol treatment of breast cancer cell lines MCF-7 (ER positive) and MDA-MB-231 (ER negative) results in apoptosis as evidenced by PARP cleavage and caspase-7 activation showing delta-tocotrienol to be an effective apoptotic inducer independent of estrogen receptor status [44]. Furthermore, gamma-tocotrienol induces apoptosis in MCF-7 and MDA-MB-231 cells through cleavage and activation of caspase-7. Further analysis revealed an activation of PERK and pIRE1 alpha that induced ER stress with the activating transcription factor 3 (ATF3) identified as the most up-regulated gene in response to gamma-tocotrienol in breast cancer cells, implicating a potential modulation of mTOR signaling [44]. By measurement of DNA laddering, MCF-7 cells (estrogen responsive) were discovered to be more susceptible than MDA-MB-435 (estrogen unresponsive) cells when treated with delta-tocopherol or alpha-, gamma-, or delta-tocotrienol [45], suggesting that the DNA damage response pathway may be modulated more effectively with tocopherols and tocotrienols in estrogen responsive breast cancer cells. In malignant mouse mammary epithelial cells treated with gamma-tocotrienol, apoptosis was found to occur by cleavage of caspase 8, but was unrelated to death receptor signaling [46]. In colon cancer cell lines HCT-116, SW480, HCT-15, and HT-29, gamma-tocopherol is superior to alpha-tocopherol at inducing apoptosis through cleavage of caspase 8 and apoptosis is not observed in nontransformed primary cells CCD-112CoN, demonstrating a preference of action on cancer cells [47]. As demonstrated in Table 1, these four colon cell lines demonstrate genetic differences among APC, COX-2, p21, and p53, suggesting that either gamma-tocopherol is working independent of these pathways in colon cancer or gamma-tocopherol may be able to work through multiple pathways to return cellular homeostasis and halt cancer progression [48-66].

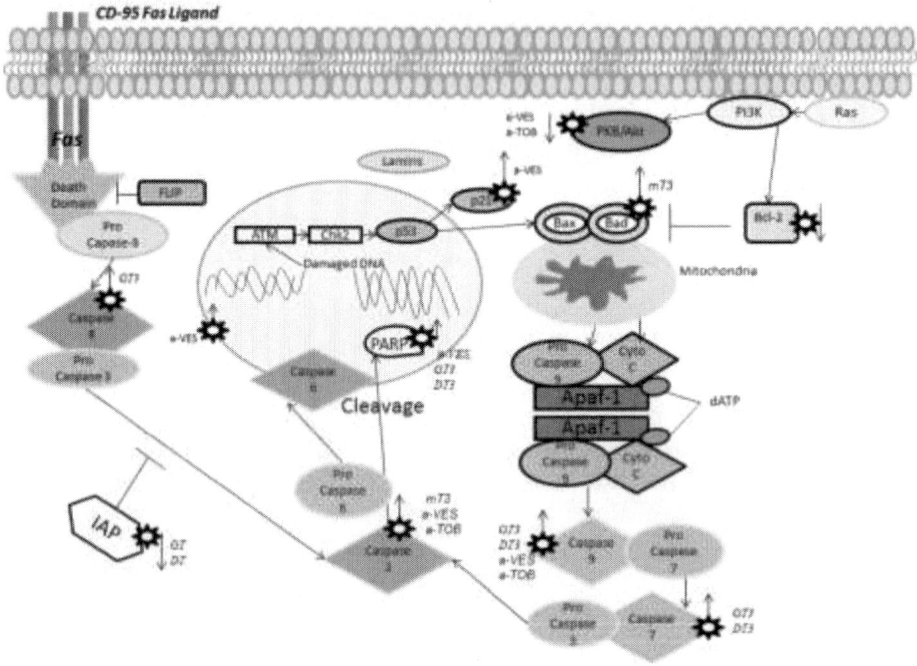

Figure 5. The signaling pathways to apoptosis and survival modulated by vitamin E isoforms. Beginning in the upper left hand corner, the death receptor pathway begins with the CD95 (Fas ligand) binding to the Fas receptor, which in turn recruits the FADD death domain. The death domain cleaves procaspase 8 to caspase 8. This cleavage can be prevented by gamma-tocotrienol (GT3). Caspase 8 binds procaspase 3 and cleaves it to caspase 3. IAP is the inhibitor of apoptosis protein, which inhibits the conversion of procaspase 3 to caspase 3. The protein expression of IAP is down regulated by gamma-tocopherol (GT) and RRR-alpha-tocopherol (AT). Caspase 3 expression is up regulated in the presence of mixed tocotrienols (mT3), alpha-tocopheryl succinate (a-VES), and alpha-tocopheryloxybutyrate (a-TOB). Caspase 3 can lead to PARP cleavage. PARP is a protein involved in DNA repair and is cleaved during apoptosis. PARP cleavage is up regulated in the presence of a-VES, GT3, and delta-tocotrienol (DT3). Damaged DNA within the cell leads to the expression of p53 in the nucleus which upregulates p21. p21 is protein that induces G0 cell cycle arrest, which can lead to apoptosis. p21 is up regulated by a-VES. In addition to the up regulation of p21 which initiates G0 cell cycle arrest, p53 expression can lead to the up regulation of Bax and Bad proteins leading to apoptosis through the intrinsic pathway. The expression of Bad is increased in the presence of mT3. Bax and Bad proteins bind to the mitochondria and induce release of cytochrome c. Cytochrome c release enables the assembly of the apoptosis activating factor -1, which leads to ATP-dependent apoptosis through the cleavage of procaspase 9 to release caspase 9. This cleavage is increased in the presence of GT3, DT3, a-VES and a-TOB. Caspase 9 cleaves procaspase 7 to caspase 7. Caspase 7 can cleave procaspsase 3 to caspsase 3, which executes apoptosis. Caspase 7 expression is deregulated in the presence of GT3 and DT3.

Further evidence of the modulation of multiple pathways is indicated by studies on human gastric adenocarcinoma SGC-7091 cells which are susceptible to mitochondria-dependent apoptosis as shown by the cleavage of PARP, caspase 3, and caspase 9 when treated with gamma-tocotrienol [67]. In reference to cellular ras status, studies on Mia PaCa-2 (ras mutant), PANC-1 (ras mutant), and BxPC-3 (WT ras) pancreatic cancer cell lines treated with delta-tocotrienol treatment results in concentration-dependent suppression of cell proliferation. This indicates the induction of apoptosis occurs irrespective of cellular ras status [68]. Similar results were found with gamma-tocotrienol [69].

Table 1. Genetic differences of selected colon cell lines from Campbell et al. [47]

Cell Line	COX-2	APC	PPAR	p21	p53
HCT-116	Inducible [48]	Normal [48, 51]	Functional [56]	Deleted [62]	WT [60]
HT-29	(+) [53]	Truncated [48, 49]	Functional [57, 58]	WT [62]	P53 mutant, nonfunctional [60, 66]
SW480	(-) [54]	Truncated [50-52]	Functional [58, 59]	Functional [63, 64]	Mutant [64]
HCT-15	(-) [53, 55]	Truncated [52]	Mutant [60, 61]	Functional [65]	Mutant [60, 61]

Apoptotic Induction by Natural Tocopherols and Tocotrienols Occurs in Animal Models

Apoptotic induction by natural tocopherols and tocotrienols is not limited to cancer cell lines, but occur in varying animal models. For example, dietary delta- and gamma-tocopherol, but not alpha-tocopherol, inhibit estrogen receptor positive mammary tumorigenesis as well as tumor multiplicity in N-methyl-N-nitrosourea-treated female Sprague-Dawley rats [70]. Rats consuming delta- and gamma-tocopherol demonstrate inhibition of the anti-apoptotic markers Bcl-2 and XIAP. In addition, a mixed tocotrienol (Tocomin® Carotech, BhD (Perak, Malaysia) containing 12-14%D-alpha-tocotrienol,1% D-beta-tocotrienol, 18-20% D-gamma-tocotrienol, 4-6% D-delta-tocotrienol, and 12-4% D-alpha-tocopherol) diet administered to transgenic adenocarcinoma mouse prostate (TRAMP) mice results in a lower incidence of tumor formation with concomitant increased expressions of pro-apoptotic proteins BAD and cleaved caspase-3 as well as a significant reduction in levels of high-grade neoplasia [71].

Natural Tocotrienols Need not be Purified to Demonstrate Apoptotic Activity

Natural tocotrienols need not be purified to demonstrate apoptotic activity. For example, the tocotrienol-rich fraction extracted from palm oil induces significant apoptosis evidenced by DNA fragmentation in LNCaP (androgen-dependent), DU145 (androgen-independent), and PC-3 (androgen-independent) prostate cancer cell lines, but not in normal PrEC or non-tumorigenic PZ-HPV-7 prostate cells [72]. The apoptosis demonstrated by treatment with the tocotrienol-rich fraction occurs irrespective of androgen receptor status and does not occur in normal prostate cancer cells. Much of the tocotrienol data has been obtained using tocotrienols found in palm oil, but delta-tocotrienol has been found in other plants. For example, examination of the bark of Brazilian Kielmeyera coriacea have rendered a delta-tocotrienol mixture which has been efficacious in treating breast, colon, leukemia, and glioblastoma cell lines through the triggering of apoptosis [43].

Synthetic Forms of Vitamin E Result in Apoptosis of Cancer Cells

Synthetic forms of vitamin E result in apoptosis of cancer cells. a-VES induces apoptosis in murine EL4 lymphoma cells as evidenced by chromatin condensation and fragmentation staining [73]. In HL-60 human leukemia cells, a-VES induces membrane translocation of Fas, cleavages of caspase-3, PARP, and lamin B, hypophosphorylation of retinoblastoma protein, and an increase in p21 (WAF1) protein, all indicative of apoptotic induction [74]. a-VES is nontoxic to normal cells and tissues, but reduces cell proliferation and induces apotosis in colon cancer xenografts in nude mice. In this case, apoptosis is triggered in p53(-/-) and p21(Waf1/Cip1(-/-)) cancer cells and exerted a cooperative proapoptotic activity with tumor necrosis factor-related apoptosis-inducing ligand (Apo2 ligand) to suppress tumor growth *in vivo* [75]. a-TEA (a nonhydrolyzable ether analog of RRR-alpha-tocopherol) and celecoxib alone and in combination were tested in MDA-MB-435 human breast cancer xenografts in nude mice for apoptotic properties. Analyses of tumor sections show that both treatments significantly enhance apoptosis (TUNEL) and significantly decrease cell proliferation (Ki-67) [76]. A comparison of the ester analog a-VES to the ether analog a-TOB in androgen-dependent LnCaP and androgen-independent PC-3 prostate cancer cells reveal that both compounds were capable of inhibiting cell growth and inducing apoptosis, although a-TOB requires twice as much to achieve the same response as a-VES. Despite the concentration differences required, both compounds share the same mechanism of targeting Akt and JNK signaling pathways through the intrinsic death pathway through caspase 9 to caspase 3. The difference in apoptotic activity between a-TOB and a-VES does not appear to be related to cellular uptake, thus future studies will need to be performed to investigate the possibility that the apoptotic disparity is a result of different kinetic mechanisms [77]. This study indicates that each vitamin E compound needs to be tested at a wide variety of concentrations to determine its efficacy in each tissue type. A comprehensive study of this kind has not been published to date.

These data demonstrate that many vitamin E compounds induce apoptosis: [1] in a wide variety of tissue types including solid tumors such as colon breast, prostate, and pancreatic as well as blood and brain tumors such as leukemias and lymphomas, and glioblastomas; [2] by a wide-variety of mechanisms including intrinsic apoptotic pathway (cleavage of caspase 9), extrinsic apoptotic pathway (cleavage of caspase 8), down regulation of anti-apoptotic factors such as Bcl-2 and XIAP, up regulation of pro-apoptotic factors such as Bad, and activation of DNA response pathway by p21, p53 and PARP cleavage; [3] irrespective of hormone status in breast and prostate cancer; [4] irrespective of ras status in pancreatic cancer; and [5] irrespective of APC, COX-2, p21, and p53 status in colorectal cancer.

Anticancer Effects of Synthetic Vitamin E Analogues Using Apoptosis as an Endpoint

In light of the apoptotic response of cancer cells to vitamin E compounds, Birringer *et al.* used apoptosis as a model of anti-neoplastic activity to examine the structure and function of natural and synthetic analogues finding that the addition of a dicarboxylic acid group through an ester link to the number 6 position of tocopherols, will enhance their apoptogenic activity compared to the natural analogue [25]. The proapoptotic activity of these compounds depends upon the unsaturation and length of the substituted dicarboxylic acid group. The shortest, least saturated dicarboxylic acid is maleate, which showed the highest apoptotic activity in cancer cells compared with succinate and glutarate analogs. Similarly, shortening the side chain of the tocotrienols from three saturated carbons to two saturated carbons resulted in higher apoptotic activity. Taken together, these data suggest that the more-water soluble agents are more effective at apoptotic induction in the carcinogenic cells.

Apoptosis is being used to test the potency of synthetic tocotrienols [19, 21]. A redox silent ether of alpha-tocotrienol, a-T3E, induces apoptosis in A549 human lung cancer cells and in aggressive malignant mesothelioma with no treatment options [22, 23]. Redox silent esters of tocotrienol have been developed that enhance the ability to prevent breast cancer proliferation and migration [20].

The Influence of Vitamin E Isoforms on Cell Cycle, Cell Proliferation, and Tumor Burden

The cell cycle is a control mechanism with specific check points designed to prevent superfluous proliferation and protect genetically instable cells from replicating damaged DNA. Aberrant cell cycle progression occurs in cancer cells resulting in excessive cell proliferation. If these cells have damaged DNA, genetic instability is advanced. By reducing the progression from G1 to S phase, excessive cell proliferation and genetic instability can be slowed. If the cell cycle is slowed long enough, differentiation or apoptosis can result, which is advantageous in the battle against cancer cells.

As demonstrated in Figure 6, cyclins regulate progression through the cell cycle. The presence of cyclins D1, D2, D3, and E result in progression from the G1 to S phase of the cell cycle. Cyclins function in conjunction with cyclin dependent kinases (cdks) to phosphorylate the retinoblastoma protein (Rb) which when bound to E2F, inhibits cell cycle progression. The activation of cdks can be prevented with cdk inhibitors resulting in cell cycle arrest. The p21 (cip) and p27 (kip) protein are inhibitors for the cyclin E's dependent kinase, cdk2. Through down-regulation of the cyclins or cdks, the cell cycle progression can be stopped, resulting in inhibition of cell growth and induction of cell death, apoptosis, and differentiation. Cancer cells are often genetically unstable due to mutations in DNA repair machinery, which leads to damaged DNA. It is imperative to stop the cell cycle at the G1 checkpoint to maintain the fidelity of the genome.

Several cell line studies demonstrate that gamma-tocopherol can prevent cell cycle progression and cell growth in cancer cells. For example, androgen-dependent, LNCaP, and androgen-independent DU-145 prostate cancer cells both demonstrate down-regulation of cyclins D1 and E after 24 hours in the presence of 25 μM gamma-tocopherol [78]. Gamma-tocopherol and its major metabolite, gamma-carboxyethyl-hydroxychroman (CEHC) down-regulate cyclin D1 and cdk4 in androgen-independent hyperproliferative PC-3 cells when treated with 25 μM gamma-tocopherol or gamma-CEHC for 24 hours [79].

This action prevents the cancer cells from progressing past the G1 checkpoint and entering S phase to replicate DNA, which may be damaged as it so frequently is during carcinogenesis.

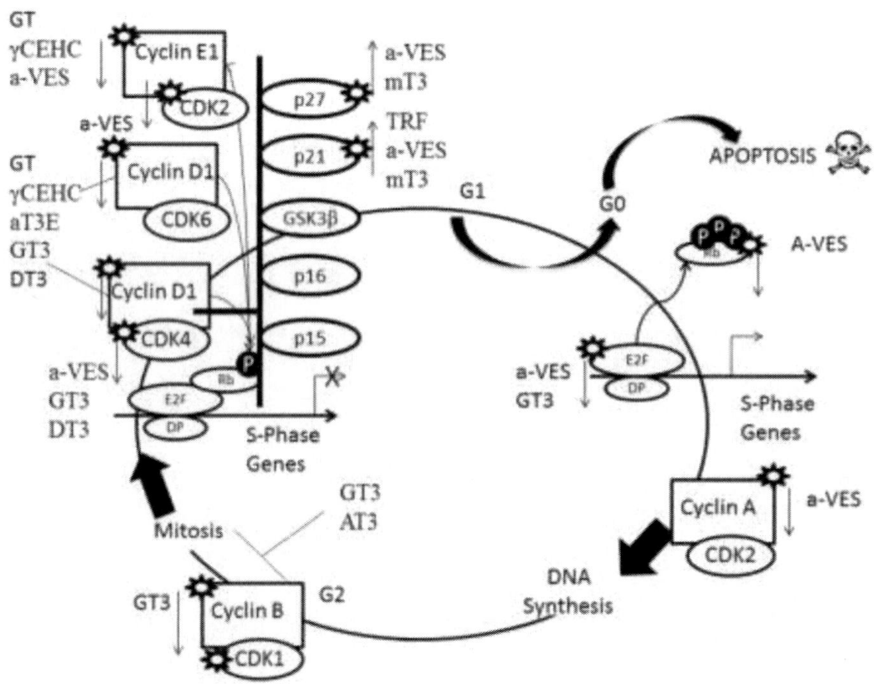

Figure 6. Vitamin E compounds are cell cycle modulators. Cells undergo mitosis and progress to G1. The G1 phase of the cell cycle is a pause that allows the cell to examine if conditions are favorable for S-phase or DNA synthesis. The key to the pause is the phosphorylation status of the retinoblastoma protein (Rb). If Rb is hypophosphorylated, then it will remain bound to the E2F/DP complex preventing cell cycle progression. Three different cyclin/cyclin dependent kinase (CDK) complexes work to phosphorylate Rb and allow for its release from the E2F/DP complex to result in cell cycle progression to DNA synthesis phase (S-phase). Vitamin E complexes gamma-tocopherol (GT), gamma-CEHC, and a-VES result in the down regulation of cyclin E. a-VES down regulates CDK4. GT, gamma-CEHC, a-T3E, gamma-tocotrienol (GT3) and delta-tocotrienol (DT3) result in the down regulation of cyclin D1. a-VES, GT3, and DT3 result in the down regulation of CDK4. In addition to the down regulation of cyclins or CDKs, specific cell cycle inhibitors can block the cyclin/CDK phosphorylation of Rb, thus inhibiting cell cycle progression. These inhibitors include: p27, p21, GSK3b, p16, and p15. a-VES upregulates p21 and p27. Palm oil's tocotrienol-rich fraction (TRF) upregulates p21. GT3 reduces the expression of E2F and Rb proteins in the cell, thus preventing the transition to S phase.

a-VES Modulates the Cell Cycle

Numerous studies demonstrate that a-VES acts through many mechanisms modulating the cell cycle in various cell and tissue types. Physiological concentrations of a-VES (20 μg/mL) result in a robust reduction of the S-phase cell population in LNCaP (androgen-dependent) and PC-3 (androgen-independent) prostate cancer cells (69% and 95%, respectively) which is accompanied by a 3-fold increase in the expression of p27 [80]. a-VES reduces Rb phosphorylation and cyclin E mRNA expression [81]. Similar data in human MDA-MB-435 ductal carcinoma cells demonstrate that a-VES modulates the cell cycle through the p21 pathway [82], while in HL-60 human leukemia cells the induction of p21 by a-VES induces monocytic differentiation [83]. The induction of monocytic differentiation results in the conversion of leukemia cells to differentiated monocytes reversing the carcinogenesis process. Further, a-VES inhibits cell proliferation in an estrogen receptor negative cell line, BT-20, through a mechanism involving cyclin A protein and negative regulation of E2F-mediated transcription [84] indicating that a-VES does not require the estrogen receptor to reduce breast cancer cell proliferation. In two different osteosarcoma cell lines, a-VES induces cell cycle arrest independent of p53 status; however, U2OS cells containing WT p53 demonstrate concentration-dependent induction of E2F1-mediated apoptosis, while the cell line with mutant p53, MG63, did not [85]. This clearly demonstrates that a-VES can induce cell cycle arrest in cancer cells in the absence of p53. In osteosarcoma cells, a-VES in the absence of p53 slows the cancer growth through cell cycle arrest; but in combination with p53, a-VES induces apoptosis of osteosarcoma cells thus reducing the number of cancer cells available. In LNCaP (androgen-dependent) prostate cancer cell line, a-VES mediates cell cycle G1/S phase arrest through the decreased expression of cell cycle regulatory proteins cyclin D1, D3, and E as well as cdk 2 and 4, but not cdk6 [81].

Cell Cycle Modulation is Also Regulated by Tocotrienols

Cell cycle modulation is not limited to the tocopherol analogs and isoforms, but is also regulated by tocotrienols. In human breast cancer cell lines MCF-7 (estrogen-dependent) and MDA-MB-231 (estrogen-independent), the tocotrienol-rich fraction treatment results in the upregulation of c-myc binding protein MM-1 and the highly basic protein (HBP) and the down regulation of interferon inducible protein 9-27 (IFITM-1) in both cell lines [86]. Modulations of these proteins influence cell cycle regulation and differentiation of tumor cells. The tocotrienol-rich fraction of palm oil induces growth arrest in human colon carcinoma cells, RKO, through the induction of p21 resulting in apoptosis [87]. Further, it reduces the proliferation of prostate cancer cells LnCaP, DU-145, and PC-3 while having no effect on PrEC (normal) and PZ-HPV-7 (non-carcinogenic) cells, through a dose-dependent G0/G1 cell cycle arrest [72]. Redox silent a-T3E was found to decrease the expression of cyclin D1 after a 40 μM treatment for 24 hours in A549 human lung cancer cells [22]. In MCF-7 breast cancer cells, growth suppression by gamma-tocotrienol results in changes in the levels of cell cycle regulatory proteins including: Rb/E2F complex, cyclin D1/cdk4, and cyclin B1/cdk1[88]. Delta-tocotrienol reduces cell growth through the loss of Rb phosphorylation, resulting in the down regulation of cyclin D1 and its regulatory partner cdk4 with concomitant reduced expression of E2F protein in the ER negative cell line MDA-MB-231 [89]. HeLa cell proliferation is inhibited by gamma- and alpha-tocotrienol treatment, which results in G2/M cell cycle arrest and the down regulation of cyclin D3, p16, and cdk6 with concomitant induction of apoptosis, as demonstrated by externalization of annexin V-targeted phosphotidyl serine [90].

Cell Cycle Intervention by Vitamin E Isoforms in Animal Models

The data for cell cycle intervention by vitamin E isoforms is not limited to cell lines. Dietary delta- and gamma-tocopherol inhibit estrogen receptor positive mammary tumorigenesis as well as tumor multiplicity in N-methyl-N-nitrosourea-treated female Sprague-Dawley rats [70]. Markers of cell proliferation (PCNA, PKCa), survival (PPAR-gamma, PTEN, p-Akt), and cell cycle (p53, p21) were affected by dietary delta- and gamma-tocopherol. In contrast, alpha-tocopherol did not decrease tumor burden or multiplicity [70]. The effect of gamma-tocopherol-enriched mixed tocopherol diet on prostate carcinogenesis was studied in the transgenic adenocarcinoma mouse prostate (TRAMP) model. The incidence of palpable tumor is significantly suppressed and a reduction in prostate intraepithelial neoplasia (PIN) development is observed without affecting the expression of the SV-40 transgene. Nrf2 (a redox sensitive transcription factor known to mediate the expression of phase II detoxifying enzymes) is significantly up-regulated following treatment with gamma-tocopherol-enriched mixed tocopherol diet [91]. Further, a mixed tocotrienol diet (Tocomin® Carotech, BhD (Perak, Malaysia) containing 12-14%D-alpha-tocotrienol,1% D-beta-tocotrienol, 18-20% D-gamma-tocotrienol, 4-6% D-delta-tocotrienol, and 12-4% D-alpha-tocopherol) applied in the TRAMP mouse model results in a lower incidence of tumor formation, reduced levels of high-grade neoplastic lesions, and a significant reduction in the average wet weight of genitourinary apparatus. The decrease in the high-grade neoplastic lesions is associated with increased expression of the cdk inhibitors p21 and p27 [71].

Many different forms of vitamin E can reduce the overburdened cell cycle in cancer cells. As demonstrated in Figure 6, these forms gamma- and delta-tocopherol, gamma-CEHC, a-TEA, a-VES, a-T3E, a-VEA, alpha-, gamma-, and delta-tocotrienol have various cell cycle targets including cyclins, cyclin-dependent kinases, and cyclin-dependent kinase inhibitors. These targets may differ depending upon tissue type and genetic make-up of the cancer cells. Cell cycle check points G1 and G2 are averted with various vitamin E isoforms and metabolites in a multitude of cancer cell lines and animal models through the modulation of cyclins, cyclin-dependent kinases, and cyclin-dependent kinase inhibitors. This aversion prevents damaged DNA from being replicated and propagated to daughter cells rendering them susceptible to carcinogenic mutations. DNA damage, a by-product and exacerbating agent of cancer, is decreased, while DNA repair is increased in the presence of vitamin E treatment. These responses to various vitamin E isoforms occur despite the hormone status, tissue type, cancer model (animal or tissue culture), or overall genetic make-up of the cancer cell. These data clearly suggest that many vitamin E isoforms have many pathways with in the cell cycle by which it can return homeostasis to damaged cells.

Non-Alpha-Tocopherol Forms of Vitamin E Reduce Tumor Burden in Animal Models

In addition to halting the cell cycle, gamma-tocopherol, a-VES, and a-TEA have demonstrated the ability to reduce tumor burden in several animal models of carcinogenesis. Tumor burden is reduced in 4-(methylnitrosamino)-1-(3-pyridyl)-1-butanone (NNK)-induced lung cancer in A/J mice using a gamma-tocopherol-rich mixture of tocopherols during the initiation stage or throughout the entire period of the experiment (by 36 or 43% respectively)

[92]. In addition, tumor multiplicity is reduced by 17.8% during the initiation stage (week 0 to 3), by 19.7% during the post-initiation stage (week 3 to 19), or by 29.3% during the entire experimental period [92]. In A/J mice tumors chemically induced with NNK plus benzo[a]pyrene (B[a]P), a dietary gamma-tocopherol-rich mixture reduces tumor multiplicity, tumor volume and tumor burden by 30, 50, and 55%, respectively [92]. In an H1299 human lung cancer cell xenograft model, dietary gamma-tocopherol-rich mixture significantly reduces tumor volume and tumor weight by 56 and 47%, respectively [92]. These data clearly demonstrate the potential of dietary gamma-tocopherol to reduce tumor burden in lung cancer. In mice with colon cancer xenografts, a-VES suppresses tumor growth by 80% [93]. MDA-MB-435 human breast cancer xenograft animals demonstrate reduced tumor volume in comparison to the control when treated with a-TEA [76].

Vitamin E Inhibits Radiation-Induced Genotoxicity

An integral part of maintaining healthy cells lies in the proper functioning of DNA repair mechanisms. DNA can be damaged by UV-radiation, cigarette smoke, genotoxic drugs, and free radicals. These agents can induce double strand breaks through the production of gamma histone 2A, family member X (g-H2AX) a factor that is critical for maintaining genomic integrity, but is also an integral part of hypoxia-driven neovascularization [94]. As DNA double strand breaks are introduced, the damaged DNA can release 8-hydroxydeoxyguanine as a marker of DNA damage. The replication of damaged DNA leads to genetic instability which, in turn, can lead to carcinogenesis. In both carcinogenesis and tumor growth animal models, a dietary administration of a gamma-tocopherol-rich mixture demonstrates lower levels of gamma H2AX and lower levels of 8-hydroxydeoxyguanine, preventing the potential of hypoxia-driven neovascularization and reducing DNA damage, respectively [92]. This demonstrates an ability of gamma-tocopherol to reduce DNA damage. a-TEA reduces UV-induced carcinogenesis in hairless SKH-1 mice [95]. Hairless SKH-1 mice were treated with a-VEA 30 minutes before or after a single minimal erythemic dose of UV light. DNA synthesis determined by 5-bromo-2'-deoxyuridine incorporation was two-fold higher after 15 hours in the untreated groups, but was not statistically different among a-VEA treatment groups (administration of a-VEA before versus administration of a-VEA after UV light dose) resulting in a delay in tumor formation for the first 20 weeks [95]. The promotion of oral cancer induced by dibenzo[a,l]pyrene-induced in Syrian hamsters was suppressed by oral gavage administration of a-VES by reducing the number of cells entering S-phase [96], while the initiation of dibenzo[a,l]pyrene-induced oral cancer in Syrian hamsters was suppressed by a-VES resulting in a reduction in DNA damage and an increase in DNA repair [96]. In human MDA-MB-435 ductal carcinoma cells, a-VES shows a dose- and time-dependent inhibition of DNA synthesis as well as a G0/G1 cell cycle arrest through the induction of p21 independent of transforming growth factor beta [97].

Epidemiological Evidence that Multiple Forms of Vitamin E, Rather than Alpha Tocopherol Alone May be Chemopreventive

Despite several decades of epidemiological research that report links between diet and cancer, few specific dietary factors have been unambiguously shown to contribute to carcinogenesis, either as a cause or a protective factor. Vitamin E has been no exception. Many retrospective case-control studies of vitamin E intake (dietary or supplemental) or serum vitamin E concentrations, as seen in Tables 2-10, have been conducted to determine the association between vitamin E and cancer outcomes with mixed results (50;65;98-161). Design limitations in these studies hinder the interpretation of the results. For example, dietary or serum levels of vitamin E were measured at or after the diagnosis of cancer making it difficult to correlate the measure with the onset of disease. In addition, dietary intake data in these studies are subject to recall-bias, as after diagnosis, cancer patients are more likely to make an effort to recall dietary intakes than the control group. The uncertainty of these results are likely to be overcome by large prospective studies over prolonged periods of times throughout various stages of the disease process. Proof of this concept is demonstrated when examining the association of serum alpha-tocopherol with colon cancer. In individual studies of small number an association of serum alpha-tocopherol with colon cancer was non-determinant, but a pooled analysis of five cohorts (including 289 cases of colorectal cancer and 1267 matched controls) a protective association was found [162]. The pooled analysis for serum alpha-tocopherol was not statistically significant ($p = 0.15$), but demonstrated a trend for an inverse relationship between serum levels of alpha-tocopherol and the risk of colorectal cancer with the matched odds ratio for the highest quartile of serum alpha-tocopherol at 0.6 (95% confidence interval 0.4 – 1.0) for colorectal cancer. While the effects were modest in this study, the observation is important as it demonstrates that measuring dietary factors may require larger populations in order to overcome the measurement errors associated with the epidemiological analytical methods.

As demonstrated in Table 11, with few exceptions, for digestive, malignant melanoma, and lung cancers [125, 148, 163], the majority of retrospective, prospective cohort, or nested case-control studies did not find statistically significant associations between pre-diagnostic serum concentations of alpha-tocopherol and the risk of developing cancer, [103, 116, 117, 149-153, 155;1, 56, 160-162, 164-170]. With respect to vitamin E dietary correlations, the type of vitamin E used in the study may be a factor in the ambiguous results. For example, in a nested case-control study in Washington County, MD [171], examining the effects of alpha-tocopherol, gamma-tocopherol and selenium on prostate cancer incidence, found that statistically significant protective associations for high levels of selenium and alpha-tocopherol were found but only when gamma-tocopherol levels were high. Men in the highest quintile of plasma gamma-tocopherol concentrations had a striking five-fold reduction in prostate cancer compared with men in the lowest quintile ($p=0.002$). This observation emphasizes the concern that supplementation with alpha-tocopherol can actually lower the gamma-tocopherol levels in plasma and tissues [4;172] thus decreasing the circulating levels of other forms of vitamin E and compromising their chemopreventive effects. In vitamin E-deficient rats, graded levels of dietary gamma-tocopherol increased alpha-tocopherol levels in several tissues [173]. Further, in a prospective study, plasma gamma-tocopherol was the only micronutrient tested with strong inverse associations for the risk of prostate cancer in two different cohorts (p=0.02 and p=0.0001) [153]. The Iowa Women's Health study showed that high intake of total vitamin E as associated with a decreased incidence of colon cancer. In this prospective study, 35,000 women between the age of 55 and 66 years of age with no previous history of cancer were enrolled.

The age-adjusted relative risk of colon cancer was highest for women in the lowest quintile of total vitamin E intake. Vitamin E was inversely related to the risk of colon cancer ($p < 0.0001$). These data suggest the possibility that combined use of several forms of vitamin E (particularly gamma-tocopherol), rather than alpha-tocopherol alone, may confer chemopreventive benefits.

Table 2. Case control studies of vitamin E and bladder cancer outcome

Exposure	*Time Period*	*Age (yr) (mean/ median) or range*	*Population*	*Odds Ratio 95% CI*	*p-trend*	*Study Type /Reference*
serum α-tocopherol	1974-1986	59	35 cases; 70 controls	0.57 (0.12-2.70)	ns	Nested [150]
serum α-tocopherol	1968-1977		15 cases; 29 controls	1.25	ns	Nested [148]
Dietary Vitamin E	1979-1985	35-90	351 cases; 855 population controls	ns	ns	Retrospective [99]
Dietary Vitamin E	1983-1986	<80	432 cases; 792 hospital and population controls	0.72 (0.48-1.09)	ns	Retrospective [100]

Table 3. Case control studies of vitamin E and brain cancer outcome

Exposure	*Time Period*	*Age (yr) (mean/ median)*	*Population*	*Odds Ratio 95% CI*	*p-trend*	*Study Type/ Reference*
serum α-tocopherol	1968-1977		18 cases; 34 controls	0.62	ns	Nested [148]
Dietary Vitamin E	1987-1991	50 (males) 49 (females)	416 cases; 409 population controls	Male: 1.68 (1.07-2.63) Female: 1.09 (0.62-1.92)	<0.01	Retrospective [102]

Table 4. Case control studies of vitamin E and breast cancer outcome

Exposure	*Time Period*	*Age (yr) (mean/ median/or range)*	*Population*	*Odds Ratio 95% CI*	*p-trend*	*Study Type/ Reference*
serum α-tocopherol	Prior to 1998	44 cases, 38 controls	44 cases 46 clinic controls with benign breast tumors	ns	ns	Retrospective [103]
serum α-tocopherol	1986-1988	64 cases, 62 controls, premeno-pausal	377 stage 1 or 2 breast cancer cases; 403 clinic controls	0.8 (0.5-1.2)	ns	Retrospective [116]
Dietary Vitamin E	1991-1994	55-64	2569 cases; 2588 hospital controls	0.75 (0.6-0.9)	<0.01	Retrospective [140]
Dietary Vitamin E	1994-1997	52 cases, 50 controls	409 cases; 515 hospital controls	1.3(0.9-1.8)	ns	Retrospective [106]
Dietary Vitamin E	1994-1997	60-69	400 cases; 515 hospital controls	0.50 (0.30-0.82)	0.009	Retrospective [107]
Dietary Vitamin E	1984-1986	20-69	834 cases; 834 community controls	0.7 (0.5-1.1)		Retrospective [108]
Dietary Vitamin E	1993-1999	55-64	289 cases; 442 hospital controls	0.37 (0.23-0.59)	<0.001	Retrospective [109]
Dietary Vitamin E	1991-1994	20-74	2569 cases; 2588 hospital controls	0.83 (0.69-1.01)		Retrospective [110]
Dietary Vitamin E	1986-1991	40-85	633 cases; 711 population controls	FH+: 0.2 (0.1-1.1) FH-: 0.4 (0.3-0.7)	ns <0.01	Retrospective [111]
Dietary Vitamin E	1991-1994	20-74	2569 cases, 2588 hospital controls	Premeno-pause: 0.80 (0.7-1.0) Postmeno-pause: 0.75 (0.6-0.9)	<0.05 <0.01	Retrospective [112]
Dietary Vitamin E	1989-1991	56 cases, 54 controls	820 cases; 1548 hospital controls	0.71 (0.48-1.05) Premeno-pause: 0.50 (0.25-1.02) Postmeno-pause: 0.85 (0.53-1.36)	0.04 0.03 ns	Retrospective [113]

Table 4. (Continued)

Exposure	*Time Period*	*Age (yr) (mean/ median/or range)*	*Population*	*Odds Ratio 95% CI*	*p-trend*	*Study Type/ Reference*
Dietary Vitamin E	1986-1991	≥40	297 white cases; 311 white population controls	0.55 (0.34-0.88)	0.03	Retrospective [115]
Dietary Vitamin E	1986-1988	64 cases, 62 controls	377 stage 1 or 2 breast cancer cases; 403 clinic controls.	0.4 (0.2-0.9)	0.02	Retrospective [116]
serum γ-tocopherol	Prior to 1998	44 cases, 38 controls	44 cases 46 clinic controls with benign breast tumors	ns	ns	Retrospective [103]
Plasma Vitamin E	Prior to 1991	25-65	48 cases; 50 hospital controls	Higher levels in cases	<0.01	Retrospective [104]
Plasma Vitamin E/cholesterol ratio	Prior to 1991	25-65	48 cases; 50 hospital controls	ns	ns	Retrospective [104]
Leukocyte vitamin E	Prior to 1991	25-65	48 cases; 50 hospital controls	Higher levels in cases	<0.01	Retrospective [104]
Erythrocyte vitamin E	Prior to 1991	25-65	48 cases; 50 hospital controls	ns	ns	Retrospective [104]
Dietery + supplemental Vitamin E	1990-1995	25-75	289 cases, 433 community controls	ns	ns	Retrospective [114]
Vitamin supplement	1986-1991	≥40	297 white cases, 311 white population controls	0.95 (0.58-1.55)	ns	Retrospective [124]
Dietary + supplemental Vitamin E	1986-1988	64 cases, 62 controls	377 stage 1 or 2 breast cancer cases, 403 clinic controls.	0.7 (0.4-1.3)	ns	Retrospective [116]

Table 5. Case control studies of vitamin E and cervical, ovarian and endometrial cancer outcomes

Exposure	*Time Period*	*Age (yr) (mean/ median)*	*Population*	*Odds Ratio 95% CI*	*p-trend*	*Cancer Site*	*Study Type/ Reference*
serum α-tocopherol	Prior to 1991		387 cases, 670 community and hospital controls	1.14 (0.6-2.1)	ns	Cervical	Retrospective [117]
serum α-tocopherol	1974-1990		50 cases, 99 controls	1.02 (0.35-2.94)	ns	Cervical	Nested [160]
serum α-tocopherol	1983-1994	33	38 cases, 116 controls	1.3 (0.4-3.3)	ns	Cervical	Nested [161]
plasma α-tocopherol	1990-1991	49	27 cases, 27 hospital controls	Lower levels in cases	<0.05	Cervical	Retrospective [118]
Serum γ-tocopherol	1990-1991	49	27 cases, 27 hospital controls	2.09 (1.1-3.9)	0.03	Cervical	Retrospective [118]
Plasma γ-tocopherol	1990-1991	49	27 cases, 27 hospital controls	ns	ns	Cervical	Retrospective [118]
Cervical tissue α-tocopherol	1990-1991	49	27 cases, 27 hospital controls	Higher in cases	<0.05	Cervical	Retrospective [118]
Cervical tissue γ-tocopherol	1990-1991	49	27 cases, 27 hospital controls	Higher in cases	<0.05	Cervical	Retrospective [118]
serum α-tocopherol	1974-1989	53	35 cases, 67 controls	3.91 (1.1-14.0)	0.04	Ovarian	Nested [149]
Dietary Vitamin E	1988-1994	62 cases, 61 controls	368 cases, 713 hospital controls	0.9	ns	Endo-metrial	Retrospective [126]
Dietary Vitamin E	1985-1993	53	35 cases, 67 controls	3.91 (1.1-14.0)	ns	Endo-metrial	Retrospective [117]

Table 6. Case control studies of vitamin E and esophageal, gastric, oral, laryngeal, pharyngeal cancer outcomes

Exposure	*Time Period*	*Age (yr) (mean/ Median or range)*	*Population*	*Odds Ratio 95% CI*	*p-trend*	*Cancer Site*	*Study Type/ Reference*
serum-α-tocopherol	1968-1977		9 cases, 16 controls	0.39	ns	Esophagus	Nested [148]
Dietary Vitamin E	1995-1997	69 cases, 68 controls	185 cases, 815 population controls	0.9 (0.5-1.6)	ns	Esophageal (adeno-carcinoma)	Retrospective [129]
Dietary Vitamin E	1995-1997	67 cases 68 control	165 cases, 815 population control	0.5 (0.2-1.0)	ns	Esophageal (squamous-cell)	Retrospective [129]
Dietary Vitamin E	1992-1994	95 cases, 132 clinic controls	0.7 (0.5-1.1)	0.13 (ns)	ns	Esophageal and gastric cardia (adeno-carcinoma)	Retrospective [130]
serum-α-tocopherol	Prior to 1989	65 cases, 59 controls	70 cases, 78 hospital or clinic controls	Lower levels in cases	0.002		Retrospective [125]
Dietary Vitamin E	1995-1997	66 cases, 68 controls	258 cases, 815 population controls	1.2 (0.8-1.7)	ns	Gastric (adeno-carcinoma)	Retrospective [129]
Dietary Vitamin E	1989-1985	40-79	74 cardia cases, 406 noncardia cases, 1067 population controls Non cardia: 0.6 (0.4-0.9)	Cardia: 0.6 (0.3-1.2) 0.05	ns	Gastric	Retrospective [131]
Dietary Vitamin E	1989-1990	57 cases, 59 controls	220 cases; 752 population controls	0.36 (0.16-0.82)	<0.001	Gastric	Retrospective [134]
Dietary Vitamin E	1975-1985	62	250 cases, 250 community controls	0.73 (0.36-1.49)	ns	Laryngeal	Retrospective [135]
Dietary Vitamin E	1992-1997	50-59	344 oral cases, 410 pharyngeal cases, 1775 hospital controls	0.44 (0.28-0.71)	<0.01	Oral and pharyngeal	Retrospective [126]
Vitamin E Supplement	Prior to 1992	55-64	133 cases, 264 hospital controls	0.4 (0.2-1.0)		Esophageal	Retrospective [128]
Serum Vitamin E	1995	58 cases, 55 controls	22 cases, 63 hospital controls	1.8 (0.6-5.0)	ns	Gastric	Retrospective [132]

Serum Vitamin E	1994-1996	64-72	51 cases, 49 control		ns	Gastric	Retrospective [133]
Vitamin E supplement	Prior to 1992	55-64	290 cases, 576 hospital controls	0.5 (0.3-0.9)		Oral	Retrospective [128]
serum α-tocopherol	1974-1990		28 cases, 112 controls	0.31	ns	Oral and pharyngeal	Nested [147]
serum α-tocopherol	1968-1977		20 cases; 37 controls	1.26	ns	Lip, oral cavity and pharynx	Nested [148]
serum α-tocopherol	1968-1977		11 cases; 17 controls	0.48	ns	Larynx	Nested [148]
Dietary+ supplemental Vitamin E	1989-1993	57	141 cases, 191 population controls	1.2 (0.6-2.3)	ns	Salivary gland	Retrospective [145]

Table 7. Case control studies of vitamin E and colon cancer outcome

Exposure	***Time Period***	***Age (yr) (mean/ median or range)***	***Population***	***Odds Ratio 95% CI***	***p-trend***	***Study Type/ Reference***
serum α-tocopherol		15-99	Pooled analysis of 289 cases and 1267 controls from 5 cohorts	0.7 (0.4-1.1)	ns	Nested [162]
serum α-tocopherol		15-99	Pooled analysis of 289 cases and 1267 controls from 5 cohorts	0.7 (0.4-1.3)	ns	Nested [162]
serum α-tocopherol		15-99	Pooled analysis of 289 cases and 1267 controls from 5 cohorts	0.6 (0.2-1.5)	ns	Nested [162]
Dietary Vitamin E	1985-1992	62 cases, 55 controls	1326 cases, 2024 hospital controls	0.63 (0.5-0.8)	<0.001	Retrospective [119]
Dietary Vitamin E	1992-1996	62 cases, 58 controls	1953 cases, 4154 hospital controls	0.63 (0.5-0.8)	<0.001	Retrospective [120]
Dietary Vitamin E	1989-1993	35-79	402 cases, 668 population controls	0.53 (0.36-0.78)		Retrospective [122]
Dietary Vitamin E	1985-1992	62 cases, 55 controls	828 cases, 2024 hospital controls	0.58 (0.42-0.81)		Retrospective [119]
Dietary Vitamin E	1991-1994	30-79	1953 cases, 2410 hospital controls	Men: 0.97 (0.68-1.40) Women: 0.90 (0.61-1.40)		Retrospective [121]
Dietary Vitamin E	1992-1996	62 cases, 58 controls	1225 cases, 4154 hospital controls	0.73 (0.6-0.9)		Retrospective [120]
Dietary Vitamin E	1985-1992	62 cases, 55 controls	498 cases, 2024 hospital controls	0.67 (0.45-0.98)	ns	Retrospective [119]

Table 7. (Continued)

Exposure	*Time Period*	*Age (yr) (mean/ median or range)*	*Population*	*Odds Ratio 95% CI*	*p-trend*	*Study Type/ Reference*
Dietary Vitamin E	1992-1996	62 cases, 58 controls	728 cases, 4154 hospital controls	1.14 (1.0-1.4)		Retrospective [120]
Dietary Vitamin E	1978-1986	64 65	277 male cases, 277 male community controls 145 female cases, 145 female community controls	1.04 (0.64-1.66) 0.75 (0.44-1.27)	ns ns	Retrospective [124]
Dietary α-tocopherol	1991-1994	30-79	1953 cases, 2410 hospital controls	Men: 0.99 (0.69-1.42); Women: 1.08 (0.71-1.62)	ns	Retrospective [121]
Dietary β-tocopherol	1991-1994	30-79	1953 cases, 2410 hospital controls	Men: 1.05 (0.77-1.42); Women: 1.14 (0.81-1.62)	ns	Retrospective [121]
Dietary γ-tocopherol	1991-1994	30-79	1953 cases, 2410 hospital controls	Men: 1.11 (0.78-1.57); Women: 1.16 (0.78-1.72)	ns	Retrospective [121]
Dietary δ-tocopherol	1991-1994	30-79	1953 cases, 2410 hospital controls	Men: 1.10 (0.79-1.53); Women: 1.12 (0.77-1.64)	ns	Retrospective [121]
Vitamin E supplement	1991-1994	30-79	1953 cases, 2410 hospital controls	Men: 0.99 (0.78-1.27); Women: 0.90 (0.69-1.16)	ns	Retrospective [121]
Dietary α-tocopherol	1989-1993	35-79	402 cases, 668 population controls	0.53 (0.36-0.78)	ns	Retrospective [122]
Vitamin E supplement	1985-1989	30-62	444 cases, 427 population controls	0.43 (0.26-0.71)	<0.001	Retrospective [123]

Table 8. Case control studies of vitamin E and lung cancer outcome

Exposure	*Time Period*	*Age (yr) (mean/ median)*	*Population*	*Odds Ratio 95% CI*	*p-trend*	*Study Type/ Reference*
serum α-tocopherol	1968-1991	58	92 cases, 83 controls	0.83 (0.33-2.07)	ns	Nested [151]
serum α-tocopherol	1974-1993	45-64	258 cases, 515 controls	0.77	ns	Nested [152]
serum α-tocopherol	1992-1999	63	108 cases, 216 controls	1.1 (0.6-2.3)	ns	Nested [65]
serum α-tocopherol	1985-1993	50-69	1144 cases in a chhort of 29133 male smokers (ATBC trial)	0.81 (0.67-0.97)	ns	Prospective [50]
Dietary Vitamin E	1993-1997	60-69	541 cases, 540 hospital controls	0.50 (0.34-0.74)	<0.001	Retrospective [137]
Serum Vitamin E	1995	57 cases, 55 controls	58 cases, 63 hospital control	0.3 (0.1-0.8)	<0.01	Retrospective [132]
Serum Vitamin E	Prior to 1990	58	59 cases, hospital and community controls	Lower levels in cases	0.04	Retrospective [136]
Supplemental Vitamin E	1982-1985	67 cases, 68 control	413 cases, 413 population controls	0.55 (0.35-0.85)		Retrospective [138]

Table 9. Case control studies of vitamin E and prostate cancer outcome

Exposure	*Time Period*	*Age (yr) (mean/ median)*	*Population*	*Odds Ratio 95% CI*	*P-trend*	*Study Type/ Reference*
serum α-tocopherol	1974-1996	54 yrs	182 cases; 364 controls	0.58 (0.31-1.06)	0.11 ns	Nested [153]
serum α-tocopherol	1971-1993	62 yrs	142 cases; 142 controls	1.4 (0.7-2.9)	0.71 ns	Nested [154]
serum α-tocopherol	1974-1986	71 yr	103 case; 103 controls	1.00 (0.29-3.45)		Nested [163]
serum α-tocopherol	1982-1995	61 cases, 62 controls	578 cases, 1294 controls	1.06 (0.76-1.48)	ns	Nested [155]
serum α-tocopherol	1985-1993	50-69	317 cases in a cohort of 29133 male smokers (ATBC trial)	No AT supplement:0.98 (0.60-1.60) AT supplement: 0.76 (0.42-1.37)	ns ns	Prospective Cohort [156]
Dietary Vitamin E	1993-1995	60 cases, 42 controls	65 cases, 132 controls recruited from blood bank	0.38 (0.09-1.68)	0.59	Retrospective [157]

Table 9. (Continued)

Exposure	*Time Period*	*Age (yr) (mean/ median)*	*Population*	*Odds Ratio 95% CI*	*P-trend*	*Study Type/ Reference*
Dietary Vitamin E	1994-1997	70-79	175 cases, 233 hospital controls	0.6 (0.3-1.1)	0.03	Retrospective [142]
Dietary Vitamin E	1994-1997	71-80	217 cases, 434 hospital and community controls	1.3 (0.9-2.0)	0.09	Retrospective [158]
Plasma α-tocopherol	1994-1998	60 cases, 42 controls	65 cases, 132 controls recruited from blood bank	1.02 (0.23-4.62)	ns	Retrospective [157]
Plasma γ-tocopherol	1993-1995	60 cases, 42 controls	65 cases, 132 controls recruited from blood bank	0.66 (0.22-1.97)	ns	Retrospective [157]
Vitamin E supplement	1993-1996	55-59 yrs	697 cases; 666 population controls	0.76 (0.54-1.08)	ns	Retrospective [143]

Table 10. Case control studies of vitamin E and skin cancer outcome

Exposure	*Time Period*	*Age (yr) (mean/ median or range)*	*Population*	*Odds Ratio 95% CI*	*p-trend*	*Cancer Type*	*Study Type /Reference*
serum α-tocopherol	1974-1992	65-74	32 cases, 64 controls	2.6 (0.7-9.2)	ns	Basal-cell skin	Nested [164]
serum α-tocopherol	1974-1992	55-64	37 case, 74 controls	1.5 (0.5-4.6)	ns	Squamous cell skin	Nested [164]
serum α-tocopherol	1974-1992	45-54	30 cases, 60 controls	2.0 (0.5-8.4)	ns	Malignant melanoma	Nested [164]
serum α-tocopherol	1968-1977		10 cases, 18 controls	0.2	<0.01	Malignant melanoma	Nested [148]
Dietary Vitamin E	1990-1992	65	46 cases, 46 clinic controls	ns	ns	Basal-cell skin	Retrospective [98]
Dietary Vitamin E	1992-1995	48 yr male and 42 yr female cases; 41 yr male and 38 yr female control	204 cases,248 dermatology clinic patients	0.6	0.03	Malignant melanoma	Retrospective [139]
Plasma α-tocopherol	1992-1995	48 yr male and 42 yr female cases and controls	204 cases, 248 dermatology clinic patients	1.0	ns	Malignant melanoma	Retrospective [139]

Table 11. Case control studies for serum α-tocopherol concentration measures and cancer outcome

Time Period	*Age (yr) (mean/ Median or range)*	*Population*	*Site of Cancer*	*Odds Ratio (95% CI)*	*P-trend*	*Type of Study/ Reference*
Prior to 1998	44 cases, 38 controls	44 cases 46 clinic controls with benign breast tumors	Breast	ns	ns	Retrospective [103]
1986-1988	64 cases, 62 controls	377 stage 1 or 2 breast cancer cases; 403 clinic controls.	Breast (menopausal)	0.8 (0.5-1.2)	ns	Retrospective [116]
Prior to 1991		387 cases; 670 community and hospital controls	Cervical	1.14 (0.6-2.1)	ns	Retrospective [117]
Prior to 1989	65 cases, 59 controls	70 cases, 78 hospital or clinic controls	Digestive (eg esophageal, gastric, biliary, colorectal and pancreatic)	Lower levels in cases	0.002	Retrospective [125]
1974-1992	65-74	32 cases, 64 controls	Basal-cell skin	2.6 (0.7-9.2)	ns	Nested [164]
1974-1986	59	35 cases, 70 controls	Bladder	0.57 (0.12-2.70)	ns	Nested [150]
1968-1977		15 cases, 29 controls	Bladder	1.25	ns	Nested [148]
1968-1977		18 cases, 34 controls	Brain	0.62	ns	Nested [148]
1974-1990		50 cases, 99 controls	Cervical	1.02(0.35-2.94)	ns	Nested [160]
1983-1994	33	38 cases, 116 controls	Cervical	1.3 (0.4-3.3)	ns	Nested [161]
1983-1994	15-99	Pooled analysis of 289 cases and 1267 controls from 5 cohorts	Colorectal	0.7 (0.4-1.1)	ns	Nested [162]
1983-1994	15-99	Pooled analysis of 206 cases and 938 controls from 5 cohorts	Colon	0.7 (0.4-1.3)	ns	Nested [162]
1983-1994	15-99	Pooled analysis of 83 cases and 329 controls from 5 cohorts	Rectal	0.6 (0.2-1.5)	ns	Nested (162)
1968-1977		9 cases, 16 controls	Esophagus	0.39	ns	Nested (148)
1968-1977		20 cases, 38 controls	Kidney	0.86	ns	Nested (148)
1968-1977		11 cases, 17 controls	Larynx	0.48	ns	Nested (148)
1968-1977		20 cases, 37 controls	Lip, oral cavity and pharynx	1.26	ns	Nested (148)

Table 11. (Continued)

Time Period	*Age (yr) (mean/ Median or range)*	*Population*	*Site of Cancer*	*Odds Ratio (95% CI)*	*P-trend*	*Type of Study/ Reference*
1968-1977		12 cases, 22 controls	Liver and gallbladder	2.23	ns	Nested (148)
1968-1991	58	92 cases, 83 controls	Lung	0.83 (0.33-2.07)	ns	Nested (151)
1968-1977		10 cases, 18 controls	Malignant melanoma	0.2	<0.01	Nested (148)
1992-1999	63	108 cases, 216 controls	Lung	1.1 (0.6-2.3)	ns	Nested (167)
1974-1992	45-54	30 cases, 60 controls	Malignant melanoma	2.0 (0.5-8.4)	ns	Nested (164)
1974-1989	53 yrs	35 cases, 67 controls	Ovarian	3.91 (1.1-14.0)	0.04	Nested (149)
1974-1996	54 yrs	182 cases, 364 controls	Prostate	0.58 (0.31-1.06)	ns	Nested (179)
1971-1993	62 yrs	142 cases, 142 controls	Prostate	1.4 (0.7-2.9)	ns	Nested (169)
1974-1986	71 yrs	103 case, 103 controls	Prostate	1.00 (0.29-3.45)		Nested (163)
1982-1995	61cases, 62 controls	578 cases, 1294 controls	Prostate	1.06 (0.76-1.48)	ns	Nested (155)
1982-1995	61cases, 62 yrs for controls	578 cases, 1294 controls	Prostate	1.06 (0.76-1.48)	ns	Nested (155)

Two additional studies, the Physicians' Health Study II and the SELECT Trial have been performed examining the potential of vitamin E to prevent cancer have been performed using 400 IU vitamin E (all-rac- alpha-tocopheryl-acetate) daily. Neither demonstrated a correlation with the reduction in cancer incidence [174-176]. The Physicians' Health Study II was a large randomized double-blind, placebo controlled factorial trial of vitamins E and C which began in 1997 and continued until 2007 containing more than 14,000 men. The outcome measures in this trial were prostate cancer and total cancer incidence. Vitamin E (all-rac-alpha-tocopheryl-acetate at 400IU/day) did not reduce the incidence of total cancer, prostate, colorectal, lung, bladder, and pancreatic cancers. Neither did this study result in significant effects on total mortality or cancer mortality. The SELECT Trial, Selenium and Vitamin E Cancer Prevention Trial began in July of 2001. It was a large Phase III, randomized placebo control trial examining the potential for selenium and vitamin E to reduce the incidence of prostate cancer with more than 35,000 men. The primary endpoint was prostate cancer incidence with secondary outcomes including: lung, colorectal and overall primary cancer incidence. The SELCT Trial found that dietary supplementation with all-rac-alpha-tocopheryl-acetate at 400IU/day enhanced the incidence for prostate cancer [176]. While these trials were conceived and carried out prior to the publication of the data concerning gamma-tocopherol, retrospective analysis would suggest that the concentration of 400 IU/day of alpha-tocopherol in these two trials likely reduced the beneficial effects of any dietary gamma-tocopherol (and perhaps other vitamin E isoforms) these patients may have taken in by lowering their tissue levels. The most compelling data that alpha-tocopherol may reduce the risk of prostate cancer came from the Alpha Tocopherol Beta Carotene (ATBC) study where doses of 50 mg all-rac-alpha-tocopheryl-acetate were administered among more than 29,000 male smokers. This demonstrated a 34% reduction in prostate cancer incidence during a 6 year follow-up. Further, in the Chinese Cancer Prevention Trial in which more than 29,000 poorly nourished residents of Linxian, China received a combined daily treatment of alpha-tocopherol (30 mg, RRR, all-rac, or a-VEA not specified), beta carotene (15 mg) and selenium (50 μg) statistically significant reductions of 9% in total mortality, 13% in cancer mortality, and 21% in gastric cancer mortality after 6 years of treatment and follow-up were experienced [177]. In both the ATBC study and Chinese Cancer Prevention Trial positive results were obtained with 20 fold lower doses of alpha-tocopherol than used in SELECT and Physicians' Health Study II, emphasizing the importance of the appropriate concentration of tocopherol to achieve positive results. Further, as smokers eliminate tocopherols faster and take up less newly absorbed tocopherols [30], the difference between the ATBC and the Chinese Prevention Trial suggest the need to increase the dose of alpha-tocopherol to compensate for the loses due to smoking is minimal (20 mg/day).

Nomura *et al.* demonstrated that serum carotenoids and gamma-tocopherol, but not alpha-tocopherol were shown to be lowest in subjects who developed areodigestive cancers (cancers of the oral cavity, sinonasal tract, larynx, pyriform sinus, pharynx, and esophagus) when compared with controls in a nested case control study that involved 6000 men of Japanese ancestry [178]. Another nested case control cohort study of 6860 Japanese American men examined between 1971 and 1975, resulted in 142 cases of men who developed prostate cancer. In these 142 cases, the serum levels of gamma-tocopherol were examined. Analysis shows that men with the highest serum levels of gamma-tocopherol have a statistically non-significant reduction in the incidence of prostate cancer (odds ratio 0.7, CI 0.3-1.5), a trend that may become significant with a larger cohort of cases to examine [168]. These data suggest that gamma-tocopherol supplementation may be required to prevent cancer, rather than alpha-tocopherol. To further demonstrate the potential of gamma-tocopherol supplementation in cancer, Ingles *et al.* assayed plasma alpha- and gamma-tocopherol concentrations in 332 subjects with colorectal adenomas and 363 control subjects. They found increasing plasma alpha-tocopherol and decreasing gamma-tocopherol levels were associated with the decreased occurrence of large (1cm or greater), but not small (less than 1 cm) adenomas. They observed a stronger trend of decreased occurrence ($p=0.02$) in large adenomas when the plasma alpha-tocopherol:gamma-tocopherol ratio was used. Subjects in the highest versus lowest quintile of plasma alpha-tocopherol: gamma-tocopherol ratio had an odds ratio of 0.36 (95% confidence interval, 0.14-0.95) for large adenomas. Since there are differences in tissue distribution and metabolism for different isoforms of vitamin E, it is conceivable that the colon tissue had higher levels of gamma-tocopherol, which may have conferred the protective effect. However, since this study did not measure tissue levels of tocopherols, the data are not conclusive, but do suggest that gamma-tocopherol plasma levels may be important in cancer prevention.

When reviewing the epidemiological data presented in Table 11, it becomes evident that serum alpha-tocopherol concentrations are not correlated with cancer. Further, supplementation of high doses of alpha-tocopherol alone is not an effective chemopreventive measure and may enhance the cancer by reducing tissue levels of other tocopherols, such as gamma-tocopherol which may be chemopreventive. In addition, these data suggest that the effects of varying concentrations of many dietary vitamin E isoforms need to be examined in animal models before making the jump to human trials. Having enough data with regard to how these compounds function in normal cells as well as at different stages of cancer will allow for a more successful outcome in clinical trials.

Vitamin E's Role in Oxidative Stress and Cancer

It is well established that vitamin E is a lipid soluble, chain breaking antioxidant and free radical scavenger [179-186]. In addition, it is established that oxidative stress and ROS play a role in the development of age-associated pathologies, including cancer [187, 188]. Taken together, these data suggest that vitamin E isoforms may reduce the oxidative stress formed during the carcinogenesis process through its antioxidant function and free radical scavenging [189]. For example, a water soluble vitamin E derivative, Trolox, diminishes the free-radical-induced up-regulation of COX-2 as well as reducing the downstream activation of p38 and extracellular signal-regulated kinase (ERK) signaling pathways, suggesting a therapeutic role of free radical scavenging [190]. F2 isoprostanes have been suggested as reliable *in vivo* markers of free radical generation and oxidative lipid damage [191-195]. Recently, plasma 8-isoprostane levels were increased during colon carcinogenesis in azoxymethane (AOM)/dextran-sulfate treated mice [196]. Gamma-tocopherol-rich diet (57% gamma-tocopherol, 24% delta-tocopherol, 13% alpha-tocopherol and 0.5% beta-tocopherol) reduces colon tumor formation and inflammation, as well as reduces the plasma levels of the proinflammatory eicosanoids of 8-isoprostane and PGE2. This suggests that the production of ROS may occur in azoxymethane (AOM)/dextran-sulfate -induced colon carcinogenesis and is reduced by dietary gamma-tocopherol [196].

Vitamin E and Aberrant Crypt Foci

AOM treatment is a commonly accepted model for the induction of aberrant crypt foci (ACF) at 16 weeks, followed by the progression to colon carcinogenesis at 32 weeks [197, 198]. This model has been used to test the ability of compounds to prevent or treat colon cancer [198-202]. The ability of many forms of vitamin E at varying concentrations to reduce the induction of ACF or reduce carcinogenesis has been tested using this model with varying results. Rats fed the AIN76A diet containing 50 IU/kg diet (control diet) of alpha-tocopherol (RRR, all-rac-, or a-VEA not specified, but likely all-rac-alpha-tocopherol) versus 200 IU/kg diet alpha-tocopherol were tested for their ability to prevent the formation ACF [203]. No significant differences were observed in the colonic proliferative index by increasing the vitamin E from 50IU/kg diet to 200 IU/kg diet, but an enhanced proliferation was observed in the prostate glands suggestive that increased alpha-tocopherol concentrations may be detrimental to prostate cancer prevention [203]. Experimental diets of varying concentations of selenium combined with various concentrations (50 mg/kg diet, 750 mg/kg diet) of vitamin E (form not specified, likely all-rac-alpha-tocopheryl-acetate) given to AOM-treated Fisher 344 rats demonstrate that selenium deficiency significantly inhibits the percentage animals with tumors (both colon adenocarcinomas and adenomas) [204]. Vitamin E at neither concentration had an effect on the development of colon carcinogenesis nor was there an interaction between selenium status and vitamin E [204]. Vitamin E (500mg/kg diet of dl-alpha-tocopheryl-acetate) did not alter the aberrant crypt formation in AOM-treated mice [205]. In fact, only three forms of tocopherol tested in this model result in a reduction in ACF or colon tumor formation. They include alpha-tocopherol at 90 mg/kg diet (unspecified form, but likely all-rac-alpha-tocopheryl-acetate) [206], RRR-gamma-tocopherol [196, 207], and a-VES [208]. Vitamin E at 90 mg/kg diet (form not specified, likely all-rac-alpha-tocopheryl-acetate) resulted in a significant decrease in the number ACF when administered within a high fat diet which presents a high risk for colorectal cancer [206]. With the exception of this study, none of the previously mentioned studies using this model demonstrates therapeutic results with alpha-tocopherol. The reason may lie within the concentration used, 90 mg/kg diet, which is lower than the alpha-tocopherol in all of the other studies presented. Further, it may be that the additional stress of testing a high fat diet, which is a risk factor for colorectal cancer, requires a slightly higher tocopherol in the diet than the standard 50 mg/kg diet found in rodent chow to provide protection against the formation of ACF. Alternatively, a high fat diet may potentiate the uptake of alpha-tocopherol into the tissues allowing for the protective effect observed. The explanation for the protective effect of alpha-tocopherol in this study needs to be explored further to understand under what conditions alpha-tocopherol becomes protective. A gamma-tocopherol rich diet (57% gamma-tocopherol, 24% delta-tocopherol, 13% alpha-tocopherol and 0.5% beta-tocopherol) reduced colon tumor formation by 55% as well as inflammation in the colon tissues using the AOM model [207]. An independent study by Ju *et al.* demonstrates reduced tumor formation and inflammation as well as reduced plasma and colonic levels of the proinflammatory eicosanoids of 8-isoprostane, LTB4, and PGE2 [196].

The Exon *et al.* study used the AOM model to tests old rats (20 months old) versus young rats (2 months old) for their susceptibility to the development of ACF in the presence or absence of a-VES [208]. The a-VES-treated group demonstrated a reduction in the development of ACF regardless of the age of the rat. Interestingly, the group with the lowest number of ACF is the old rats treated with a-VES, not the young a-VES-treated group nor the young or old untreated groups. The reason for this outcome may lie within the concentrations of tocopherol in the colon tissue and in the serum from these rats. Treatment with a-VES increased the colon tissue levels of alpha-tocopherol by 2 fold in the young and old rats; however the levels of gamma-tocopherol were also increased in both treatment groups. The young, untreated rats have undetectable levels of gamma-tocopherol, but the young animals treated with a-VES result in a 4 fold increase of gamma-tocopherol in their colon tissues. Despite the concentration increase in the young rats, the old rats had significantly higher concentrations of gamma-tocopherol in their colon tissues compared with the young counterparts (old no a-VES = 19.83 ±4.67, old + a-VES = 29.68 ±6.52 compared with young no a-VES = below detectable limits, young a-VES = 3.78 ± 0.31), suggesting that gamma-tocopherol may be required in an aging population to protect tissues from age-related diseases such as cancer. The serum tocopherol concentrations in the young and old rats treated with a-VES are also increased compared to their untreated counterparts. There was also an increase in serum gamma-tocopherol. Neither the old or young rats had detectable levels of gamma-tocopherol in their serum, but the final concentration was 2.16 ± 0.23 in the old rats versus 1.19 ±0.05 nmol/ml serum in the young rats. This study was the first to find detectable levels of a-VES in the tissues of animals. The results in this study suggest that a-VES is transported to tissues and is converted to alpha-tocopherol, thus increasing tissue levels of alpha-tocopherol and perhaps allowing for an increase in tissue uptake and maintenance of gamma-tocopherol which allow for additional protection of colonic tissues.

Tocopherol isoforms are not alone in their ability to prevent ACF formation in the AOM model, red palm oil (with the vitamin E content of alpha-tocotrienol-29%, gamma-tocotrienol-28%, delta-tocotrienol-14%, and alpha-tocopherol -28%) substituted for soybean oil in standard rat chow reduce ACF foci and ACF formation [209] and enhance the activity of glutathione-S-transferase in the liver.

Some Vitamin E Isoforms May Exert Anticancer Effects by Non-Redox Mechanisms

If the action on ROS is the sole activity of vitamin E in cancer, then alpha-tocopherol should have a greater effect on the inhibition of proliferation and apoptosis in cancer cell lines by virtue of the additional methyl groups on the phenolic ring lending it superior antioxidant activity. However, data presented earlier in this chapter demonstrate that gamma-tocopherol and other forms of vitamin E including redox silent isoforms are superior to alpha-tocopherol at inhibiting cancer cell proliferation, reducing tumor burden, and inducing cell cycle arrest where alpha-tocopherol is ineffective [20, 47, 210-213]. These data suggest that the role of vitamin E in carcinogenesis may occur through mechanisms in addition to the redox pathways. Gamma-tocopherol can be nitrated at the five carbon position in the presence of nitric oxide to form 5-nitro-gamma-tocopherol proving to be a more effective trapping agent of nitrogen species having a greater effect on apoptosis compared with alpha-tocopherol when reactive nitrogen species are involved [5, 214, 215]. As previously discussed in this chapter, however, isoforms of vitamin E other than alpha-tocopherol have superior effects on the inhibition of proliferation and apoptosis in cancer cells, thus it is possible that vitamin E isoforms have an indirect antioxidant activity through signal transduction to modulate the expression of antioxidant enzymes. For example, Barve, *et al.* has shown that a mixed tocopherol diet that exceeded 60% gamma-tocopherol results in suppression of prostate carcinogenesis through the increased expression of antioxidant enzymes such as catalase, superoxide dismutase, glutathione peroxidase, heme-oxygenase-1, and phase II detoxifying enzymes [91]. This hypothesis is further supported by the fact that gamma-tocopheryl quinone induces an adaptive response in PC-12 cells via up-regulation of intracellular GSH synthesis and activation of ATF4 [216]. Hsieh *et al.* discovered that breast cancer cells exposed to alpha-, gamma-, and delta-tocotrienols result in differential suppression of proliferation as well as altered expression in the oxidative stress enzymes glutathione peroxidase, catalase, thioredoxin, and NRF2 [217]. In a cell model of human breast cancer,

MCF-10A epithelial cells, 4-hydroxyestradiol treatment results in the accumulation of ROS, decreasing the GSH/GSSG ratio and MnSOD protein levels which is suggestive of oxidative stress [218]. This treatment concomitantly changes the levels of DNA repair proteins, BRCA1 and PARP-1. Gamma-tocopherol treatment suppresses the 4-hydroxyestradiol-induced increases in redox markers, as well as increasing the GSH/GSSG ratio (by reducing the level of GSSG) and MnSOD protein expression. Alpha-tocopherol treatment did not exert a significant effect on the redox makers, but rather up regulated the protein expression of BRCA1 and PARP-1. The combined data in this section suggests that vitamin E isoforms other that alpha-tocopherol (a-VES, gamma-tocopherol , alpha-, gamma-, delta-tocotrienol, and gamma-tocopheryl quinone) suppress oxidative stress by scavenging free radicals as well as by up regulating oxidative stress enzymes through signal transduction. Gamma-tocopherol may have a dual role in cancer prevention and treatment through the scavenging of nitrogen species as well as regulating oxidative stress enzymes [5, 214, 215, 217].

The Potential for Vitamin E Isoforms to be Used as Adjuvant Chemotherapy

Oncologists attempt to improve survival rates for patients with malignancies with a wide variety of treatments including combination therapy with or without radiation therapy. Dietary antioxidants at high doses induce differentiation, inhibit proliferation, and apoptosis depending upon the dose and type of antioxidant, treatment schedule and type of tumor cells without producing similar effects on most normal cells *in vitro* and *in vivo* [219, 220]. The concept is that the antioxidants would prevent free radical damage to normal tissues while allowing the cancer cells to be damaged by the chemotherapy; however some argue that chemotherapeutic agents use ROS to damage the cancer cells. For this reason, the concept of using antioxidants in combination with chemotherapy has been proposed and debated [221-228]. Many of these debates have referred to vitamin E solely as an antioxidant, but it is important to remember that not all vitamin E isoforms are antioxidants. The synthetic isoforms that having an ether attached at carbon number 6 are redox silent; therefore any effect that is observed with these isoforms is not due to antioxidant activity, but occurs through a signal transduction mechanism rendering any antioxidant objection to using them as adjuvant chemotherapeutic agents mute.

Some Vitamin E Isoforms Demonstrate an Ability to Enhance the Antiproliferative Effects of Chemotherapy in Cancer Cell Lines

Select vitamin E isoforms have been tested in cell lines and demonstrate the ability to enhance the antiproliferative effects of chemotherapy. For example, a-VES was tested in three human osteosarcoma cell lines. Cells containing wild type p53 in the presence of a-VES demonstrate a transition from S phase to G2 phase and sensitization to methotrexate enhancing the cell death of cancer cells [229]. The overexpression of HER-2 receptor contributes to the malignant transformation of breast cancer cells. a-TOB (a redox silent vitamin E) inhibits the activation of HER-2 receptor in the MDA-MB-453 breast cancer cell line and enhances the cytotoxic effects of adriamycin at doses less than the IC50 [230]. In combination with 13-cis-retinoic acid and interferon-alpha 2a, all-rac-alpha-tocopherol results in the inhibition of cell growth and cell cycle progression in five different head and neck cancer cell lines [231]. Depending upon the concentration used, in conjunction with adriamycin, a-VES results in synergistic or additive growth inhibition of human prostate cancer cells, DU-145 when compared to treatment with either agent alone [232]. Doses of a-VES larger than the a-VES IC50 result in synergy, while does smaller than a-VES IC50 result in an additive growth inhibition [232]. In a human breast cancer xenograft model, the combination of dietary a-TEA (redox silent, 300mg/kg body weight) plus trastuzumab (a Her2/neu antibody) results in faster tumor regression and more tumor-free animals than trastuzumab alone [233]. In a xenograft tumor model of ovarian cancer, a-TEA was administered alone (as a liposomal aerosol that was deposited in the respiratory tract the mice each day) and in combination with cisplatin (administered by weekly intraperitoneal injections). A significant reduction in cell proliferation of transplanted cis-platin resistant ovarian tumors ($p<0.001$), tumor burden, as well as lung and lymph metastases was observed in the subcutaneous transplanted tumors treated with a-TEA + cisplatin compared with the controls and the individual treatments [234]. Further, apoptosis was increased in the combined treatment compared with that of the controls [234].

Some Vitamin E Isoforms Reduce the Harmful Side Effects of Chemotherapeutic Agents

Select vitamin E isoforms can reduce some of the harmful side effects of chemotherapeutic agents. For example, platinum agents such as cisplatin, carboplatin, and oxaliplatin results in chemotherapy that is severely limited by peripheral neurotoxicity through oxidative stress. This painful side effect has been reported in 90% of patients receiving cumulative doses higher than 300 mg/m^2 and reduced by treatment with alpha-tocopherol (RRR, all-rac, or a-VEA not specified, specified purchase from Sigma-Aldrich, Milan, Italy) in an animal study [235]. In a randomized-placebo controlled trial, a-VEA (300 mg Ephynal, Roche, Milan, Italy) provided neuroprotection against cisplatin-induced neuropathy when administered in a 300 mg oral dose 4 days before the start of cisplatin treatment and continued for 3 months following [236]. A combination treatment of cisplatin and daily oral administration of alpha-tocopherol (RRR, all-rac, or a-VEA not specified, specified purchase from Merck, Darmstadt, Germany) at a concentration of 4.3mg/kg body weight results in an increase in survival of animals over those treated with cisplatin alone (3.3 mg/kg body weight) [237]. The results from this study show that alpha-tocopherol supplementation does not alter the cisplatin antitumor efficacy, but increases the survival of the cisplatin-treated animals and protects the animals from cisplatin-induced lipoperoxidation, as well as from cisplatin-induced neurotoxicity.

Tamoxifen is an anti-estrogen used in the treatment of breast cancer where hemolytic anemia is a known side-effect. Low concentrations of a-TEA prevent tamoxifen incorporation into thc crythrocytc membrane thereby reducing the hemolytic effect of tamoxifen [238]. Patients with advanced hepatocellular carcinoma (HCC) have been shown to benefit from tamoxifen treatment. Results from studies on the human hepatoblastoma cell line HepG2 provide evidence that estrogen-receptor-alpha-independent antiproliferative actions of tamoxifen in HCC are mediated by the suppression of telomerase activity [239]. Alpha-tocopherol (RRR, all-rac, nor a-VEA was specified, neither was the supplier specified) diminished the effects of tamoxifen on telomerase activity [240].

Cells have the ability to transport small molecules such as chemotherapeutic agents out of the cytoplasm reducing their effectiveness for cancer cells and make the cells drug-resistant. This occurs through the action of an ATP-dependent pump known as multidrug resistant 1 (MDR1). Gamma-tocopheryl quinone and delta-tocopheryl quinone are cytotoxic and effective at inducing apoptosis in multidrug resistant lymphoma, leukemia, and breast cancer cells [241]. Further, a-VES reduces adriamycin efflux by inhibition of the MDR1 transporter [242].

Radiation therapy can be very effective in the treatment of many types of cancer by damaging the DNA of the cancer cells beyond repair and sending them into apoptosis. However, radiation therapy leads to the reduction in red blood cells also known as cytopenia. Several forms of vitamin E demonstrate radioprotective effects. For example, alpha-tocopherol (RRR) demonstrates radioprotective efficacy in a CD2F21 male mouse model system at 400 IU/kg body weight against lethal doses of cobalt-60 radiation [243]. Gamma-tocotrienol (400 mg/kg body weight) demonstrates protection from 12Gy doses of cobalt-60 radiation used to treat PC-3 prostate cancer tumors in nude mice [244]. Alpha-tocopherol, a-VES, and gamma-tocotrienol demonstrate radioprotective efficacy through induction of hematopoietic cytokines when administered subcutaneously 24 hr before irradiation [245, 246]. Gamma-tocotrienol provides a 90% recovery of radiation-induced depletion of progenitor cells in sub-lethally irradiated mice and preserved the self-renewal capability of human stem cells by preventing persistent DNA damage in these cells, increasing white blood cells, neutrophil counts, and increasing cytokines and chemokines such as: G-CSF, IL-1alpha, IL-1beta, IL-6, IL-12, p70, IL-17, MIP-1alpha, and PKC levels [247, 248]. In light of this evidence, vitamin E isoforms may be beneficial as adjuvant chemotherapy agents for some cancers. More work needs to be done in this area to determine the efficacy of different vitamin E isoforms and determine effective concentration ranges to work with different chemotherapy agents.

Vitamin E Isoforms Modulate Major Regulatory Elements Involved in Inflammation

One of the earliest hypotheses with regard to the cause of cancer was made by Rudolf Virchow in 1863 as he observed the lymphocytes in neoplastic tissues and detected chronic inflammation. He suggested that chronic inflammation was the cause of cancer. Experiments today are proving his hypothesis to be true [249, 250]. NFκβ is a major regulatory factor of inflammation and appears to be involved in cancer [251]. In many cancers, NFκβ is over expressed and in some cancer is constitutively active rendering inflammation constant. NFκβ is a transcription factor that regulates a number of genes, including cyclooxygenase-2 (COX-2). The up regulation COX-2 is associated with reduced survival in a number of epithelial cancers [7-10].

Vitamin E isoforms can reverse the immunological dysregulation that may allow for chronic inflammation. For example, nitration of gamma-tocopherol increases under inflammatory conditions [252], gamma-tocopherol traps mutagenic electrophiles of NO [214], and supplementation with gamma-tocopherol inhibits protein nitration and ascorbate oxidation in rats with inflammation [215]. Rat lung cells depleted of vitamin E, results in a shift of protein kinase C from the cytosol to the membranes indicating that deficiency of vitamin E in the lung induces a reversible immunological dysregulation that may predispose the lung to develop acute or chronic inflammation [215].

Gamma-tocotrienol was first shown to decrease the transcriptional activity of NFκβ in neoplastic +SA (highly malignant) mouse mammary epithelial cells by suppressing the activation of Iκβ kinase-alpha/beta [253]. Later it was shown that gamma-tocotrienol inhibits TNF-alpha-mediated activation of NFκβ by inhibiting TNF associated factor 1 (TAK-1)[254]. Gamma-tocopherol and gamma-tocotrienol decrease the activity of NFκβ in PC-3 prostate cancer cells [210, 255]. Gamma-tocopherol-mediated reduction of NFκβ was found to be dependent upon PPAR gamma and arachidonic acid (AA) metabolism, while gamma-tocotrienol-mediated reduction of NFκβ occurs through the reduction of TGFβ2, a known cause of NFκβ constitutive activation in cancer cells [256].

In microglial cells, alpha-tocopherol down regulates the inflammatory response through NFκβ, Erk 1/2, and p38 MAPK [257]. In activated human monocytes, alpha-tocopherol inhibits the release of the proinflammatory cytokine, IL-1 beta, via inhibition of the 5-lipoxygenase pathway [258].

Products of AA metabolism, in particular, prostaglandin (PG)E(2) are over expressed in colon cancer cells as a major product of COX-2. In peritoneal macrophages isolated and cultured from mice fed 30 ppm or 500 ppm all-rac-alpha-tocopheryl-acetate in their diet for 30 days reduced LPS-stimulated production of PGE (2) demonstrating reduced COX-2 activity, but had no effect on COX-2 mRNA and protein levels indicating a post-translational regulation of COX-2 by vitamin E [259]. RRR Tocopherols (alpha, gamma, delta, beta) were tested in culture using peritoneal macrophages isolated and cultured from mice fed the standard diet and resulted in effective in inhibition of COX-2 activity, with varying degrees of inhibition depending upon tocopherol isoform and concentration employed [260, 261]. For example to achieve a similar level of PGE (2) inhibition 50 μM of alpha-tocopherol was required to equal 25 μM gamma-tocopherol or 1. 25 μM of delta-tocopherol [260]. Similar results were found in murine RAW264.7 macrophages and IL-1beta treated A549 human lung cancer cells when testing alpha-tocopherol, gamma-tocopherol, and gamma-tocopherol metabolite gamma-CEHC(2,7,8-trimethyl-2-(beta-carboxyethyl)-6-hydroxychroman) [6]. Gamma-tocopherol and gamma-CEHC reduced PGE2 formation in both lipopolysaccharide-stimulated RAW264.7 macrophages and IL-1beta-treated A549 lung cancer cells. Alpha-tocopherol at 50 μM had a modest effect on PGE2 production in lipopolysaccharide-stimulated RAW264.7 macrophages; however did not have an effect on the inhibition of COX-2 activity in IL-1beta-activated A549 lung cancer cells [6]. As described previously by Wu *et al.*, the inhibitory effects of gamma-tocopherol and gamma-CEHC stemmed from their inhibition of COX-2 activity, rather than affecting protein expression or substrate availability, and appeared to be independent of antioxidant activity [6]. The inhibitory potency of gamma-tocopherol and gamma-CEHC is diminished by an increase in AA concentration, suggesting that they might compete with AA at the active site of COX-2 [6]. Taken together these findings indicate that gamma- and delta-tocopherol isoforms as well as gamma-CEHC, but not alpha-tocopherol possess anti-inflammatory activities that are important for cancer treatment and prevention.

Vitamin E Isoforms Modulate Pathways Involved in Metastasis

Tissues contain cells that work in concert to maintain normal physiology including both cellular positional identity and number. Malignant cancer cells have lost these restraints and can migrate or metastasize from the site of the primary tumor, enter the lymphatic vessels or bloodstream and seed into distant organs. Metastasis is the last step in tumor progression, and once it occurs, the cancer is more difficult to treat. For metastasis to happen genetic alterations occur that not only confer a selective growth advantage, but also allow for up regulation of genes that begin the process of degrading the basal lamina or extracellular matrix. Some of these genes include the matrix metalloproteinase (MMP) family. Many MMP family members are up regulated during the carcinogenesis process. Integrins are proteins that span the lipid bilayer and receive signals from the extracellular matrix. Integrin signaling is known to activate MMPs. In normal cells, negative feedback of integrin/protease binding is required to prevent the excessive degradation of the ECM. However in cancer cells some integrins are significantly up regulated which are expressed at very low levels in normal cells, providing this negative feedback. These integrins include: alpha v beta3, alpha5beta1, and alphavbeta6. The tumor metastasis in human prostate cancer cell lines PC-3 and DU-145 cells associated with MMPs and this process is inhibited by a-VES in a matrigel assay [262]. alpha (1-6), beta1, and alpha v integrins (significantly up regulated in cancer cells) are less expressed at the cell surface of human erythroleukemia cell (HEL) after alpha-tocopherol treatment, but not beta-tocopherol treatment suggesting that alpha-tocopherol was performing this function by a mechanism other than its antioxidant function [263]. Leptin-induced enhanced proliferation and increase in MMP-2 expression in human aortic smooth muscle cell (HASMC) was abolished by vitamin E (form not specified) [264].

Angiogenesis, the formation of new capillaries from existing microvessels, plays a role in cancer by providing a route for the cancer cells to enter to the blood stream and metastasize as well as providing nutrition for tumor growth. Some important proangiogenic factors include: basic fibroblast growth factor (BFGF), fibroblast growth factor 1 (FGF1), and vascular endothelial growth factor (VEGF). It is well-known that VEGF regulates angiogenesis by binding to vascular endothelial growth factor receptor (VEGFR). Tocotrienols inhibit both the proliferation and tube formation of bovine aortic endothelial cells, with delta-tocotrienol appearing to have the highest activity [265]. Delta-tocotrienol reduces the VEGF-stimulated tube formation by human umbilical vein endothelial cells. Moreover, delta-tocotrienol inhibited the new blood vessel formation on the growing chick embryo chorioallantoic membrane (assay for *in vivo* angiogenesis) [265]. Orally administered tocotrienol suppressed the tumor cell-induced angiogenesis in the mouse dorsal air sac assay. Based on DNA microarray analysis, the antiangiogenic effect of tocotrienol was attributable in part to regulation of intracellular VEGF signaling (phospholipase C-gamma and protein kinase C) [265]. In the cell culture experiments, delta-tocotrienol reduced the VEGF-stimulated tube formation by human umbilical vein endothelial cells (HUVEC) [266]. DNA chip analysis revealed that delta-tocotrienol specifically down regulates the expression of VEGF receptor (VEGFR) in endothelial cells [266] thus blocking the intracellular signaling of VEGF, resulting in the inhibition of angiogenesis.

Connective tissue growth factor (CTGF) stimulates the synthesis of extracellular matrix. In cancer cells, the extracellular matrix is degraded, allowing for invasion of cancer cells into lymph and surrounding tissues. An up regulation of CTGF would assist in preventing the degradation of the extracellular matrix. The expression of the CTGF gene was analyzed by gene expression arrays. RRR-alpha-tocopherol, but not RRR-beta-tocopherol was found to induce gene expression by 1.8-fold [267], suggesting that alpha-tocopherol is acting through a mechanism other than antioxidant activity. Similar results were obtained by RT-PCR (1. 7-fold) and at the protein level (1.4-fold) [267]. The stimulation of CTGF by RRR-alpha-tocopherol may lead to synthesis of extracellular matrix components that are ordinarily degraded during carcinogenesis. This process may slow the process of carcinogenesis.

Using MDA-MB-435 human breast cancer xenografts in nude mice, a-TEA or celecoxib (1250 mg/kg diet) alone and in combination results in significantly reducing lung and lymph metastases compared to the control [76]. a-TEA and a-TEA + celecoxib (1250) treatments significantly reduced blood vessel density of the tumors as demonstrated by CD-31 staining in comparison to control. For many tumors, the vascular density can provide a prognostic indicator of metastatic potential, with highly vascular primary tumors having a higher incidence of metastasis than poorly vascular tumors.

Vitamin E Isoforms Modulate Ras Levels Resulting in Cell Cycle Arrest and Apoptosis

Ras proteins have the role of controlling the activity of several critical signaling pathways that regulate normal cell proliferation. The transcriptional induction of cyclin D1 by growth factors is dependent upon the Ras/Raf-1/MEK/Erk pathway. Point mutations in ras in codons 12, 13, and 61 of the three ras genes (H-ras, K-ras, and N-ras) convert them to oncogenes. In K-ras, the mutations accumulate as carcinogenesis progresses [268]. These mutations result in the maintenance of ras in the active state allowing or propagating carcinogenesis in a number of cancer cell types including: pancreatic, colon, lung, thyroid, and myeloid leukemia. This over expression of ras not only up regulates the expression of the cell cycle through cyclin D1, but also results in an inhibitory effect on p21 through the expression of c-myc. This expression of c-myc also influences the apoptosis pathway by allowing for the over expression the pro-apoptotic protein, Bcl-2.

Investigating the effects of dietary iron, alpha-tocopherol and gamma-tocopherol play on oxidative stress and ras in the colon, Stone *et al.* was the first to find that the levels of ras-p21 were significantly lower in rats fed the gamma-tocopherol diets compared with rats fed the alpha-tocopherol diets [41]. The effect alpha-and gamma-tocopherol have on levels of ras could be advantageous in the reduction of ras activity in cancer cells.

a-VES inhibits growth and reduces the expression of c-myc, N-myc and H-ras specific mRNAs in murine neuroblastoma cells (NBP2) by reducing the expression of c-myc, N-myc, and H-ras in neuroblastoma (NBP2) cells in culture [269]. Similar results using a-VES were obtained with B-16 melanoma cells [270]. Treatment of A549 lung cancer cells with 40 μM

6-O-carboxypropyl-alpha-tocotrienol (a synthetic form of alpha-tocotrienol that is redox silent) results in suppression of ras farnesylation, as well as ras and rhoA prenylation, causing an accumulation of cells in the G1 phase of the cell-cycle and the subsequent induction of apoptosis to A549 lung cancer cells [22]. It is important to note that the redox silence of a-T3E indicates that the reduction of ras levels in cancer cells by vitamin E isoforms is not occurring as a result of free radical scavenging.

Vitamin E Modulates the Master Fat Regulatory Element, Peroxisome Proliferator Activator Receptor, (PPAR)

PPAR gamma is a promising molecular target for cancer prevention. Up regulation of PPAR gamma activity is anticarcinogenic through its effects on downstream genes that affect cellular proliferation, apoptosis, and differentiation. The thiazolidine drugs are powerful PPAR gamma ligands. As seen in Figure 7, vitamin E compounds have structural similarity to the thiazolidine, troglitazone.

The ability of vitamin E to up regulate PPAR gamma was first tested in colon cancer cell lines [27]. It was discovered that gamma-tocopherol has superior ability to up regulate mRNA and protein expression compared with alpha-tocopherol. It was later discovered that gamma-tocopherol up regulates AA metabolism through a PPAR dependent mechanism in prostate cancer cells [210] leading to the inhibition of cellular proliferation.

Tocopherols are not the only vitamin E family members that regulate carcinogenesis proliferation through PPAR gamma. Tocotrienols are also involved in PPAR gamma regulation and co-modulate transforming growth factor beta 2 (TGFβ2) [255, 271].

Receptor Tyrosine Kinase Activity is Modulated by Redox Silent Forms of Vitamin E as Well as Naturally occuring Vitamin E forms

Tyrosine kinases are enzymes that transfer a phosphate group from ATP to the hydroxy group of tyrosine residues on signal transduction molecules. The transfer of phosphate ultimately leads to signal transduction of fundamental processes such as the cell cycle, proliferation, differentiation, motility, and cell death or survival.

Due to their abnormal up regulation in many cancer cells, tyrosine kinase inhibitors are being examined for their potential to prevent and treat cancer. Two major tyrosine receptor kinases involved in carcinogenesis are protein kinase B (PKB/Akt) and protein kinase C (PKC).

PKB is a serine-threonine kinase encoded by the Akt gene. Akt activation by phosphorylation is associated with poor outcome in endocrine-treated breast cancer and drives progression of breast cancer [272]. PKB is activated by phosphatidylinositol 3-kinase-dependent kinase (PI3K) and can regulate the progression of the cell cycle, the activation of NFκβ, as well as protein translation through the mTOR pathway. Vitamin E isoforms play a role in the regulation of PKB; for example, 4 μM gamma-tocotrienol reduces growth more than 50% compared with untreated controls in neoplastic +SA mammary epithelial cells with a concomitant decrease in levels of activated PI3K and PKB with a reduction in phosphorylated-PKB activity [253].

A comparison of a-VES and a-TOB performed in two human prostate cancer cell lines, LNCaP and PC-3, shows that a-VES and a-TOB share the same mechanism of targeting the PKB and JNK signaling and activating the intrinsic cell death cascade though caspase 9. In addition, a-VES and a-TOB may act at the membrane level to interfere with PKB phosphorylation [273]. The phosphorylation of PKB is inhibited in HMC-1 human mastocytoma cell line, MCF-7 human breast cancer cell line, and U937 human myeloid leukemia cell line using 50 μM alpha-tocopherol, gamma-tocopherol, beta-tocopherol or delta-tocopherol [274].

The reduction in the phosphorylation of PKB results in reduced activity as demonstrated by the concomitant reduction of GSK alpha/beta phosphorylation as well as suppressed translocation of PKB to the membrane [274]. Tocotrienol-rich palm oil fraction inhibits PI3K/PKB mitogenic signaling resulting from reduction in ERK1/ERK2 MAPK and is dependent upon cAMP signaling in EGF-dependent preneoplastic CL-S1 mouse mammary cells [275].

Protein kinase C (PKC) is a tyrosine receptor kinase involved in the signal transduction pathways for cell proliferation, cell cycle, cytoskeletal organization, cell migration, differentiation, apoptosis and angiogenesis. PKC over expression has been associated with malignant transformations in several cell lines including breast [276], lung [277], gastric carcinomas, [278] and, ovarian carcinomas [278]. In 1988, Azzi *et al.* first reported that all-rac-alpha-tocopherol, (in addition to its antioxidant activity) was capable of inhibiting PKC activity in brain [279]. a-VES demonstrates the ability to inhibit PKC in human neutrophils [280]. Alpha-tocopherol (form not specified (Xu *et al.*, 2001), RRR-alpha-tocopherol(Meier and King, 2000), form not specified (Freedman *et al.*, 2000)) reduced the plasma levels of PKC and nitric oxide synthase in diabetic rats, in diabetes *in vivo* and *in vitro* and in platelets [281-283]. a-VES induces activation of PKC and PKC-dependent hypophosphorylation of Rb, which results in induction of apoptosis [284]. PKC activity is crucial for post-translational up regulation of telomerase activity. In HepG2 cells, a tamoxifen-induced suppression of the total PKC activity (cytosolic and membrane-bound) was observed. Alpha-tocopherol diminished the effects of tamoxifen on PKC activity as well as on telomerase activity suggesting that the tamoxifen-induced decrease of telomerase activity in HepG2 cells is mediated post-translationally via suppression of PKC activity [240]. The initial event in EGF-receptor mitogenic-signalling is PKC activation. Normal mammary epithelial cells isolated from midpregnant BALB/c mice grown in primary culture, and maintained on serum-free media containing 10 ng/mL EGF as a mitogen were treated with growth inhibitory doses of delta-tocopherol (100 μM), alpha-tocotrienol (50 μM), or gamma- or delta-tocotrienol (10 μM) which result in inhibition of EGF-induced PKC-alpha activation as determined by its translocation from the cytosolic to membrane fraction [285]. a-VES demonstrates ability to induce apoptosis through inhibition of PKC by increasing activity of protein phosphatase 2A (PP2A) resulting in a gain- or loss-of-function bcl-2 mutants which implies modulation of bcl-2 activity by PKC/PP2A as a mitochondrial target of a-VES-induced proapoptotic signals [93].

Many vitamin E compounds have an effect on tyrosine kinase enzymes other than PKB and PKC. Malignant mesothelioma is an aggressive cancer with no effective treatment options. In a chemoresistant cell line (H28), a-T3E (a redox silent analogue of alpha-tocotrienol) inhibited cell growth through inhibition of the epidermal growth factor receptor (EGFR) as well as the inactivation of Src [23]. In pancreatic cancer cell lines (Panc-28, MIA PaCa-2, Panc-1, and BxPC-3) gamma- and delta-tocotrienol induced cell death by greater than 50% in all cell lines through the down regulation of the tyrosine kinase ErbB-2 [69]. The over expression of ErbB-2 receptor is also central to the malignant transformation of breast cancer. a-TOB causes induction of apoptosis in MDA-MB-453 cells that over express the ErbB-2 receptor and reduces levels of activated ErbB-2 receptor and PKB [286].

Vitamin E Compounds Modulate Proteins Involved in the Sphingolipid and Cholesterol Metabolism

Eukaryotic cells obtain cholesterol either by receptor-mediated endocytosis of lipoprotein cholesterol via the low-density lipoprotein receptor (LDL-R) or by *de novo* synthesis, catalyzed by HMGCoA reductase at the rate-limiting step. The scavenger receptor class B type I (SR-BI) mediates the selective uptake of cholesterol and cholesteryl ester (CE) from high density lipoprotein (HDL) into cells. Regulations of the SR-BI include induction by hormones via cAMP-activated protein kinase A. Vitamin E has a major effect on the expression of SR-BI in rat liver. The feeding of a vitamin E depleted diet to male wistar rats for 38-40 days results in an 11-fold increase in the SR-BI protein level in the liver. Upon feeding the repleted animals with an alpha-tocopherol-enriched diet (form not specified, 400 mg/kg diet) for two days prior to testing, the increased concentration of SR-BI seen in the absence of dietary vitamin E was readily reversed with concomitant down regulation of PKC. These results are consistent with the view that the cellular level of vitamin E exerts a tight control over the expression of SR-BI with potential involvement of PKC [287]. A blend of delta-tocotrienol and lovastatin synergistically suppressed the proliferation of human pancreatic cells MIA Paca-2 through the HMGCoA reductase pathway demonstrating reduction in the mevalonate pathway through HMGCoA reductase may have potential in pancreatic cancer therapy [68].

In five different head and neck squamous cell carcinoma (HNSCC) in and a solid tumor xenograft model, a-VES inhibits cell growth and induced apoptosis in each of the five the HNSCC cell lines tested [288]. By increasing time of exposure to a-VES, an increase of ceramide, sphingomyelinase activity, caspase-3, and p53 levels and a decrease in proapoptotic and inflammatory proteins such as NFκβ, Bcl-2, and Bcl-XL occurs. Tumor growth in the xenograft model was slowed with i.p. administration of a-VES. The induction of enzymes involved in ceramide metabolism by a-VES suggests that ceramide-mediated apoptosis may expand therapeutic strategies in the treatment of carcinoma [288].

Conclusion

Vitamin E compounds have the potential to inhibit cancer cell proliferation and induce apoptosis in a number of different tissue types and a variety of genetic backgrounds. These compounds can exert their effects through a number of different pathways including cell survival, apoptosis, proliferation, fat metabolism, inflammation, oncogene expression all of which are dysregulated in carcinogenesis. As with all vitamins, vitamin E isoforms have the potential to regulate a number of different pathways and maintain cellular homeostasis. The clinical trials performed to date demonstrate that alpha-tocopherol alone may not be as effective at inhibiting carcinogenesis as a combination of isoforms. The major work that needs to be performed prior to any next large clinical trial is to determine: (1) which compounds should be used and under what circumstances they should be employed; (2) what genetic backgrounds are most suitable and which compounds work in synergy and; (3) what concentrations will be most effective. This will require preliminary data in animals. Understanding the limitations of each vitamin E family member, the concentration dependence of their activity and the conditions under which they are able to work together is imperative for designing a potential clinical trial to test their efficacy. Each vitamin E family member does not exist in nature independent of the others, which suggests that each has a role in the homeostasis of cellular function. Therefore, each needs to be examined alone and in combination to establish their potential role in cancer therapy and prevention.

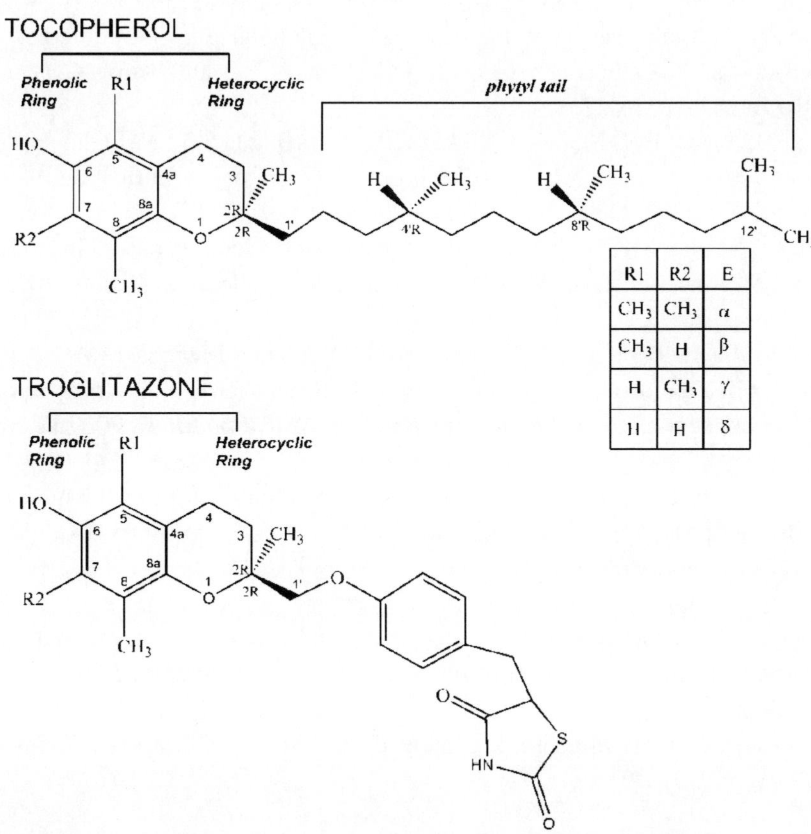

Figure 7. The PPAR ligand troglitazone is structurally similar to the tocopherol.

References

[1] Ames B. DNA damage from micronutrient deficiencies is likely to be a major cause of cancer. *Mutat. Res.,* 2001;475:7-20.

[2] Evans HM, Bishop KS. On The Existence of a Hitherto Unrecognized Dietary Factor Essential For Reproduction. *Science,* 1922 Dec 8;56(1458):650-1.

[3] Vatassery GT, Johnson GJ, Krezowski AM. Changes in vitamin E concentrations in human plasma and platelets with age. *J. Am. Coll. Nutr.,* 1983;2(4):369-75.

[4] Handelman GJ, Machlin LJ, Fitch K, Weiter JJ, Dratz EA. Oral alpha-tocopherol supplements decrease plasma gamma-tocopherol levels in humans. *J. Nutr.,* 1985 Jun;115(6):807-13.

[5] Cooney RV, Franke AA, Harwood PJ, Hatch-Pigott V, Custer LJ, Mordan LJ. Gamma-tocopherol detoxification of nitrogen dioxide: superiority to alpha-tocopherol. *Proc. Natl. Acad. Sci. USA,* 1993;90:1771-5.

[6] Jiang Q, Elson-Schwab I, Courtemanche C, Ames BN. gamma-tocopherol and its major metabolite, in contrast to alpha-tocopherol, inhibit cyclooxygenase activity in macrophages and epithelial cells. *Proc. Natl. Acad. Sci. USA,* 2000;97:11494-9.

[7] Soumaoro LT, Uetake H, Higuchi T, Takagi Y, Enomoto M, Sugihara K. Cyclooxygenase-2 expression: a significant prognostic indicator for patients with colorectal cancer. *Clin. Cancer Res.,* 2004 Dec 15;10(24):8465-71.

[8] Richardsen E, Uglehus RD, Due J, Busch C, Busund LT. COX-2 is overexpressed in primary prostate cancer with metastatic potential and may predict survival. A comparison study between COX-2, TGF-beta, IL-10 and Ki67. *Cancer Epidemiol.,* 2010 Jun;34(3):316-22.

[9] Jana D, Sarkar DK, Maji A, Chikkala BR, Hassanujjaman S, Mukhopadhyay M, *et al.* Can cyclo-oxygenase-2 be a useful prognostic and risk stratification marker in breast cancer? *J. Indian. Med. Assoc.,* 2012 Jul;110(7):429-33.

[10] Lee JY, Myung SK, Song YS. Prognostic role of cyclooxygenase-2 in epithelial ovarian cancer: A meta-analysis of observational studies. *Gynecol. Oncol.,* 2013 Jun;129(3): 613-9.

[11] Yu W, Jia L, Park SK, Li J, Gopalan A, Simmons-Menchaca M, *et al.* Anticancer actions of natural and synthetic vitamin E forms: RRR-alpha-tocopherol blocks the anticancer actions of gamma-tocopherol. *Mol. Nutr. Food Res.,* 2009 Dec;53(12):1573-81.

[12] Stauble B, Boscoboinik D, Tasinato A, Azzi A. Modulation of activator protein-1 (AP-1) transcription factor and protein kinase C by hydrogen peroxide and D-alpha-tocopherol in vascular smooth muscle cells. *Eur. J. Biochem.,* 1994 Dec 1;226(2):393-402.

[13] Thomas CE, McLean LR, Parker RA, Ohlweiler DF. Ascorbate and phenolic antioxidant interactions in prevention of liposomal oxidation. *Lipids,* 1992 Jul;27(7): 543-50.

[14] Chan AC. Partners in defense, vitamin E and vitamin C. *Can J. Physiol. Pharmacol.,* 1993 Sep;71(9):725-31.

[15] Stoyanovsky DA, Goldman R, Darrow RM, Organisciak DT, Kagan VE. Endogenous ascorbate regenerates vitamin E in the retina directly and in combination with exogenous dihydrolipoic acid. *Curr. Eye Res.*, 1995 Mar;14(3):181-9.

[16] Guo Q, Packer L. Ascorbate-dependent recycling of the vitamin E homologue Trolox by dihydrolipoate and glutathione in murine skin homogenates. *Free Radic. Biol. Med.*, 2000 Aug;29(3-4):368-74.

[17] Kagan VE, Kuzmenko AI, Shvedova AA, Kisin ER, Li R, Martin I, *et al.* Direct evidence for recycling of myeloperoxidase-catalyzed phenoxyl radicals of a vitamin E homologue, 2,2,5,7,8-pentamethyl-6-hydroxy chromane, by ascorbate/dihydrolipoate in living HL-60 cells. *Biochim. Biophys. Acta.*, 2003 Mar 17;1620(1-3):72-84.

[18] Nagaoka S, Kakiuchi T, Ohara K, Mukai K. Kinetics of the reaction by which natural vitamin E is regenerated by vitamin C. *Chem. Phys. Lipids,* 2007 Mar;146(1):26-32.

[19] Elnagar AY, Wali VB, Sylvester PW, El Sayed KA. Design and preliminary structure-activity relationship of redox-silent semisynthetic tocotrienol analogues as inhibitors for breast cancer proliferation and invasion. *Bioorg. Med. Chem.*, 2010 Jan 15;18(2):755-68.

[20] Behery FA, Elnagar AY, Akl MR, Wali VB, Abuasal B, Kaddoumi A, *et al.* Redox-silent tocotrienol esters as breast cancer proliferation and migration inhibitors. *Bioorg. Med. Chem.,* 2010 Nov 15;18(22):8066-75.

[21] Behery FA, Akl MR, Ananthula S, Parajuli P, Sylvester PW, El Sayed KA. Optimization of tocotrienols as antiproliferative and antimigratory leads. *Eur. J. Med. Chem.,* 2013 Jan;59:329-41.

[22] Yano Y, Satoh H, Fukumoto K, Kumadaki I, Ichikawa T, Yamada K, *et al.* Induction of cytotoxicity in human lung adenocarcinoma cells by 6-O-carboxypropyl-alpha-tocotrienol, a redox-silent derivative of alpha-tocotrienol. *Int. J. Cancer,* 2005 Jul 10;115(5):839-46.

[23] Kashiwagi K, Virgona N, Harada K, Kido W, Yano Y, Ando A, *et al.* A redox-silent analogue of tocotrienol acts as a potential cytotoxic agent against human mesothelioma cells. *Life Sci.,* 2009 May 8;84(19-20):650-6.

[24] Kashiwagi K, Harada K, Yano Y, Kumadaki I, Hagiwara K, Takebayashi J, *et al.* A redox-silent analogue of tocotrienol inhibits hypoxic adaptation of lung cancer cells. Biochem Biophys Res Commun 2008 Jan 25;365(4):875-81.

[25] Birringer M, EyTina JH, Salvatore BA, Neuzil J. Vitamin E analogues as inducers of apoptosis: structure-function relation. *Br. J. Cancer,* 2003 Jun 16;88(12):1948-55.

[26] Traber MG, Arai H. Molecular mechanisms of vitamin E transport. *Annu. Rev. Nutr.,* 1999;19:343-55.

[27] Campbell SE, Stone WL, Whaley SG, Qui M, Krishnan K. Gamma tocopherol upregulates peroxisome proliferator activated receptor (PPAR) gamma expression in SW 480 human colon cancer cell lines. *BMC Cancer,* 2003;3(25).

[28] Gao R, Stone WL, Huang T, Papas AM, Qui M. The uptake of tocopherols by RAW 264.7 macrophages. *Nutr. J.,* 2002 Oct 15;1(1):2.

[29] Proteggente AR, Turner R, Majewicz J, Rimbach G, Minihane AM, Kramer K, *et al.* Noncompetitive plasma biokinetics of deuterium-labeled natural and synthetic alpha-tocopherol in healthy men with an apoE4 genotype. *J. Nutr.,* 2005 May;135(5):1063-9.

[30] Jeanes YM, Hall WL, Proteggente AR, Lodge JK. Cigarette smokers have decreased lymphocyte and platelet alpha-tocopherol levels and increased excretion of the gamma-

tocopherol metabolite gamma-carboxyethyl-hydroxychroman (gamma-CEHC). *Free Radic. Res., 2004* Aug;38(8):861-8.

[31] Jeanes YM, Hall WL, Ellard S, Lee E, Lodge JK. The absorption of vitamin E is influenced by the amount of fat in a meal and the food matrix. *Br. J. Nutr.,* 2004 Oct;92 (4):575-9.

[32] Hall WL, Jeanes YM, Lodge JK. Hyperlipidemic subjects have reduced uptake of newly absorbed vitamin E into their plasma lipoproteins, erythrocytes, platelets, and lymphocytes, as studied by deuterium-labeled alpha-tocopherol biokinetics. *J. Nutr.,* 2005 Jan;135(1):58-63.

[33] Sontag TJ, Parker RS. Cytochrome P450 omega-hydroxylase pathway of tocopherol catabolism. Novel mechanism of regulation of vitamin E status. *J. Biol. Chem.,* 2002 Jul 12; 277(28):25290-6.

[34] Parker RS, Swanson JE. A novel 5'-carboxychroman metabolite of gamma-tocopherol secreted by HepG2 cells and excreted in human urine. *Biochem. Biophys. Res. Commun.,* 2000 Mar 16;269(2):580-3.

[35] Swanson JE, Ben RN, Burton GW, Parker RS. Urinary excretion of 2,7, 8-trimethyl-2-(beta-carboxyethyl)-6-hydroxychroman is a major route of elimination of gamma-tocopherol in humans. *J. Lipid Res.,* 1999 Apr;40(4):665-71.

[36] Parker RS, Sontag TJ, Swanson JE. Cytochrome P4503A-dependent metabolism of tocopherols and inhibition by sesamin. *Biochem. Biophys. Res Commun.,* 2000 Nov 2;277(3):531-4.

[37] Sontag TJ, Parker RS. Influence of major structural features of tocopherols and tocotrienols on their omega-oxidation by tocopherol-omega-hydroxylase. *J. Lipid Res.,* 2007 May;48(5):1090-8.

[38] Bardowell SA, Stec DE, Parker RS. Common variants of cytochrome P450 4F2 exhibit altered vitamin E-{omega}-hydroxylase specific activity. *J. Nutr.,* 2010 Nov;140(11): 1901-6.

[39] Bardowell SA, Ding X, Parker RS. Disruption of P450-mediated vitamin E hydroxylase activities alters vitamin E status in tocopherol supplemented mice and reveals extra-hepatic vitamin E metabolism. *J. Lipid Res.,* 2012 Dec;53(12):2667-76.

[40] Bardowell SA, Duan F, Manor D, Swanson JE, Parker RS. Disruption of mouse cytochrome p450 4f14 (Cyp4f14 gene) causes severe perturbations in vitamin E metabolism. *J. Biol. Chem.,* 2012 Jul 27;287(31):26077-86.

[41] Stone WL, Papas AM, LeClair IO, Qui M, Ponder T. The influence of dietary iron and tocopherols on oxidative stress and ras-p21 levels in the colon. *Cancer Detect. Prev.,* 2002;26(1):78-84.

[42] Frank J, Budek A, Lundh T, Parker RS, Swanson JE, Lourenco CF, *et al.* Dietary flavonoids with a catechol structure increase alpha-tocopherol in rats and protect the vitamin from oxidation in vitro. *J. Lipid Res.,* 2006 Dec;47(12):2718-25.

[43] de Mesquita ML, Araujo RM, Bezerra DP, Filho RB, de Paula JE, Silveira ER, *et al.* Cytotoxicity of delta-tocotrienols from Kielmeyera coriacea against cancer cell lines. *Bioorg. Med. Chem.,* 2011 Jan 1;19(1):623-30.

[44] Patacsil D, Tran AT, Cho YS, Suy S, Saenz F, Malyukova I, *et al.* Gamma-tocotrienol induced apoptosis is associated with unfolded protein response in human breast cancer cells. *J. Nutr. Biochem.,* 2012 Jan;23(1):93-100.

[45] Yu W, Simmons-Menchaca M, Gapor A, Sanders BG, Kline K. Induction of apoptosis in human breast cancer cells by tocopherols and tocotrienols. *Nutr. Cancer,* 1999;33(1):26-32.

[46] Shah S, Sylvester PW. Tocotrienol-induced caspase-8 activation is unrelated to death receptor apoptotic signaling in neoplastic mammary epithelial cells. *Exp. Biol. Med.,* (Maywood) 2004 Sep;229(8):745-55.

[47] Campbell SE, Stone WL, Lee S, Whaley S, Yang H, Qui M, *et al.* Comparative effects of RRR-alpha- and RRR-gamma-tocopherol on proliferation and apoptosis in human colon cancer cell lines. *BMC Cancer,* 2006 Jan 17;6:13.

[48] Glinghammar B, Rafter J. Colonic luminal contents induce cyclooxygenase 2 transcription in human colon carcinoma cells. *Gastroenterology,* 2001;120:401-10.

[49] Lipkin M, Yang K, Edelmann W, Newmark H, Fan KH, Risio M, *et al.* Inherited and acquired risk factors in colonic neoplasia and modulation by chemopreventive interventions. *J. Cell Biochem.,* 1996;25S:136-41.

[50] Yang J, Zhang W, Evans PM, Chen X, He X, Liu C. Adenomatous polyposis coli (APC) differentially regulates beta-catenin phosphorylation and ubiquitination in colon cancer cells. *J. Biol. Chem.,* 2006 Jun 30;281(26):17751-7.

[51] Schneikert J, Grohmann A, Behrens J. Truncated APC regulates the transcriptional activity of beta-catenin in a cell cycle dependent manner. *Hum. Mol. Genet.,* 2007 Jan 15;16(2):199-209.

[52] Heinen CD, Richardson D, White R, Groden J. Microsatellite instability in colorectal adenocarcinoma cell lines that have full-length adenomatous polyposis coli protein. *Cancer Res.,* 1995 Nov 1;55(21):4797-9.

[53] Grosch S, Tegeder I, Niederberger E, Brautigam L, Geisslinger G. COX-2 independent induction of cell cycle arrest and apoptosis in colon cancer cells by the selective COX-2 inhibitor celecoxib. *FASEB J.,* 2001;15(14):2742-4.

[54] Lev-Ari S, Maimon Y, Strier L, Kazanov D, Arber N. Down-regulation of prostaglandin E2 by curcumin is correlated with inhibition of cell growth and induction of apoptosis in human colon carcinoma cell lines. *J. Soc. Integr. Oncol.,* 2006;4(1):21-6.

[55] Androulakis XM, Muga SJ, Chen F, Koita Y, Toure B, Wargovich MJ. Chemopreventive effects of Khaya senegalensis bark extract on human colorectal cancer. *Anticancer. Res.,* 2006 May;26(3B):2397-405.

[56] Koga H, Sakisaka S, Harada M, Takagi T, Hanada S, Taniguchi E, *et al.* Involvement of p21(WAF1/Cip1), p27(Kip1), and p18(INK4c) in troglitazone-induced cell-cycle arrest in human hepatoma cell lines. *Hepatology,* 2001;33:1087-97.

[57] Wang J, Lv X, Shi J, Hu X, DU Y. Troglitazone induced apoptosis via PPARgamma activated POX-induced ROS formation in HT29 cells. *Biomed. Environ. Sci.,* 2011 Aug;24(4):391-9.

[58] Rohrl C, Kaindl U, Koneczny I, Hudec X, Baron DM, Konig JS, *et al.* Peroxisome-proliferator-activated receptors gamma and beta/delta mediate vascular endothelial growth factor production in colorectal tumor cells. *J. Cancer Res. Clin. Oncol.,* 2011 Jan;137(1):29-39.

[59] Behrens J. Control of beta-catenin signaling in tumor development. *Ann. NY Acad. Sci.,* 2000;910:21-35.

[60] Russo P, Malacarne D, Falugi C, Trombino S, O'Connor PM. RPR-115135, a farnesyltransferase inhibitor, increases 5-FU- cytotoxicity in ten human colon cancer cell lines: role of p53. *Int. J. Cancer,* 2002 Jul 20;100(3):266-75.

[61] Bottone FG, Jr., Baek SJ, Nixon JB, Eling TE. Diallyl disulfide (DADS) induces the antitumorigenic NSAID-activated gene (NAG-1) by a p53-dependent mechanism in human colorectal HCT 116 cells. *J. Nutr.,* 2002 Apr;132(4):773-8.

[62] Hinnebusch BF, Meng S, Wu JT, Archer SY, Hodin RA. The effects of short-chain fatty acids on human colon cancer cell phenotype are associated with histone hyperacetylation. *J. Nutr.,* 2002 May;132(5):1012-7.

[63] Chidambara Murthy KN, Jayaprakasha GK, Patil BS. The natural alkaloid berberine targets multiple pathways to induce cell death in cultured human colon cancer cells. Eur *J. Pharmacol.,* 2012 Aug 5;688(1-3):14-21.

[64] Li CY, Huang WF, Wang QL, Wang F, Cai E, Hu B, *et al.* Crocetin induces cytotoxicity in colon cancer cells via p53-independent mechanisms. *Asian Pac. J. Cancer Prev.,* 2012;13(8):3757-61.

[65] Kim JA, Park KS, Kim HI, Oh SY, Ahn Y, Oh JW, *et al.* Troglitazone activates p21Cip/WAF1 through the ERK pathway in HCT15 human colorectal cancer cells. *Cancer Lett.,* 2002 May 28;179(2):185-95.

[66] Glinghammar B, Inoue H, Rafter JJ. Deoxycholic acid causes DNA damage in colonic cells with subsequent induction of caspases, COX-2 promoter activity and the transcription factors NF-kB and AP-1. *Carcinogenesis,* 2002 May;23(5):839-45.

[67] Sun W, Xu W, Liu H, Liu J, Wang Q, Zhou J, *et al.* gamma-Tocotrienol induces mitochondria-mediated apoptosis in human gastric adenocarcinoma SGC-7901 cells. *J. Nutr. Biochem.,* 2009 Apr;20(4):276-84.

[68] Hussein D, Mo H. d-delta-Tocotrienol-mediated suppression of the proliferation of human PANC-1, MIA PaCa-2, and BxPC-3 pancreatic carcinoma cells. *Pancreas,* 2009 May;38(4):e124-e136.

[69] Shin-Kang S, Ramsauer VP, Lightner J, Chakraborty K, Stone W, Campbell S, *et al.* Tocotrienols inhibit AKT and ERK activation and suppress pancreatic cancer cell proliferation by suppressing the ErbB2 pathway. *Free Radic. Biol. Med.,* 2011 Sep 15;51(6):1164-74.

[70] Smolarek AK, So JY, Burgess B, Kong AN, Reuhl K, Lin Y, *et al.* Dietary administration of delta- and gamma-tocopherol inhibits tumorigenesis in the animal model of estrogen receptor-positive, but not HER-2 breast cancer. *Cancer Prev. Res.,* (Phila) 2012 Nov;5(11):1310-20.

[71] Barve A, Khor TO, Reuhl K, Reddy B, Newmark H, Kong AN. Mixed tocotrienols inhibit prostate carcinogenesis in TRAMP mice. *Nutr. Cancer,* 2010;62(6):789-94.

[72] Srivastava JK, Gupta S. Tocotrienol-rich fraction of palm oil induces cell cycle arrest and apoptosis selectively in human prostate cancer cells. *Biochem. Biophys. Res. Commun.,* 2006 Jul 28;346(2):447-53.

[73] Yu W, Sanders BG, Kline K. RRR-alpha-tocopheryl succinate inhibits EL4 thymic lymphoma cell growth by inducing apoptosis and DNA synthesis arrest. *Nutr. Cancer,* 1997;27(1):92-101.

[74] Bang OS, Park JH, Kang SS. Activation of PKC but not of ERK is required for vitamin E-succinate-induced apoptosis of HL-60 cells15. *Biochem. Biophys. Res. Commun.,* 2001 Nov 9;288(4):789-97.

[75] Weber T, Lu M, Andera L, Lahm H, Gellert N, Fariss MW, *et al.* Vitamin E succinate is a potent novel antineoplastic agent with high selectivity and cooperativity with tumor necrosis factor-related apoptosis-inducing ligand (Apo2 ligand) in vivo. *Clin. Cancer Res.,* 2002 Mar;8(3):863-9.

[76] Zhang S, Lawson KA, Simmons-Menchaca M, Sun L, Sanders BG, Kline K. Vitamin E analog alpha-TEA and celecoxib alone and together reduce human MDA-MB-435-FL-GFP breast cancer burden and metastasis in nude mice. *Breast Cancer Res. Treat.,* 2004 Sep;87(2):111-21.

[77] Wu Y, Zu K, Ni J, Yeh S, Kasi D, James NS, *et al.* Cellular and molecular effects of alpha-tocopheryloxybutyrate: lessons for the design of vitamin E analog for cancer prevention. *Anticancer Res.,* 2004 Nov;24(6):3795-802.

[78] Gysin R, Azzi A, Visarius T. gamma-Tocopherol inhibits human cancer cell cycle progression and cell proliferation by down-regulation of cyclins. *FASEB J.,* 2002 Dec 1;16(14):1952-4.

[79] Galli F, Stabile AM, Betti M, Conte C, Pistilli A, Rende M, *et al.* The effect of [alpha]- and [gamma]-tocopherol and their carboxyethyl hydroxychroman metabolites on prostate cancer cell proliferation. *Archives of Biochemistry and Biophysics*, 2004 Mar 1;423(1):97-102.

[80] Venkateswaran V, Fleshner NE, Klotz LH. Modulation of cell proliferation and cell cycle regulators by vitamin E in human prostate carcinoma cell lines. *J. Urol.,* 2002 Oct;168(4 Pt 1):1578-82.

[81] Ni J, Chen M, ZHANG Y, Li R, Huang J, Yeh S. Vitamin E succinate inhibits human prostate cancer cell growth via modulating cell cycle regulatory machinery. *Biochem. Biophys. Res. Commun.,* 2003 Jan 10;300(2):357-63.

[82] You H, Yu W, Munoz-Medellin D, Brown PH, Sanders BG, Kline K. Role of extracellular signal-regulated kinase pathway in RRR-alpha-tocopheryl succinate-induced differentiation of human MDA-MB-435 breast cancer cells. *Mol. Carcinog.,* 2002 Apr;33(4):228-36.

[83] Lee JK, Jung JC, Chun JS, Kang SS, Bang OS. Expression of p21WAF1 is dependent on the activation of ERK during vitamin E-succinate-induced monocytic differentiation. *Mol. Cells,* 2002 Feb 28;13(1):125-9.

[84] Turley JM, Ruscetti FW, Kim SJ, Fu T, Gou FV, Birchenall-Roberts MC. Vitamin E succinate inhibits proliferation of BT-20 human breast cancer cells: increased binding of cyclin A negatively regulates E2F transactivation activity22. *Cancer Res.,* 1997 Jul 1;57(13):2668-75.

[85] Alleva R, Benassi MS, Tomasetti M, Gellert N, Ponticelli F, Borghi B, *et al.* Alpha-tocopheryl succinate induces cytostasis and apoptosis in osteosarcoma cells: the role of E2F1. *Biochem. Biophys. Res. Commun.,* 2005 Jun 17;331(4):1515-21.

[86] Nesaretnam K, Ambra R, Selvaduray KR, Radhakrishnan A, Canali R, Virgili F. Tocotrienol-rich fraction from palm oil and gene expression in human breast cancer cells. *Ann. NY Acad. Sci.,* 2004 Dec;1031:143-57.

[87] Agarwal MK, Agarwal ML, Athar M, Gupta S. Tocotrienol-rich fraction of palm oil activates p53, modulates Bax/Bcl2 ratio and induces apoptosis independent of cell cycle association. *Cell Cycle,* 2004 Feb;3(2):205-11.

[88] Hsieh TC, Elangovan S, Wu JM. gamma-Tocotrienol controls proliferation, modulates expression of cell cycle regulatory proteins and up-regulates quinone reductase NQO2 in MCF-7 breast cancer cells. *Anticancer. Res.,* 2010 Jul;30(7):2869-74.

[89] Elangovan S, Hsieh TC, Wu JM. Growth inhibition of human MDA-mB-231 breast cancer cells by delta-tocotrienol is associated with loss of cyclin D1/CDK4 expression and accompanying changes in the state of phosphorylation of the retinoblastoma tumor suppressor gene product. *Anticancer Res.,* 2008 Sep;28(5A):2641-7.

[90] Wu SJ, Ng LT. Tocotrienols inhibited growth and induced apoptosis in human HeLa cells through the cell cycle signaling pathway. *Integr. Cancer Ther.,* 2010 Mar;9(1):66-72.

[91] Barve A, Khor TO, Nair S, Reuhl K, Suh N, Reddy B, *et al.* Gamma-tocopherol-enriched mixed tocopherol diet inhibits prostate carcinogenesis in TRAMP mice. *Int. J. Cancer,* 2009 Apr 1;124(7):1693-9.

[92] Lu G, Xiao H, Li GX, Picinich SC, Chen YK, Liu A, *et al.* A gamma-tocopherol-rich mixture of tocopherols inhibits chemically induced lung tumorigenesis in A/J mice and xenograft tumor growth. *Carcinogenesis,* 2010 Apr;31(4):687-94.

[93] Neuzil J, Weber T, Schroder A, Lu M, Ostermann G, Gellert N, *et al.* Induction of cancer cell apoptosis by alpha-tocopheryl succinate: molecular pathways and structural requirements. *FASEB J.,* 2001 Feb;15(2):403-15.

[94] Economopoulou M, Langer HF, Celeste A, Orlova VV, Choi EY, Ma M, *et al.* Histone H2AX is integral to hypoxia-driven neovascularization. *Nat. Med.,* 2009 May;15(5): 553-8.

[95] Berton TR, Conti CJ, Mitchell DL, Aldaz CM, Lubet RA, Fischer SM. The effect of vitamin E acetate on ultraviolet-induced mouse skin carcinogenesis. *Mol. Carcinog.,* 1998 Nov;23(3):175-84.

[96] Schwartz J, Baker V, Larios E, Desai D, Amin S. Inhibition of experimental tobacco carcinogen induced head and neck carcinogenesis. *Oral. Oncol.,* 2004 Jul;40(6):611-23.

[97] Yu W, Sanders BG, Kline K. RRR-alpha-tocopheryl succinate induction of DNA synthesis arrest of human MDA-MB-435 cells involves TGF-beta-independent activation of p21Waf1/Cip1. *Nutr. Cancer*, 2002;43(2):227-36.

[98] Sahl WJ, Glore S, Garrison P, Oakleaf K, Johnson SD. Basal cell carcinoma and lifestyle characteristics. *Int. J. Dermatol.,* 1995 Jun;34(6):398-402.

[99] Vena JE, Graham S, Freudenheim J, Marshall J, Zielezny M, Swanson M, *et al.* Diet in the epidemiology of bladder cancer in western New York. *Nutr. Cancer,* 1992;18(3): 255-64.

[100] Riboli E, Gonzalez CA, Lopez-Abente G, Errezola M, Izarzugaza I, Escolar A, *et al.* Diet and bladder cancer in Spain: a multi-centre case-control study. *Int. J. Cancer,* 1991 Sep 9;49(2):214-9.

[101] Giles GG, McNeil JJ, Donnan G, Webley C, Staples MP, Ireland PD, *et al.* Dietary factors and the risk of glioma in adults: results of a case-control study in Melbourne, Australia. *Int. J. Cancer,* 1994 Nov 1;59(3):357-62.

[102] Hu J, La Vecchia C, Negri E, Chatenoud L, Bosetti C, Jia X, *et al.* Diet and brain cancer in adults: a case-control study in northeast China. *Int. J. Cancer,* 1999 Mar 31;81(1):20-3.

[103] Yeum KJ, Ahn SH, Rupp de Paiva SA, Lee-Kim YC, Krinsky NI, Russell RM. Correlation between carotenoid concentrations in serum and normal breast adipose

tissue of women with benign breast tumor or breast cancer. *J. Nutr.,* 1998 Nov;128(11): 1920-6.

[104] Gerber M, Richardson S, Salkeld R, Chappuis P. Antioxidants in female breast cancer patients. *Cancer Invest.,* 1991;9(4):421-8.

[105] Negri E, La Vecchia C, Franceschi S, D'Avanzo B, Talamini R, Parpinel M, *et al.* Intake of selected micronutrients and the risk of breast cancer. *Int. J. Cancer,* 1996 Jan 17;65(2):140-4.

[106] Richardson S, Gerber M, Cenee S. The role of fat, animal protein and some vitamin consumption in breast cancer: a case control study in southern France. *Int. J. Cancer,* 1991 Apr 22;48(1):1-9.

[107] Ronco A, De Stefani E, Boffetta P, Deneo-Pellegrini H, Mendilaharsu M, Leborgne F. Vegetables, fruits, and related nutrients and risk of breast cancer: a case-control study in Uruguay. *Nutr. Cancer,* 1999;35(2):111-9.

[108] Yuan JM, Wang QS, Ross RK, Henderson BE, Yu MC. Diet and breast cancer in Shanghai and Tianjin, China. *Br. J. Cancer,* 1995 Jun;71(6):1353-8.

[109] Levi F, Pasche C, Lucchini F, La Vecchia C. Dietary intake of selected micronutrients and breast-cancer risk. *Int. J. Cancer,* 2001 Jan 15;91(2):260-3.

[110] Mezzetti M, La Vecchia C, Decarli A, Boyle P, Talamini R, Franceschi S. Population attributable risk for breast cancer: diet, nutrition, and physical exercise. *J. Natl. Cancer,* Inst 1998 Mar 4;90(5):389-94.

[111] Ambrosone CB, Marshall JR, Vena JE, Laughlin R, Graham S, Nemoto T, *et al.* Interaction of family history of breast cancer and dietary antioxidants with breast cancer risk (New York, United States). *Cancer Causes Control.,* 1995 Sep;6(5):407-15.

[112] Braga C, La Vecchia C, Negri E, Franceschi S, Parpinel M. Intake of selected foods and nutrients and breast cancer risk: an age- and menopause-specific analysis. *Nutr. Cancer,* 1997;28(3):258-63.

[113] Bohlke K, Spiegelman D, Trichopoulou A, Katsouyanni K, Trichopoulos D. Vitamins A, C and E and the risk of breast cancer: results from a case-control study in Greece. *Br. J. Cancer,* 1999 Jan;79(1):23-9.

[114] Mannisto S, Alfthan G, Virtanen M, Kataja V, Uusitupa M, Pietinen P. Toenail selenium and breast cancer-a case-control study in Finland. *Eur. J. Clin. Nutr.,* 2000 Feb;54(2):98-103.

[115] Freudenheim JL, Marshall JR, Vena JE, Laughlin R, Brasure JR, Swanson MK, *et al.* Premenopausal breast cancer risk and intake of vegetables, fruits, and related nutrients. *J. Natl. Cancer Inst.,* 1996 Mar 20;88(6):340-8.

[116] London SJ, Stein EA, Henderson IC, Stampfer MJ, Wood WC, Remine S, *et al.* Carotenoids, retinol, and vitamin E and risk of proliferative benign breast disease and breast cancer. *Cancer Causes Control,* 1992 Nov;3(6):503-12.

[117] Potischman N, Herrero R, Brinton LA, Reeves WC, Stacewicz-Sapuntzakis M, Jones CJ, *et al.* A case-control study of nutrient status and invasive cervical cancer. II. Serologic indicators. *Am. J. Epidemiol.,* 1991 Dec 1;134(11):1347-55.

[118] Peng YM, Peng YS, Childers JM, Hatch KD, Roe DJ, Lin Y, *et al.* Concentrations of carotenoids, tocopherols, and retinol in paired plasma and cervical tissue of patients with cervical cancer, precancer, and noncancerous diseases. *Cancer Epidemiol. Biomarkers Prev.,* 1998 Apr;7(4):347-50.

[119] Ferraroni M, La Vecchia C, D'Avanzo B, Negri E, Franceschi S, Decarli A. Selected micronutrient intake and the risk of colorectal cancer. *Br. J. Cancer,* 1994 Dec;70(6): 1150-5.

[120] La Vecchia C, Braga C, Negri E, Franceschi S, Russo A, Conti E, *et al.* Intake of selected micronutrients and risk of colorectal cancer. *Int. J. Cancer,* 1997 Nov 14;73 (4): 525-30.

[121] Slattery ML, Edwards SL, Anderson K, Caan B. Vitamin E and colon cancer: is there an association? *Nutr. Cancer,* 1998;30(3):201-6.

[122] Ghadirian P, Lacroix A, Maisonneuve P, Perret C, Potvin C, Gravel D, *et al.* Nutritional factors and colon carcinoma: a case-control study involving French Canadians in Montreal, Quebec, Canada. *Cancer,* 1997 Sep 1;80(5):858-64.

[123] White E, Shannon JS, Patterson RE. Relationship between vitamin and calcium supplement use and colon cancer. *Cancer Epidemiol. Biomarkers Prev.,* 1997 Oct;6 (10): 769-74.

[124] Freudenheim JL, Graham S, Marshall JR, Haughey BP, Wilkinson G. A case-control study of diet and rectal cancer in western New York. *Am. J. Epidemiol.,* 1990 Apr;131 (4): 612-24.

[125] Charpiot P, Calaf R, Di Costanzo J, Romette J, Rotily M, Durbec JP, *et al.* Vitamin A, vitamin E, retinol binding protein (RBP), and prealbumin in digestive cancers. *Int. J. Vitam Nutr. Res.*, 1989;59(4):323-8.

[126] Negri E, La Vecchia C, Franceschi S, Levi F, Parazzini F. Intake of selected micronutrients and the risk of endometrial carcinoma. *Cancer,* 1996 Mar 1;77(5):917-23.

[127] Goodman MT, Wilkens LR, Hankin JH, Lyu LC, Wu AH, Kolonel LN. Association of soy and fiber consumption with the risk of endometrial cancer. *Am. J. Epidemiol.,* 1997 Aug 15;146(4):294-306.

[128] Barone J, Taioli E, Hebert JR, Wynder EL. Vitamin supplement use and risk for oral and esophageal cancer. *Nutr. Cancer,* 1992;18(1):31-41.

[129] Terry P, Lagergren J, Ye W, Nyren O, Wolk A. Antioxidants and cancers of the esophagus and gastric cardia. *Int. J. Cancer,* 2000 Sep 1;87(5):750-4.

[130] Zhang ZF, Kurtz RC, Yu GP, Sun M, Gargon N, Karpeh M, Jr., *et al.* Adenocarcinomas of the esophagus and gastric cardia: the role of diet. *Nutr. Cancer*, 1997;27(3):298-309.

[131] Ekstrom AM, Serafini M, Nyren O, Hansson LE, Ye W, Wolk A. Dietary antioxidant intake and the risk of cardia cancer and noncardia cancer of the intestinal and diffuse types: a population-based case-control study in Sweden. *Int. J. Cancer,* 2000 Jul 1;87 (1): 133-40.

[132] Kumagai Y, Pi JB, Lee S, Sun GF, Yamanushi T, Sagai M, *et al.* Serum antioxidant vitamins and risk of lung and stomach cancers in Shenyang, China. *Cancer Lett.,* 1998 Jul 17;129(2):145-9.

[133] Battisti C, Formichi P, Tripodi SA, Vindigni C, Roviello F, Federico A. Vitamin E serum levels and gastric cancer: results from a cohort of patients in Tuscany, Italy. *Cancer Lett.,* 2000 Apr 3;151(1):15-8.

[134] Lopez-Carrillo L, Lopez-Cervantes M, Ward MH, Bravo-Alvarado J, Ramirez-Espitia A. Nutrient intake and gastric cancer in Mexico. *Int. J. Cancer,* 1999 Nov 26;83(5):601-5.

[135] Freudenheim JL, Graham S, Byers TE, Marshall JR, Haughey BP, Swanson MK, *et al.* Diet, smoking, and alcohol in cancer of the larynx: a case-control study. *Nutr. Cancer,* 1992;17(1):33-45.

[136] LeGardeur BY, Lopez A, Johnson WD. A case-control study of serum vitamins A, E, and C in lung cancer patients. *Nutr. Cancer,* 1990;14(2):133-40.

[137] Stefani ED, Boffetta P, Deneo-Pellegrini H, Mendilaharsu M, Carzoglio JC, Ronco A, *et al.* Dietary antioxidants and lung cancer risk: a case-control study in Uruguay. *Nutr. Cancer,* 1999;34(1):100-10.

[138] Mayne ST, Janerich DT, Greenwald P, Chorost S, Tucci C, Zaman MB, *et al.* Dietary beta carotene and lung cancer risk in U.S. nonsmokers. *J. Natl. Cancer Inst.,* 1994 Jan 5;86(1):33-8.

[139] Stryker WS, Stampfer MJ, Stein EA, Kaplan L, Louis TA, Sober A, *et al.* Diet, plasma levels of beta-carotene and alpha-tocopherol, and risk of malignant melanoma. *Am. J. Epidemiol.,* 1990 Apr;131(4):597-611.

[140] Negri E, Franceschi S, Bosetti C, Levi F, Conti E, Parpinel M, *et al.* Selected micronutrients and oral and pharyngeal cancer. *Int. J. Cancer,* 2000 Apr 1;86(1):122-7.

[141] Gridley G, McLaughlin JK, Block G, Blot WJ, Winn DM, Greenberg RS, *et al.* Diet and oral and pharyngeal cancer among blacks. *Nutr. Cancer,* 1990;14(3-4):219-25.

[142] Deneo-Pellegrini H, De Stefani E, Ronco A, Mendilaharsu M. Foods, nutrients and prostate cancer: a case-control study in Uruguay. *Br. J. Cancer,* 1999 May;80(3-4):591-7.

[143] Kristal AR, Stanford JL, Cohen JH, Wicklund K, Patterson RE. Vitamin and mineral supplement use is associated with reduced risk of prostate cancer. *Cancer Epidemiol. Biomarkers Prev.,* 1999 Oct;8(10):887-92.

[144] Wolk A, Gridley G, Niwa S, Lindblad P, McCredie M, Mellemgaard A, *et al.* International renal cell cancer study. VII. Role of diet. *Int. J. Cancer,* 1996 Jan 3;65(1): 67-73.

[145] Horn-Ross PL, Morrow M, Ljung BM. Diet and the risk of salivary gland cancer. *Am. J. Epidemiol., 1997* Jul 15;146(2):171-6.

[146] D'Avanzo B, Ron E, La Vecchia C, Francaschi S, Negri E, Zleglar R. Selected micronutrient intake and thyroid carcinoma risk. *Cancer,* 1997 Jun 1;79(11):2186-92.

[147] Zheng W, Blot WJ, Diamond EL, Norkus EP, Spate V, Morris JS, *et al.* Serum micronutrients and the subsequent risk of oral and pharyngeal cancer. *Cancer Res.,* 1993 Feb 15;53(4):795-8.

[148] Knekt P, Aromaa A, Maatela J, Alfthan G, Aaran RK, Nikkari T, *et al.* Serum micronutrients and risk of cancers of low incidence in Finland. *Am. J. Epidemiol.,* 1991 Aug 15;134(4):356-61.

[149] Helzlsouer KJ, Alberg AJ, Norkus EP, Morris JS, Hoffman SC, Comstock GW. Prospective study of serum micronutrients and ovarian cancer. *J. Natl. Cancer Inst.,* 1996 Jan 3;88(1):32-7.

[150] Helzlsouer KJ, Comstock GW, Morris JS. Selenium, lycopene, alpha-tocopherol, beta-carotene, retinol, and subsequent bladder cancer. *Cancer Res.,* 1989 Nov 1;49(21): 6144-8.

[151] Knekt P, Marniemi J, Teppo L, Heliovaara M, Aromaa A. Is low selenium status a risk factor for lung cancer? *Am. J. Epidemiol.,* 1998 Nov 15;148(10):975-82.

[152] Comstock GW, Alberg AJ, Huang HY, Wu K, Burke AE, Hoffman SC, *et al.* The risk of developing lung cancer associated with antioxidants in the blood: ascorbic acid, carotenoids, alpha-tocopherol, selenium, and total peroxyl radical absorbing capacity. *Cancer Epidemiol. Biomarkers Prev.,* 1997 Nov;6(11):907-16.

[153] Huang HY, Alberg AJ, Norkus EP, Hoffman SC, Comstock GW, Helzlsouer KJ. Prospective study of antioxidant micronutrients in the blood and the risk of developing prostate cancer. *Am. J. Epidemiol.,* 2003 Feb 15;157(4):335-44.

[154] Nomura AM, Stemmermann GN, Heilbrun LK, Salkeld RM, Vuilleumier JP. Serum vitamin levels and the risk of cancer of specific sites in men of Japanese ancestry in Hawaii. *Cancer Res.,* 1985 May;45(5):2369-72.

[155] Gann PH, Ma J, Giovannucci E, Willett W, Sacks FM, Hennekens CH, *et al.* Lower prostate cancer risk in men with elevated plasma lycopene levels: results of a prospective analysis. *Cancer Res.,* 1999 Mar 15;59(6):1225-30.

[156] Hartman TJ, Albanes D, Pietinen P, Hartman AM, Rautalahti M, Tangrea JA, *et al.* The association between baseline vitamin E, selenium, and prostate cancer in the alpha-tocopherol, beta-carotene cancer prevention study. *Cancer Epidemiol. Biomarkers Prev.,* 1998 Apr;7(4):335-40.

[157] Lu QY, Hung JC, Heber D, Go VL, Reuter VE, Cordon-Cardo C, *et al.* Inverse Associations between Plasma Lycopene and Other Carotenoids and Prostate Cancer. *Cancer Epidemiology Biomarkers & Prevention,* 2001 Jul 1;10(7):749-56.

[158] Ramon JM, Bou R, Romea S, Alkiza ME, Jacas M, Ribes J, *et al.* Dietary fat intake and prostate cancer risk: a case-control study in Spain. *Cancer Causes Control,* 2000 Sep; 11 (8):679-85.

[159] Wald NJ, Boreham J, Hayward JL, Bulbrook RD. Plasma retinol, beta-carotene and vitamin E levels in relation to the future risk of breast cancer. *Br. J. Cancer,* 1984 Mar;49(3):321-4.

[160] Batieha AM, Armenian HK, Norkus EP, Morris JS, Spate VE, Comstock GW. Serum micronutrients and the subsequent risk of cervical cancer in a population-based nested case-control study. *Cancer Epidemiol. Biomarkers Prev.,* 1993 Jul;2(4):335-9.

[161] Lehtinen M, Luostarinen T, Youngman LD, Anttila T, Dillner J, Hakulinen T, *et al.* Low levels of serum vitamins A and E in blood and subsequent risk for cervical cancer: interaction with HPV seropositivity. *Nutr. Cancer*, 1999;34(2):229-34.

[162] Longnecker MP, Martin-Moreno JM, Knekt P, Nomura AM, Schober SE, Stahelin HB, *et al.* Serum alpha-tocopherol concentration in relation to subsequent colorectal cancer: pooled data from five cohorts. *J. Natl. Cancer Inst.,* 1992 Mar 18;84(6):430-5.

[163] Menkes MS, Comstock GW, Vuilleumier JP, Helsing KJ, Rider AA, Brookmeyer R. Serum beta-carotene, vitamins A and E, selenium, and the risk of lung cancer. *N. Engl. J. Med.,* 1986 Nov 13;315(20):1250-4.

[164] Breslow RA, Alberg AJ, Helzlsouer KJ, Bush TL, Norkus EP, Morris JS, *et al.* Serological precursors of cancer: malignant melanoma, basal and squamous cell skin cancer, and prediagnostic levels of retinol, beta- carotene, lycopene, alpha-tocopherol, and selenium. *Cancer Epidemiol. Biomarkers Prev.,* 1995 Dec;4(8):837-42.

[165] Dorgan JF, Sowell A, Swanson CA, Potischman N, Miller R, Schussler N, *et al.* Relationships of serum carotenoids, retinol, alpha-tocopherol, and selenium with breast cancer risk: results from a prospective study in Columbia, Missouri (United States). *Cancer Causes Control*, 1998 Jan;9(1):89-97.

[166] Ratnasinghe D, Tangrea JA, Forman MR, Hartman T, Gunter EW, Qiao YL, *et al.* Serum tocopherols, selenium and lung cancer risk among tin miners in China. *Cancer Causes Control,* 2000 Feb;11(2):129-35.

[167] Burney PG, Comstock GW, Morris JS. Serologic precursors of cancer: serum micronutrients and the subsequent risk of pancreatic cancer. *Am. J. Clin. Nutr.,* 1989 May;49(5):895-900.

[168] Nomura AM, Stemmermann GN, Lee J, Craft NE. Serum micronutrients and prostate cancer in Japanese Americans in Hawaii. *Cancer Epidemiol. Biomarkers Prev.,* 1997 Jul;6(7):487-91.

[169] Hsing AW, Comstock GW, Abbey H, Polk BF. Serologic precursors of cancer. Retinol, carotenoids, and tocopherol and risk of prostate cancer. *J. Natl. Cancer Inst.,* 1990 Jun 6;82(11):941-6.

[170] Woodson K, Tangrea JA, Barrett MJ, Virtamo J, Taylor PR, Albanes D. Serum alpha-tocopherol and subsequent risk of lung cancer among male smokers. *J. Natl. Cancer Inst.,* 1999 Oct 20;91(20):1738-43.

[171] Helzlsouer KJ, Huang HY, Alberg AJ, Hoffman S, Burke A, Norkus EP, *et al.* Association between alpha-tocopherol, gamma-tocopherol, selenium, and subsequent prostate cancer. *J. Natl. Cancer Inst.,* 2000 Dec 20;92(24):2018-23.

[172] Baker H, Handelman GJ, Short S, Machlin LJ, Bhagavan HN, Dratz EA, *et al.* Comparison of plasma alpha and gamma tocopherol levels following chronic oral administration of either all-rac-alpha-tocopheryl acetate or RRR-alpha-tocopheryl acetate in normal adult male subjects. *Am. J. Clin. Nutr.,* 1986 Mar;43(3):382-7.

[173] Clement M, Bourre JM. Graded dietary levels of RRR-g-tocopherol induce a marked increase in concentrations of a-and g-tocopherol in nervous tissues, heart and muscle of vitamin E deficient rats. *Biochimica et Biophysica Acta,* 2003;1334:173-81.

[174] Gaziano JM, Glynn RJ, Christen WG, Kurth T, Belanger C, MacFadyen J, *et al.* Vitamins E and C in the prevention of prostate and total cancer in men: the Physicians' Health Study II randomized controlled trial. *JAMA,* 2009 Jan 7;301(1):52-62.

[175] Lippman SM, Klein EA, Goodman PJ, Lucia MS, Thompson IM, Ford LG, *et al.* Effect of Selenium and Vitamin E on Risk of Prostate Cancer and Other Cancers: The Selenium and Vitamin E Cancer Prevention Trial (SELECT). *JAMA: The Journal of the American Medical Association,* 2009 Jan 7;301(1):39-51.

[176] Klein EA, Thompson IM, Jr., Tangen CM, Crowley JJ, Lucia MS, Goodman PJ, *et al.* Vitamin E and the risk of prostate cancer: the Selenium and Vitamin E Cancer Prevention Trial (SELECT). *JAMA,* 2011 Oct 12;306(14):1549-56.

[177] Blot WJ, Li JY, Taylor PR, Guo W, Dawsey S, Wang GQ, *et al.* Nutrition intervention trials in Linxian, China: supplementation with specific vitamin/mineral combinations, cancer incidence, and disease-specific mortality in the general population. *J. Natl. Cancer Inst., 1993* Sep 15;85(18):1483-92.

[178] Nomura AM, Ziegler RG, Stemmermann GN, Chyou PH, Craft NE. Serum micronutrients and upper aerodigestive tract cancer. *Cancer Epidemiol. Biomarkers Prev.,* 1997 Jun;6(6):407-12.

[179] Burton GW, Joyce A, Ingold KU. First proof that vitamin E is major lipid-soluble, chain-breaking antioxidant in human blood plasma. Lancet 1982 Aug 7;2(8293):327.

[180] Burton GW, Cheeseman KH, Doba T, Ingold KU, Slater TF. Vitamin E as an antioxidant in vitro and in vivo. *Ciba Found Symp.,* 1983;101:4-18.
[181] Burton GW, Joyce A, Ingold KU. Is vitamin E the only lipid-soluble, chain-breaking antioxidant in human blood plasma and erythrocyte membranes? *Arch. Biochem. Biophys., 1983* Feb 15;221(1):281-90.
[182] Burton GW, Foster DO, Perly B, Slater TF, Smith IC, Ingold KU. Biological antioxidants. *Philos. Trans R Soc. Lond B Biol. Sci.,* 1985 Dec 17;311(1152):565-78.
[183] Burton GW, Cheng SC, Webb A, Ingold KU. Vitamin E in young and old human red blood cells. *Biochim. Biophys. Acta.,* 1986 Aug 7;860(1):84-90.
[184] Packer L. Protective role of vitamin E in biological systems. *Am. J. Clin. Nutr.,* 1991 Apr;53(4 Suppl):1050S-5S.
[185] Burton GW. Vitamin E: molecular and biological function. *Proc. Nutr. Soc.,* 1994 Jul; 53 (2): 251-62.
[186] Buettner GR. The pecking order of free radicals and antioxidants: lipid peroxidation, alpha-tocopherol, and ascorbate. *Arch. Biochem. Biophys.,* 1993 Feb 1;300(2):535-43.
[187] Sohal RS, Orr WC. The redox stress hypothesis of aging. *Free Radic. Biol. Med.,* 2012 Feb 1;52(3):539-55.
[188] Sohal RS, Weindruch R. Oxidative stress, caloric restriction, and aging. *Science,* 1996 Jul 5;273(5271):59-63.
[189] Traber MG. Vitamin E regulatory mechanisms. *Annu. Rev. Nutr.,* 2007;27:347-62.
[190] Cui Y, Kim DS, Park SH, Yoon JA, Kim SK, Kwon SB, *et al.* Involvement of ERK AND p38 MAP kinase in AAPH-induced COX-2 expression in HaCaT cells. *Chem. Phys. Lipids, 2004* Apr;129(1):43-52.
[191] Morrow JD, Awad JA, Kato T, Takahashi K, Badr KF, Roberts LJ, *et al.* Formation of novel non-cyclooxygenase-derived prostanoids (F2-isoprostanes) in carbon tetrachloride hepatotoxicity. An animal model of lipid peroxidation. *J. Clin. Invest.,* 1992 Dec;90(6):2502-7.
[192] Morrow JD, Moore KP, Awad JA, Ravenscraft MD, Marini G, Badr KF, *et al.* Marked overproduction of non-cyclooxygenase derived prostanoids (F2-isoprostanes) in the hepatorenal syndrome. *J. Lipid Mediat.,* 1993 Mar;6(1-3):417-20.
[193] Morrow JD, Minton TA, Badr KF, Roberts LJ. Evidence that the F2-isoprostane, 8-epi-prostaglandin F2 alpha, is formed in vivo. *Biochim. Biophys. Acta.,* 1994 Jan 3;1210(2): 244-8.
[194] Morrow JD, Minton TA, Mukundan CR, Campbell MD, Zackert WE, Daniel VC, *et al.* Free radical-induced generation of isoprostanes in vivo. Evidence for the formation of D-ring and E-ring isoprostanes. *J. Biol. Chem.,* 1994 Feb 11;269(6):4317-26.
[195] Lynch SM, Morrow JD, Roberts LJ, Frei B. Formation of non-cyclooxygenase-derived prostanoids (F2-isoprostanes) in plasma and low density lipoprotein exposed to oxidative stress in vitro. *J. Clin. Invest.,* 1994 Mar;93(3):998-1004.
[196] Ju J, Hao X, Lee MJ, Lambert JD, Lu G, Xiao H, *et al.* A gamma-tocopherol-rich mixture of tocopherols inhibits colon inflammation and carcinogenesis in azoxymethane and dextran sulfate sodium-treated mice. *Cancer Prev. Res.,* (Phila) 2009 Feb;2(2):143-52.
[197] McLellan EA, Bird RP. Aberrant crypts: potential preneoplastic lesions in the murine colon. *Cancer Res.,* 1988 Nov 1;48(21):6187-92.

[198] Reddy BS. Colon carcinogenesis models for chemoprevention studies. *Hematol. Oncol, Clin. North Am.,* 1998;12(5):963-73.

[199] Reddy BS. Studies with the azoxymethane-rat preclinical model for assessing colon tumor development and chemoprevention. *Environ. Mol. Mutagen.,* 2004;44(1):26-35.

[200] Reddy BS, Wang CX, Kong AN, Khor TO, Zheng X, Steele VE, *et al.* Prevention of azoxymethane-induced colon cancer by combination of low doses of atorvastatin, aspirin, and celecoxib in F 344 rats. *Cancer Res.,* 2006 Apr 15;66(8):4542-6.

[201] Reddy BS, Hirose Y, Lubet R, Steele V, Kelloff G, Paulson S, *et al.* Chemoprevention of Colon Cancer by Specific Cyclooxygenase-2 Inhibitor, Celecoxib, Administered during Different Stages of Carcinogenesis. Cancer Research, 2000 Jan 1;60(2):293-7.

[202] Reddy BS. Novel Approaches to the Prevention of Colon Cancer by Nutritional Manipulation and Chemoprevention. *Cancer Epidemiol. Biomarkers Prev.,* 2000 Mar 1;9(3):239-47.

[203] Yao K, Latta M, Bird RP. Modulation of colonic aberrant crypt foci and proliferative indexes in colon and prostate glands of rats by vitamin E. *Nutr. Cancer,* 1996;26:99-109.

[204] Reddy BS, Tanaka T. Interactions of selenium deficiency, vitamin E, polyunsaturated fat, and saturated fat on azoxymethane-induced colon carcinogenesis in male F344 rats. *J. Natl. Cancer Inst.,* 1986 Jun;76(6):1157-62.

[205] Chung H, Wu D, Han SN, Gay R, Goldin B, Bronson RE, *et al.* Vitamin E Supplementation Does Not Alter Azoxymethane-Induced Colonic Aberrant Crypt Foci Formation in Young or Old Mice. *J. Nutr.,* 2003 Feb 1;133(2):528-32.

[206] Shivapurkar N, Tang Z, Frost A, Alabaster O. Inhibition of progression of aberrant crypt foci and colon tumor development by vitamin E and beta-carotene in rats on a high-risk diet. *Cancer Lett.,* 1995;91:125-32.

[207] Newmark HL, Huang MT, Reddy BS. Mixed tocopherols inhibit azoxymethane-induced aberrant crypt foci in rats. *Nutr. Cancer,* 2006;56(1):82-5.

[208] Exon JH, South EH, Taruscio TG, Clifton GD, Fariss MW. Chemopreventive effect of dietary d-alpha-tocopheryl succinate supplementation on precancer colon aberrant crypt formation and vitamin E analogue levels in young and old rats. *Nutr. Cancer,* 2004;49 (1):72-80.

[209] Boateng J, Verghese M, Chawan CB, Shackelford L, Walker LT, Khatiwada J, *et al.* Red palm oil suppresses the formation of azoxymethane (AOM) induced aberrant crypt foci (ACF) in Fisher 344 male rats. *Food Chem. Toxicol.,* 2006 Oct;44(10):1667-73.

[210] Campbell SE, Musich PR, Whaley SG, Stimmel JB, Leesnitzer LM, Dessus-Babus S, *et al.* Gamma Tocopherol Upregulates the Expression of 15-S-HETE and Induces Growth Arrest Through a PPAR Gamma-Dependent Mechanism in PC-3 Human Prostate Cancer Cells. *Nutrition and Cancer,* 2009;61(5):649-62.

[211] Prasad KN, Kumar B, Yan XD, Hanson AJ, Cole WC. Alpha-tocopheryl succinate, the most effective form of vitamin E for adjuvant cancer treatment: a review. *J. Am. Coll. Nutr., 2003* Apr;22(2):108-17.

[212] Guan F, Li G, Liu AB, Lee MJ, Yang Z, Chen YK, *et al.* delta- and gamma-tocopherols, but not alpha-tocopherol, inhibit colon carcinogenesis in azoxymethane-treated F344 rats. *Cancer Prev. Res.,* (Phila) 2012 Apr;5(4):644-54.

[213] Moyad MA, Brumfield SK, Pienta KJ. Vitamin E, alpha- and gamma-tocopherol, and prostate cancer. *Semin. Urol. Oncol.,* 1999;17:85-90.

[214] Christen S, Woodall AA, Shigenaga MK, Southwell-Keely PT, Duncan MW, Ames BN. gamma-tocopherol traps mutagenic electrophiles such as NO(X) and complements alpha-tocopherol: physiological implications. *Proc. Natl. Acad. Sci. USA,* 1997;94: 3217-22.

[215] Jiang Q, Lykkesfeldt J, Shigenaga MK, Shigeno ET, Christen S, Ames BN. gamma-tocopherol supplementation inhibits protein nitration and ascorbate oxidation in rats with inflammation. *Free Radic. Biol. Med.,* 2002 Dec 1;33(11):1534-42.

[216] Ogawa Y, Saito Y, Nishio K, Yoshida Y, Ashida H, Niki E. Gamma-tocopheryl quinone, not alpha-tocopheryl quinone, induces adaptive response through up-regulation of cellular glutathione and cysteine availability via activation of ATF4. *Free Radic. Res.*, 2008 Jul;42(7):674-87.

[217] Hsieh TC, Elangovan S, Wu JM. Differential suppression of proliferation in MCF-7 and MDA-MB-231 breast cancer cells exposed to alpha-, gamma- and delta-tocotrienols is accompanied by altered expression of oxidative stress modulatory enzymes. *Anticancer Res.,* 2010 Oct;30(10):4169-76.

[218] Lee EJ, Oh SY, Kim MK, Ahn SH, Son BH, Sung MK. Modulatory effects of alpha- and gamma-tocopherols on 4-hydroxyestradiol induced oxidative stresses in MCF-10A breast epithelial cells. *Nutr. Res. Pract.,* 2009;3(3):185-91.

[219] Prasad KN, Cole WC, Kumar B, Prasad KC. Scientific rationale for using high-dose multiple micronutrients as an adjunct to standard and experimental cancer therapies. *J. Am. Coll Nutr., 2001* Oct;20(5 Suppl):450S-63S.

[220] Prasad KN, Cole WC, Kumar B, Che PK. Pros and cons of antioxidant use during radiation therapy. *Cancer Treat Rev.,* 2002 Apr;28(2):79-91.

[221] Ladas E, Kelly KM. The antioxidant debate. Explore (NY) 2010 Mar;6(2):75-85.

[222] Galland L. Antioxidants and chemotherapy. *Altern. Ther. Health Med.,* 2007 Sep;13(5): 13.

[223] Simone CB, Simone NL, Simone V, Simone CB. Antioxidants and other nutrients do not interfere with chemotherapy or radiation therapy and can increase kill and increase survival, Part 2. *Altern. Ther. Health Med.,* 2007 Mar;13(2):40-7.

[224] Simone CB, Simone NL, Simone V, Simone CB. Antioxidants and other nutrients do not interfere with chemotherapy or radiation therapy and can increase kill and increase survival, part 1. *Altern. Ther. Health Med.,* 2007 Jan;13(1):22-8.

[225] Moss RW. Should patients undergoing chemotherapy and radiotherapy be prescribed antioxidants? *Integr. Cancer Ther.,* 2006 Mar;5(1):63-82.

[226] Block KI. Antioxidants and cancer therapy: furthering the debate. *Integr. Cancer Ther.,* 2004 Dec;3(4):342-8.

[227] Borek C. Dietary antioxidants and human cancer. *Integr. Cancer Ther.,* 2004 Dec;3(4): 333-41.

[228] Ladas EJ, Jacobson JS, Kennedy DD, Teel K, Fleischauer A, Kelly KM. Antioxidants and cancer therapy: a systematic review. *J. Clin. Oncol.,* 2004 Feb 1;22(3):517-28.

[229] Alleva R, Benassi MS, Pazzaglia L, Tomasetti M, Gellert N, Borghi B, *et al.* Alpha-tocopheryl succinate alters cell cycle distribution sensitising human osteosarcoma cells to methotrexate-induced apoptosis. *Cancer Lett.,* 2006 Feb 8;232(2):226-35.

[230] Nishikawa K, Satoh H, Hirai A, Suzuzki K, Asano R, Kumadaki I, *et al.* alpha-Tocopheryloxybutyric acid enhances necrotic cell death in breast cancer cells treated with chemotherapy agent. *Cancer Lett.,* 2003 Nov 10;201(1):51-6.

[231] Zhang X, Chen ZG, Khuri FR, Shin DM. Induction of cell cycle arrest and apoptosis by a combined treatment with 13-cis-retinoic acid, interferon-alpha2a, and alpha-tocopherol in squamous cell carcinoma of the head and neck. *Head Neck,* 2007 Apr;29(4):351-61.

[232] Ripoll EA, Rama BN, Webber MM. Vitamin E enhances the chemotherapeutic effects of adriamycin on human prostatic carcinoma cells in vitro. *J. Urol.,* 1986 Aug;136(2): 529-31.

[233] Hahn T, Bradley-Dunlop DJ, Hurley LH, Von-Hoff D, Gately S, Mary DL, *et al.* The vitamin E analog, alpha-tocopheryloxyacetic acid enhances the anti-tumor activity of trastuzumab against HER2/neu-expressing breast cancer. *BMC Cancer,* 2011;11:471.

[234] Anderson K, Lawson KA, Simmons-Menchaca M, Sun L, Sanders BG, Kline K. Alpha-TEA plus cisplatin reduces human cisplatin-resistant ovarian cancer cell tumor burden and metastasis. *Exp. Biol. Med.,* (Maywood) 2004 Dec;229(11):1169-76.

[235] Di Cesare ML, Zanardelli M, Failli P, Ghelardini C. Oxaliplatin-induced neuropathy: oxidative stress as pathological mechanism. Protective effect of silibinin. *J. Pain,* 2012 Mar;13(3):276-84.

[236] Pace A, Giannarelli D, Galie E, Savarese A, Carpano S, Della GM, *et al.* Vitamin E neuroprotection for cisplatin neuropathy: a randomized, placebo-controlled trial. *Neurology,* 2010 Mar 2;74(9):762-6.

[237] Leonetti C, Biroccio A, Gabellini C, Scarsella M, Maresca V, Flori E, *et al.* Alpha-tocopherol protects against cisplatin-induced toxicity without interfering with antitumor efficacy. *Int. J. Cancer,* 2003 Mar 20;104(2):243-50.

[238] Cruz Silva MM, Madeira VM, Almeida LM, Custodio JB. Hemolysis of human erythrocytes induced by tamoxifen is related to disruption of membrane structure. *Biochim. Biophys. Acta.,* 2000 Mar 15;1464(1):49-61.

[239] Brandt S, Heller H, Schuster KD, Grote J. Tamoxifen induces suppression of cell viability and apoptosis in the human hepatoblastoma cell line HepG2 via down-regulation of telomerase activity. *Liver Int.,* 2004 Feb;24(1):46-54.

[240] Brandt S, Heller H, Schuster KD, Grote J. The tamoxifen-induced suppression of telomerase activity in the human hepatoblastoma cell line HepG2: a result of post-translational regulation. *J. Cancer Res. Clin. Oncol.,* 2005 Feb;131(2):120-8.

[241] Jones KH, Liu JJ, Roehm JS, Eckel JJ, Eckel TT, Stickrath CR, *et al.* Gamma-tocopheryl quinone stimulates apoptosis in drug-sensitive and multidrug-resistant cancer cells. *Lipids,* 2002 Feb;37(2):173-84.

[242] Zhang X, Peng X, Yu W, Hou S, Zhao Y, Zhang Z, *et al.* Alpha-tocopheryl succinate enhances doxorubicin-induced apoptosis in human gastric cancer cells via promotion of doxorubicin influx and suppression of doxorubicin efflux. *Cancer Lett.,* 2011 Aug 28;307(2):174-81.

[243] Kumar KS, Srinivasan V, Toles R, Jobe L, Seed TM. Nutritional approaches to radioprotection: vitamin E. *Mil. Med.,* 2002 Feb;167(2 Suppl):57-9.

[244] Kumar KS, Raghavan M, Hieber K, Ege C, Mog S, Parra N, *et al.* Preferential radiation sensitization of prostate cancer in nude mice by nutraceutical antioxidant gamma-tocotrienol. *Life Sci.,* 2006 Mar 27;78(18):2099-104.

[245] Singh VK, Shafran RL, Jackson WE, III, Seed TM, Kumar KS. Induction of cytokines by radioprotective tocopherol analogs. *Exp. Mol. Pathol.,* 2006 Aug;81(1):55-61.

[246] Ghosh SP, Kulkarni S, Hieber K, Toles R, Romanyukha L, Kao TC, *et al.* Gamma-tocotrienol, a tocol antioxidant as a potent radioprotector. *Int. J. Radiat. Biol.,* 2009 Jul; 85 (7): 598-606.

[247] Kulkarni S, Ghosh SP, Satyamitra M, Mog S, Hieber K, Romanyukha L, *et al.* Gamma-tocotrienol protects hematopoietic stem and progenitor cells in mice after total-body irradiation. *Radiat. Res.,* 2010 Jun;173(6):738-47.

[248] Kulkarni SS, Cary LH, Gambles K, Hauer-Jensen M, Kumar KS, Ghosh SP. Gamma-tocotrienol, a radiation prophylaxis agent, induces high levels of granulocyte colony-stimulating factor. *Int. Immunopharmacol.,* 2012 Dec;14(4):495-503.

[249] Hagemann T, Balkwill F, Lawrence T. Inflammation and cancer: a double-edged sword. *Cancer Cell,* 2007 Oct;12(4):300-1.

[250] Kulbe H, Thompson R, Wilson JL, Robinson S, Hagemann T, Fatah R, *et al.* The inflammatory cytokine tumor necrosis factor-alpha generates an autocrine tumor-promoting network in epithelial ovarian cancer cells. *Cancer Res.,* 2007 Jan 15;67(2): 585-92.

[251] Shishodia S, Aggarwal BB. Nuclear factor-[kappa]B: a friend or a foe in cancer? *Biochemical Pharmacology,* 2004 Sep 15;68(6):1071-80.

[252] Christen S, Jiang Q, Shigenaga MK, Ames BN. Analysis of plasma tocopherols alpha-, gamma-, and 5-nitro-gamma in rats with inflammation by HPLC coulometric detection. *J. Lipid Res.,* 2002 Nov 1;43(11):1978-85.

[253] Shah SJ, Sylvester PW. Gamma-tocotrienol inhibits neoplastic mammary epithelial cell proliferation by decreasing Akt and nuclear factor kappaB activity. *Exp. Biol. Med.,* (Maywood) 2005 Apr;230(4):235-41.

[254] Ahn KS, Sethi G, Krishnan K, Aggarwal BB. gamma-Tocotrienol Inhibits Nuclear Factor-kappa B Signaling Pathway through Inhibition of Receptor-interacting Protein and TAK1 Leading to Suppression of Antiapoptotic Gene Products and Potentiation of Apoptosis. *Journal of Biological Chemistry,* 2007 Jan 5;282(1):809-20.

[255] Campbell SE, Rudder B, Phillips RB, Whaley SG, Stimmel JB, Leesnitzer LM, *et al.* gamma-Tocotrienol induces growth arrest through a novel pathway with TGFbeta2 in prostate cancer. *Free Radic. Biol. Med.,* 2011 May 15;50(10):1344-54.

[256] Lu T, Burdelya LG, Swiatkowski SM, Boiko AD, Howe PH, Stark GR, *et al.* Secreted transforming growth factor beta-2 activates NF-kappaB, blocks apoptosis, and is essential for the survival of some tumor cells. *Proc. Natl. Acad. Sci. USA,* 2004;101: 7112-7.

[257] Egger T, Schuligoi R, Wintersperger A, Amann R, Malle E, Sattler W. Vitamin E (alpha-tocopherol) attenuates cyclo-oxygenase 2 transcription and synthesis in immortalized murine BV-2 microglia. *Biochem. J.,* 2003 Mar 1;370(Pt 2):459-67.

[258] Devaraj S, Jialal I. Alpha-tocopherol decreases interleukin-1 beta release from activated human monocytes by inhibition of 5-lipoxygenase. *Arterioscler Thromb. Vasc. Biol.,* 1999 Apr;19(4):1125-33.

[259] Beharka AA, Wu D, Serafini M, Meydani SN. Mechanism of vitamin E inhibition of cyclooxygenase activity in macrophages from old mice: role of peroxynitrite. *Free Radic. Biol. Med., 2002* Mar 15;32(6):503-11.

[260] Wu D, Meydani M, Beharka AA, Serafini M, Martin KR, Meydani SN. In vitro supplementation with different tocopherol homologues can affect the function of immune cells in old mice. *Free Radic. Biol. Med.,* 2000 Feb 15;28(4):643-51.

[261] Wu D, Hayek MG, Meydani S. Vitamin E and macrophage cyclooxygenase regulation in the aged. *J. Nutr.,* 2001 Feb;131(2):382S-8S.

[262] Zhang M, Altuwaijri S, Yeh S. RRR-alpha-tocopheryl succinate inhibits human prostate cancer cell invasiveness. *Oncogene,* 2004 Apr 15;23(17):3080-8.

[263] Breyer I, Azzi A. Differential inhibition by alpha- and beta-tocopherol of human erythroleukemia cell adhesion: role of integrins. *Free Radic. Biol. Med.,* 2001 Jun 15;30 (12): 1381-9.

[264] Li L, Mamputu JC, Wiernsperger N, Renier G. Signaling pathways involved in human vascular smooth muscle cell proliferation and matrix metalloproteinase-2 expression induced by leptin: inhibitory effect of metformin. *Diabetes,* 2005 Jul;54(7):2227-34.

[265] Miyazawa T, Tsuzuki T, Nakagawa K, Igarashi M. Antiangiogenic potency of vitamin E. *Ann. NY Acad. Sci.,* 2004 Dec;1031:401-4.

[266] Nakagawa K, Eitsuka T, Inokuchi H, Miyazawa T. DNA chip analysis of comprehensive food function: inhibition of angiogenesis and telomerase activity with unsaturated vitamin E, tocotrienol. *Biofactors,* 2004;21(1-4):5-10.

[267] Villacorta L, Graca-Souza AV, Ricciarelli R, Zingg JM, Azzi A. Alpha-tocopherol induces expression of connective tissue growth factor and antagonizes tumor necrosis factor-alpha-mediated downregulation in human smooth muscle cells. *Circ. Res.,* 2003 Jan 10;92(1):104-10.

[268] Span M, Moerkerk PTM, De Goeli AFPM, Arends JW. A detailed analysis of K-ras point mutations in relation to tumor progression and survival in colorectal cancer patients. *Int. J. Cancer,* 1996 Jun 21;69(3):241-5.

[269] Cohrs RJ, Torelli S, Prasad KN, Edwards-Prasad J, Sharma OK. Effect of vitamin E succinate and a cAMP-stimulating agent on the expression of c-myc and N-myc and H-ras in murine neuroblastoma cells. *Int. J. Dev. Neurosci.,* 1991;9(2):187-94.

[270] Prasad KN, Cohrs RJ, Sharma OK. Decreased expressions of c-myc and H-ras oncogenes in vitamin E succinate induced morphologically differentiated murine B-16 melanoma cells in culture. *Biochem. Cell Biol.,* 1990 Nov;68(11):1250-5.

[271] Campbell SE, Whaley SG, Phillips R, Aggarwal BB, Stimmel JB, Leesnitzer LM, *et al.* Gamma tocotrienol and prostate cancer: the regulation of two independent pathways to potentiate cell growth inhibtion and apoptosis. *Journal of Oil Palm Research,* 2008; Special Issue(October, 2008):33-43.

[272] Spears M, Cunningham CA, Taylor KJ, Mallon EA, Thomas JS, Kerr GR, *et al.* Proximity ligation assays for isoform-specific Akt activation in breast cancer identify activated Akt1 as a driver of progression. *J. Pathol.,* 2012 Aug;227(4):481-9.

[273] Wu Y, Zu K, Ni J, Yeh S, Kasi D, James NS, *et al.* Cellular and molecular effects of alpha-tocopheryloxybutyrate: lessons for the design of vitamin E analog for cancer prevention. *Anticancer. Res.,* 2004 Nov;24(6):3795-802.

[274] Kempna P, Reiter E, Arock M, Azzi A, Zingg JM. Inhibition of HMC-1 mast cell proliferation by vitamin E: involvement of the protein kinase B pathway. *J. Biol. Chem.,* 2004 Dec 3;279(49):50700-9.

[275] Sylvester PW, Nachnani A, Shah S, Briski KP. Role of GTP-binding proteins in reversing the antiproliferative effects of tocotrienols in preneoplastic mammary epithelial cells. *Asia Pac. J. Clin.Nutr.,* 2002;11 Suppl 7:S452-S459.

[276] Carey I, Williams CL, Ways DK, Noti JD. Overexpression of protein kinase C-alpha in MCF-7 breast cancer cells results in differential regulation and expression of alphavbeta3 and alphavbeta5. *Int. J. Oncol.,* 1999 Jul;15(1):127-36.

[277] Bae KM, Wang H, Jiang G, Chen MG, Lu L, Xiao L. Protein kinase C epsilon is overexpressed in primary human non-small cell lung cancers and functionally required for proliferation of non-small cell lung cancer cells in a p21/Cip1-dependent manner. *Cancer Res.,* 2007 Jul 1;67(13):6053-63.

[278] Galgano MT, Conaway M, Spencer AM, Paschal BM, Frierson HF, Jr. PRK1 distribution in normal tissues and carcinomas: overexpression and activation in ovarian serous carcinoma. *Hum. Pathol.,* 2009 Oct;40(10):1434-40.

[279] Mahoney CW, Azzi A. Vitamin E inhibits protein kinase C activity. *Biochem. Biophys. Res. Commun., 1988* Jul 29;154(2):694-7.

[280] Chan SS, Monteiro HP, Schindler F, Stern A, Junqueira VB. Alpha-tocopherol modulates tyrosine phosphorylation in human neutrophils by inhibition of protein kinase C activity and activation of tyrosine phosphatases. *Free Radic. Res.,* 2001 Dec; 35 (6):843-56.

[281] Xu X, Chen P, Wu X, Feng X, Wang Q, Zhang L. [Renal protective effects of vitamin E in diabetic rats]. *Zhonghua Nei Ke Za Zhi,* 2001 May;40(5):321-4.

[282] Meier M, King GL. Protein kinase C activation and its pharmacological inhibition in vascular disease. *Vasc. Med.,* 2000;5(3):173-85.

[283] Freedman JE, Li L, Sauter R, Keaney JF, Jr. alpha-Tocopherol and protein kinase C inhibition enhance platelet-derived nitric oxide release. *FASEB J.,* 2000 Dec;14(15): 2377-9.

[284] Bang OS, Park JH, Kang SS. Activation of PKC but not of ERK is required for vitamin E-succinate-induced apoptosis of HL-60 cells. *Biochem. Biophys. Res. Commun.,* 2001 Nov 9;288(4):789-97.

[285] Sylvester PW, McIntyre BS, Gapor A, Briski KP. Vitamin E inhibition of normal mammary epithelial cell growth is associated with a reduction in protein kinase C (alpha) activation. *Cell Prolif.,* 2001 Dec;34(6):347-57.

[286] Akazawa A, Nishikawa K, Suzuki K, Asano R, Kumadaki I, Satoh H, *et al.* Induction of apoptosis in a human breast cancer cell overexpressing ErbB-2 receptor by alpha-tocopheryloxybutyric acid. *Jpn. J. Pharmacol.,* 2002 Aug;89(4):417-21.

[287] Witt W, Kolleck I, Fechner H, Sinha P, Rustow B. Regulation by vitamin E of the scavenger receptor BI in rat liver and HepG2 cells. *J. Lipid Res.,* 2000 Dec;41 (12):2009-16.

[288] Gu X, Song X, Dong Y, Cai H, Walters E, Zhang R, *et al.* Vitamin E succinate induces ceramide-mediated apoptosis in head and neck squamous cell carcinoma in vitro and in vivo. *Clin. Cancer Res.,* 2008 Mar 15;14(6):1840-8.

In: Free Radicals
Editor: Bill Stone

ISBN: 978-1-63117-177-2

Chapter IV

Glutaredoxin in Cancer Development, Progression, Chemo-Resistance and Clinical Applications

Ying Qu[1], Xiaojiang Cui[1] and Ninghui Cheng[*2]
[1]Department of Surgery, Department of Obstetrics and Gynecology,
Women's Cancer Institute, Samuel Oschin Comprehensive Cancer Institute,
Cedars-Sinai Medical Center, Los Angeles, CA, US
[2]Department of Pediatrics and Children's Nutrition Research Center,
Baylor College of Medicine, Houston, TX, US

Abstract

The Glutaredoxin (Grx) proteins, coupled with glutathione and glutathione reductase, constitute a major antioxidant system that counteracts the effects of oxidative stress in the cell. Grx proteins regulate diverse cellular functions and play an essential role in redox homeostasis. Abnormal regulation of Grx levels and/or activity has been shown in many human cancers. Recent discoveries have revealed that Grxs are important players in modulating malignant behaviors of cancer cells including uncontrolled growth, epithelial–mesenchymal transition (EMT), migration/invasion, and chemo-resistance. This chapter summarizes the current findings of Grxs in cancer biology and treatment. It describes the role and signaling pathways of Grxs in cancer with a special focus on tumorigenesis and therapy-resistance. It concludes that Grxs may serve as therapeutic targets in cancer treatment and their role in cancer warrants further investigation.

Keywords: glutaredoxin, cancer, survival, metastasis, chemotherapy, resistance

---

[*] Corresponding author: Ninghui Cheng, Department of Pediatrics and Children's Nutrition Research Center, Baylor College of Medicine, Houston, TX 77030, Email: ncheng@bcm.tmc.edu.

Abbreviations

Grx: Glutaredoxin
EMT: epithelial–mesenchymal transition
ROS: reactive oxygen species
GSH: glutathione
RNRs: ribonucleoside diphosphate reductases
NTD: N-terminal domain
FasL: Fas ligand
MnSOD: manganese superoxide dismutase
TrxR1: thioredoxin reductase 1
Trx: thioredoxin
H_2O_2: hydrogen peroxide
GSS: glutathionylation
TGFβ: transforming growth factor-beta
ICAM-1: intercellular adhesion molecule-1
NF-κB: nuclear factor of kappa light polypeptide gene enhancer in B-cells
IKK: inhibitor of nuclear factor kappa-B kinase
CDDP: cis-diamminedichloroplatinum
LDH: lactate dehydrogenase

1. The Glutaredoxin System

Glutaredoxins (Grxs) are ubiquitous small heat-stable oxidoreductases that are conserved in both prokaryotes and eukaryotes [1-2]. Grxs, as part of the antioxidant system, play a central role in redox signaling, metabolism and scavenging of reactive oxygen species (ROS) that are important for both normal health and diseases as well (Figure 1). The classical dithiol Grxs contain a conserved active site sequence, namely –Cys-Pro-Tyr-Cys- [1]. In addition to this redox center, Grxs possess a binding site for glutathione (GSH) [3]. Grxs were first identified acting as electron donors to modulate the activity of ribonucleoside diphosphate reductases (RNRs) that play an important function in DNA synthesis [4-5]. When coupled with GSH and glutathione reductase in the presence of NADPH, Grxs can also catalyze the reduction of protein disulfides and of GSH-protein mixed disulfides via a dithiol or monothiol mechanism [6-7] (Figure 2), suggesting that these proteins are essential in regulating redox state of target proteins in diverse cellular processes [2, 8]. Grxs can be divided into three major groups with dithiol (Cys-X-X-Cys), monothiol (Cys-X-X-Ser), and CC-type (Cys-Cys-X-Cys or Cys-Cys-X-Ser) motifs depending on the number of active site Cys residues [9-10]. The last group has been only identified in green photosynthetic organisms, such as plants [10].

Dithiol Grxs have been extensively studied since the bacterial Grxs were discovered about forty years ago and shown to regulate diverse cellular processes [2, 4, 9] (See more details in the following sections). In contrast, monothiol Grxs were discovered quite recently and have been less characterized. Monothiol Grxs were initially identified in yeast (Grx3, 4, and 5) [11]. Yeast Grx5 encodes a mitochondrial monothiol Grx [12], whereas Grx3 and Grx4 can function in both cytoplasm and nuclei [13-15]. This group of monothiol Grxs is also conserved across organisms and has now been identified in bacteria, malarial parasites, fungi, plants, zebrafish, mice, and humans [16-21]. Monothiol Grxs can be further classified as single- and multi-domain monothiol Grxs (Figure 3).

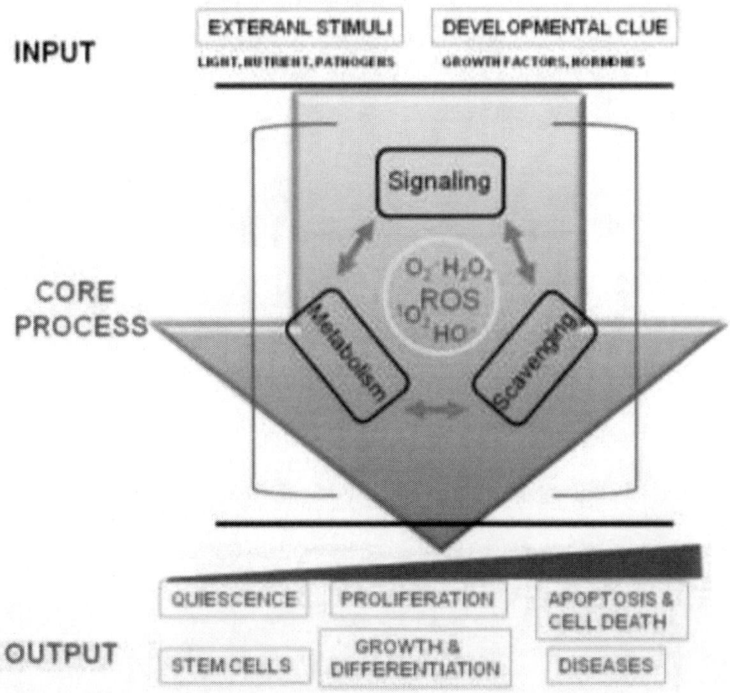

Figure 1. Reactive oxygen species (ROS)-mediated signaling network. The heart of the system is a core process, comprising ROS production and metabolism, scavenging, redox signaling that are tightly coupled to each other. Grxs are thought to play a central role in this core process that interfaces with two sets of components: two input modules that come from either external stimuli, such as light, temperature, nutrient, toxins, and pathogens or developmental cues including growth factors and hormones. The output of the core process is translated to ROS levels that regulate various cellular processes and determine cell fates, normal growth and differentiation, and pathogenesis.

Unlike dithiol Grxs that can act as thioreductases in reversible glutathionylation [22], whether monothiol Grxs catalyze protein deglutathionylation remains to be determined. Several recent studies suggest that monothiol Grxs may be able to deglutathionylate disulfides and/or GSH-protein mixed disulfides in different species [11, 23-25]. Specifically, Zaffagnini *et al.* recently reported that a CGFS-type monothiol Grx from *Chlamydomonas reinhardtii* could be reduced by photoreduced ferredoxin and ferredoxin-thioredoxin reductase in the chloroplast under light and was able to efficiently catalyze A(4)-glyceraldehyde-3-phosphate dehydrogenase deglutathionylation, whereas cytosolic and chloroplastic thioredoxins were inefficient [26]. This finding provides experimental evidence that glutathionylated A(4)-glyceraldehyde-3-phosphate dehydrogenase is the first physiological substrate identified for a CGFS-typc Grx [26]. Interestingly, bacterial Grx4, unlike other previously characterized Grxs, can serve as a substrate for thioredoxin reductase instead of NADPH/glutathione reductase [27]. Together, those studies suggest that monothiol Grxs have distinct functions compared to dithiol Grxs.

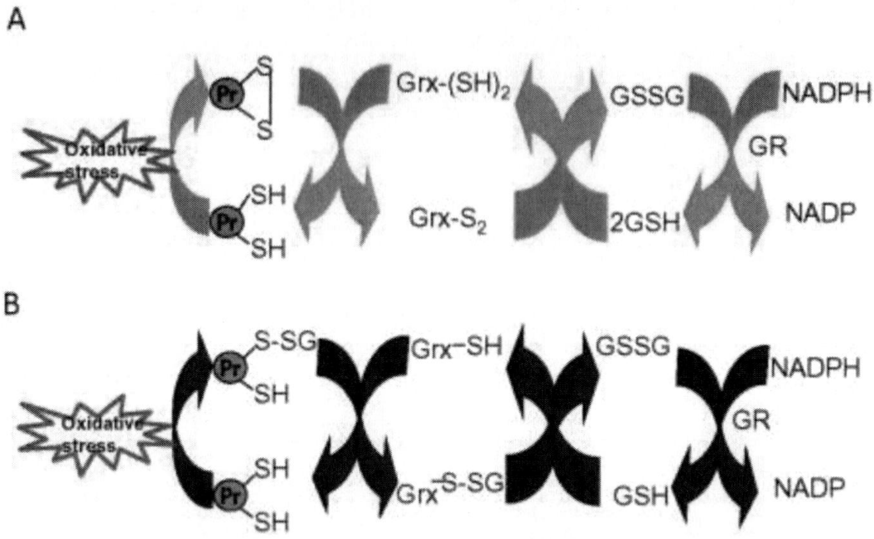

Figure 2. The catalytic mechanism of the glutaredoxin systems. Dithiol (A) and monothiol (B) catalytic mechanisms have been proposed for the glutaredoxin system. In the glutaredoxin action, electrons are received from reduced nicotinamide adenine dinucleotide phosphate (NADPH) and transferred to glutathione reductase (GR), then glutathione (GSH), and relayed to glutaredoxins (Grxs). Grxs then reduce disulfide bonds in target proteins (Pr) caused by oxidative stress.

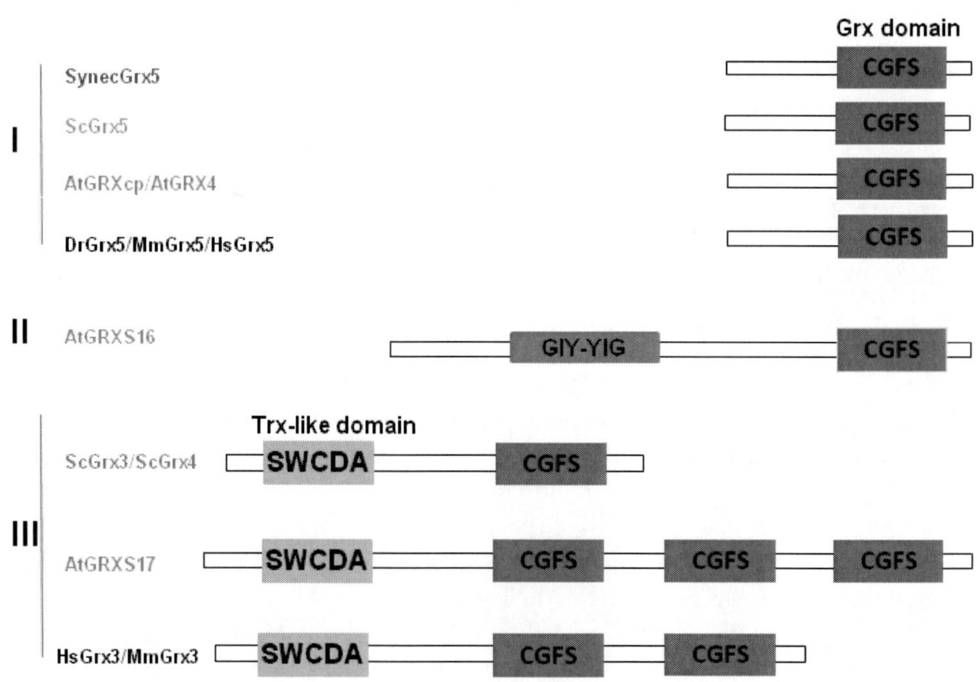

Figure 3. Structure of CGFS-type monothiol glutaredoxins from different organisms. The green boxes indicate Grx domains with "CGFS" motifs; the blue boxes indicate a unique GIY-YIG endonuclease domain in AtGRXS16; the orange boxes indicate the N-terminal Trx-like domains. At represents *Arabidopsis thaliana*, Dr is *Danio rerio*, Hs is *Homo sapiens*, Mm is *Mus musculus*, Sc is *Saccharomyces cerevisiae*, Synec is *Synechocystis*.

Recently, the human mitochondrial dithiol Grx2 has been identified as an iron-sulfur cluster protein, in which Grx2 binds a [2Fe-2S] cluster that bridges two Grx2 molecules through two structural Cys residues to form a Grx2 dimer [28]. Structure-function analyses also indicate that poplar dithiol Grx C1, like human Grx2, contains a [2Fe–2S] cluster in the holo form [29-30]. This [2Fe-2S] cluster is proposed to act as a redox sensor for the activation of Grx under stress conditions [31]. Compared to dithiol Grxs, biochemical analysis indicates that the vast majority of monothiol Grxs are able to bind a Fe-S cluster in the dimer form [32]. Only a few structures of monothiol Grxs have been determined [33-37]. The structures of two monothiol Grxs, *Escherichia coli* Grx4 and the Trx-like domain of yeast Grx3, have been reported. However, the active-site motif regions are not visible or are partially disordered in two of these monothiol Grx structures [33-34]. The structure of poplar GrxS12 has recently been determined [38]. This enzyme possesses an unusual monothiol CSYS active-site sequence and is similar to yeast ScGrx6 which contains the CSYS motif [38-39]. In contrast to some other monothiol Grxs, GrxS12 does not incorporate an iron–sulfur cluster in its original form, whereas bacterial Grx4, Arabidopsis AtGRXcp (AtGRXS14), and human Grx5 have been shown to bind an iron–sulfur cluster in their homodimeric forms [35-38]. It has been proposed that monothiol Grx dimers function in Fe-S cluster biogenesis in both prokaryotes and eukaryotes and serve as a carrier to deliver the intact Fe–S cluster to the apoproteins [35. 40-42] or form a [2Fe–2S] cluster–ligand complex to mediate signaling events in the cell [43].

Grxs are known to be involved in DNA synthesis through modulating RNR activity [9]. A recent study implicates that activation of phage T4 intron endonuclease, I-TevI, is redox-dependent and regulated by Grx1, suggesting that there may be a link between endonuclease activity and redox homeostasis [44]. Most significantly, Liu *et al.* reported that a chloroplastic monothiol glutaredoxin, AtGRXS16, from *Arabidopsis thaliana*, comprises two distinct functional domains, an N-terminal domain (NTD) with GlyIleTyr-TyrIleGly (GIY-YIG) endonuclease motif and a C-terminal Grx module, to coordinate Fe-S cluster biosynthesis and DNA cleavage in chloroplasts [45]. This study further demonstrated that these two functional domains were negatively regulated through the formation of an intramolecular disulfide bond [45]. Given the emerging evidence that Fe–S clusters may be essential components of diverse nucleic acid processing machinery [46-47] and may also be critical for DNA damage recognition [48-50], these findings unravel a novel manner of regulation for Grxs and provide insight into a mechanistic link between redox regulation and Fe-S cluster-mediated DNA metabolism in the cell.

The mammalian glutaredoxins: There are four members of Grxs that have been discovered in mammals: Grx1, Grx2, Grx3 (also known as PICOT and TXNL2), and Grx5. The 12 kDa dithiol Grx1 possesses Cys-Pro-Tyr-Cys active site and is mainly localized in the cytosol, but also can be located in the nucleus [51], mitochondria [52], and secreted from the cell [53]. Unlike Grx1, the 14 kDa dithiol Grx2 possesses Cys-Ser-Tyr-Cys active site and is located in mitochondria, but its cancer-specific isoforms show different subcellular localizations [54]. The 38 kDa monothiol Grx3 is a multi-domain protein that contains an N-terminal Trx-like domain with the active site motif Ala-Pro-Gln-Cys and two repeated C-terminal monothiol Grx domains with the active site Cys-Gly-Phe-Ser (Figure 3). It is localized in the cytosol and the nucleus [55]. The 17kDa monothiol Grx5 is localized in mitochondria and harbors the same active site motif of Grx3. Among the four human Grxs, Grx1 and Grx2 have been studied more comprehensively than the other two members, Grx3 and Grx5. Generally, Grxs can function as electron donors, catalyze reversible glutathionylation, and participate in iron metabolism [9]. Grx2 [56], Grx3 [57], and Grx5 [37] are able to bind [2Fe-2S] clusters. An earlier finding shows that Grx expression and activity can be induced by tumor promoters such as phorbol ester 12-O-tetradecanoylphorbol-13-acetate (TPA) in mouse models, suggesting a role of Grx in tumorigenesis [58]. Studies on Grxs have been directed more towards human diseases, including cancer (Figure 4). However, the role of this family in the process of carcinogenesis and the potential applications in therapeutic approaches by targeting Grxs await further exploration. This chapter will update the current understanding of Grxs in human cancers and offer insights for future directions.

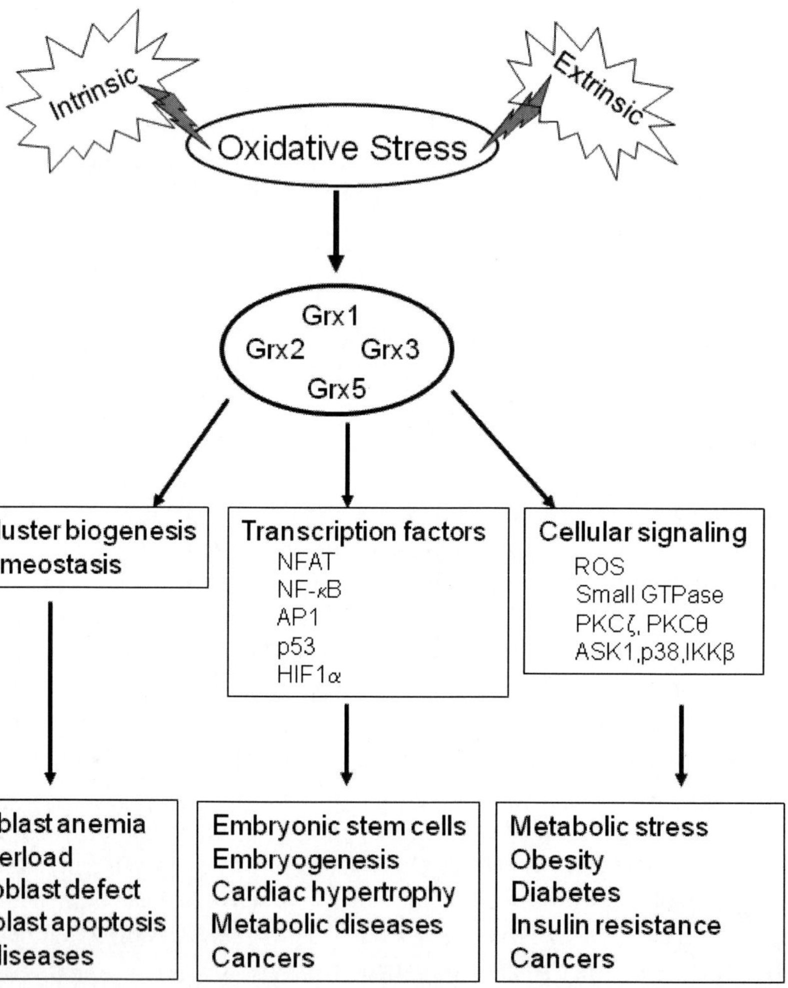

Figure 4. Mammalian Grx systems play a central role in normal human health and disruption of their systems is closely linked to many human diseases. Grxs have crucial functions in Fe-S cluster assembly and iron regulation in the cell and critical in the pathogenesis of anemia and bone diseases [73, 119-120]. Grxs are able to modulate the activity of many transcription factors that control both physiological and pathological processes [63, 75, 77, 121-123]. Furthermore, the Grx systems regulate many cellular signaling pathways that are essential for the development of metabolic disorders and cancer [16, 53, 124-125].

2. Grxs in Cancer Development

2.1. Expression of Grxs in Human Cancers

The expression of Grxs in cancers has been widely investigated. An immune-histochemical analysis performed by Nakamura *et al.* [59] reveals an increased expression of Grx1 in 90% of pancreatic cancer tissues. In a screening of 588 genes by differential hybridization of a human cDNA microarray, upregulation of Grx1 has been found in basal cell carcinoma tissues [60]. Grx1 and Grx2 expression have been found to be correlated with the degree of differentiation in non-small lung adenocarcinoma [61]. Grx2 mRNA levels are elevated in breast, colon and lung cancer tissues and Grx5 mRNA levels are elevated in lung cancers [62]. Grx3 protein is found to be dramatically increased in lung and colon cancers, while the levels of other Grxs are relatively unaltered [62]. Similarly, Ohayon *et al.* reveal that Grx3 expression is increased in Hodgkin's lymphoma/Reed Sternberg cells [63]. Another study reported by Qu *et al.* [64] shows that the levels of Grx3 are elevated in breast cancers and are correlated with patient survival and metastasis to the lung and brain. These findings suggest that Grx3 has a positive role in supporting/promoting tumor cell growth and/or survival. There is also contradictory finding which shows downregulation of Grx1 in malignant gallbladder tissues [65]. Nevertheless, increased Grxs levels were found to be associated with cancers in the majority of studies.

2.2. Cancer Specific Isoforms and Subcellular Localizations

Cancer specific isoforms of Grx members have been recently discovered. Grx2 has long been established as a mitochondrial oxidoreductase and is suggested to play a critical role in protection against apoptotic stimuli. Recent discoveries by Lönn *et al.* show that Grx2b and Grx2c, which are derived from alternative transcription initiation and splicing [54], are enzymatically active isoforms of Grx2 whose expression is restricted to the testes in normal tissues, but broadly expressed in various cancer cell lines [66]. Unlike Grx2a, Grx2b and Grx2c show both cytosolic and nuclear localization. Their novel findings provide evidence for the presence and functions of Grx isoforms. Although the role of these isoforms in tumorgenesis and/or progression needs further investigation, targeting cancer-cell-specific isoforms is a prospective strategy for an effective and secure therapy against cancer.

Besides its well-known cytosolic localization, Grx1 is also localized in the inter-membrane space of mitochondria [52]. This differs from Grx2a, which is localized exclusively in the mitochondrial matrix. The role of Grx1 in mitochondria is correlated with SOD activity [67]. Grx2 is pivotal in reversible interactions of protein thiols with the mitochondrial glutathione pool and protects cells from apoptosis and oxidant damage [68-70]. The localization and presence of cancer-specific Grx isoforms may also provide novel mechanisms involving tumorigenesis and progression. More detailed investigations on the mechanisms of Grxs subcellular distribution and/or translocation may provide new insights into better understanding cancer and new clues for therapeutic strategies in cancer therapy.

2.3 The Role of Grxs in Cancer Cell Proliferation and Survival

ROS can act in dual roles as inhibitors or accelerators of malignant transformation. Elevated oxidative status has been observed in many types of cancer cells due in part to their high metabolic rate. On the other hand, many tumor cells possess stronger antioxidative defense mechanisms to counterbalance excessive ROS, maintain their redox status, and thus suppress apoptosis [71]. As one of the major antioxidant systems, the Grx system protects cancer cells from oxidative stress-induced apoptosis and enables them to better adapt/utilize stress. Anathy *et al.* show that stimulation with the Fas ligand (FasL) induces S-glutathionylation of Fas, and thereby induces and amplifies apoptosis through caspase-dependent degradation of Grx1 [72]. This apoptosis can be attenuated by overexpression of Grx1 [72]. Grx5 also protects cells from apoptosis induced by oxidative stress [74]. Grx5 deficiency reduces manganese superoxide dismutase (MnSOD) activity and increases caspase activity [73]. Human Grx2 has been shown to protect HeLa cells from oxidative stress-induced apoptosis [69] by preventing the release of cytochrome c [70]. In particular, Grx2 prevented loss of cardiolipin, the phospholipid anchoring cytochrome c to the inner mitochondrial membrane. In Hela cells, the Grx system plays a backup role to keep Trx1 reduced in conditions that lack of thioredoxin reductase 1 (TrxR1) and thus prevents ROS accumulation as well as subsequent cell death [74].

Knockdown of Grxs show severe phenotypes; however, only Grx3-knockout mice are embryonically lethal [75]. Grx3 inhibits apoptosis through its role in cell activation-associated signaling pathways or in the cellular response to stress signals [55]. Consistent with its role in anti-apoptosis, the expression of Grx3 showed significant positive correlation with Survivin [62], which is a known anti-apoptotic factor and is positively correlated with tumor stage in lung cancer [76]. Qu *et al.* also showed an anti-apoptotic effect of Grx3 in breast cancer cells. Grx3 knockdown increased intracellular ROS levels and decreased the GSH/GSSG ratio, thereby inhibiting cell growth and survival [64]. Impaired cell proliferation caused by Grx3 depletion was observed in another study, which further showed that Grx3 depletion rendered cell cycle arrest at G2/M phase and cytokinesis failure [77]. In summary, Grxs can regulate cancer cell growth through inhibiting apoptosis and controlling cell cycle progression.

2.4. Reversible Glutathionylation of Cancer-Associated Proteins by Grxs

Glutaredoxin acts either as a dithiol protein disulfide reductase, similar to thioredoxin (Trx), or as a catalyst for the reduction of mixed disulfides of glutathionylated proteins [22] (Figure 2). This process is also called deglutathionylation, which is exclusively catalyzed by Grxs. Glutathionylation is often considered to be a process that protects sensitive cysteinyl residues from irreversible oxidation [22, 78]. In addition to this protective effect, glutathionylation also results in protein-specific functional changes during the regulation of signaling mediators.

Grxs are known to regulate the activity of many proteins through reversible glutathionylation, such as Ras, Fas, ASK1, NF-κB, and procaspase-3, all of which play important roles in the process of tumorigenesis [79]. Glutathionylation is one of the common types of post-translational regulation of protein functions which can be both activating and suppressing. The glutathionylation of Ras (GSS-Ras) activates this oncoprotein, leading to the downstream phosphorylation of AKT, p38, as well as increased cell proliferation [80]. Grx1 overexpression decreases GSS-Ras and inhibits its activity [80]. On the other hand, glutathionylation can inhibit protein functions as well. AKT undergoes disulfide bond formation between Cys-297 and Cys-311 under stress, which subsequently causes dephosphorylation at Thr-308 and Ser-473 and loss of function [81]. Grx1 can directly regulate AKT activity through reducing oxidized AKT by deglutathionylation accordance with GSH. Overexpression of Grx protects cells from hydrogen peroxide (H_2O_2)-induced apoptosis by regulating the redox state of AKT [81]. Grx1 participates in the deglutathionylation of Sirt1, a redox-sensitive deacetylase which regulates p53 activity and plays critical role in tumorigenesis [82]. Grx5 appears to function in the reversal of glutathionylation as well. Kim *et al.* showed that Grx5 could reduce oxidized tumor suppressor PTEN caused by oxidative stress such as H_2O_2 *in vitro* [83].

NF-κB is another redox-sensitive transcriptional factor that is critical in tumor development and progression. Qanungo's group first reported that Grx1-dependent S-glutathionylation of p65-NF-κB in hypoxic pancreatic cancer cells suppressed NF-κB activity and induced apoptosis [84]. Qu *et al.* also discovered that S-glutathionylation of NF-κB under Grx3-depletion-induced severe oxidative stress suppresses its activity [64]. Therefore, the reversible glutathionylation catalyzed by Grxs plays both promoting and inhibiting roles in cancer which also reflects the delicacy of the Grxs and ROS in modulating the activity of key signaling pathways.

2.5. The Role of Grxs in the Cancer Microenvironment

Tumor microenvironment is critical not only in supporting tumor cell growth, but also in reprogramming tumor cells to develop malignant features [85-86]. In 1995, a study by Rubartelli *et al.* showed that reduced extracellular conditions caused by extracellular Trx inhibit HepG2 cell growth [87]. Their finding suggests a critical role of secreted antioxidant proteins in regulating tumor cell biology and reveals a novel mechanism linking intracellular redox status with extracellular redox status and the modulation of cell functions [88-89]. Grx1 and Grx2 can also be secreted and detected in human plasma by ELISA [90]. The secretion of Grx1 and its presence in plasma suggests extracellular functions. Björnstedt *et al.* discovered that extracellular Grx can function as a reductant for the selenium-dependent peroxidase [91]. Grx1 plays an important role in both autocrine and paracrine pro-inflammatory responses [53]. Extracellular Grx1 is a potential redox modulatory protein that regulates extracellular homeostasis of glutathionylated proteins and GSH [92]. Lundberg *et al.* analyzed intra- and extracellular Grx levels in different cell lines, and showed that Grx was found in all cell lines tested and in the extracellular media of several cell lines [90]. It is possible that secreted Grxs play a role in regulating the redox status of the tumor microenvironment. Currently, the role of secreted Grxs in cancer is largely unknown.

3. Grxs in Cancer Metastasis and Therapy Resistance

3.1. Grxs in Cancer Metastasis

ROS is considered to be a double-edged sword in regulating cell motility in human cancer cells. EMT, which promotes tumor progression, is regulated by ROS [93]. Grxs are scavengers of ROS, and can play positive and negative roles in regulating EMT and metastasis. A moderate increase of ROS promotes tumorigenesis by activating tumor-promoting signaling pathways, but a more drastic increase of ROS inhibits tumor formation and progression [94-95]. Elevation of ROS is concomitant with some EMT signaling pathways. Transforming growth factor-beta (TGFβ) is a cytokine important in inducing EMT in cancer cells. A study reported by Lee *et al.* showed that the loss of Grx1 expression is required for TGFβ induced EMT in H-Ras transformed mammary epithelial cells [62]. On the other hand, other studies have shown that up-regulation of Grx1 is concomitant with NF-κB activation, induction of intercellular adhesion molecule-1 (ICAM-1) [78] and interleukin-6 [53], and activation of IKK activity [53]. Grx3 knockdown increases intracellular ROS levels, reverses EMT, and suppresses metastasis in breast cancer cells through oxidative inhibition of NF-κB activity [64], a well-known transcription factor critical for tumor development and progression. This observation is consistent with previous findings that Grx1 modulates the inhibitory effects of H_2O_2 on IKK-β and NF-κB through deglutathionylation [96]. The contradictions seem to imply that the role of Grx as a metastasis promoter or inhibitor is cellular-context dependent and needs further detailed investigation.

3.2. The Role of Grxs in Therapy Resistance

In general, ROS generated from mitochondria is higher in cancer cells than in normal cells [97]. It is agreed that increased ROS production is a common feature associated with cancer cells [97]. The vast majority of the agents or modalities used to kill cancer cells, such as radiotherapy, chemotherapy and targeted therapies, act either directly or indirectly by generating ROS to block key steps in the cell cycle and apoptosis induction. The classic antitumor drugs such as Cisplatin and Adriamycin appear to produce ROS at excessive levels, causing oxidative stress, which in turn may cause cellular damage. It was also found that the effectiveness of ROS-generating agents, including Paclitaxel and other chemotherapy drugs, in various cancer cell lines varies widely because the antioxidant capacities of those cell lines are different [98]. Thus, as the major cellular defense system that protects cells against oxidative stress, high levels of Grxs in cancer cells may play a critical role in drug resistance, thus making them potential targets for cancer treatment.

3.3. Grx Levels and Drug Sensitivity

Previous findings have provided links between Grx levels and drug resistance in cancer cells. High Grx levels are concomitant with resistance to different chemotherapeutic drugs.

Grx is overexpressed in Adriamycin-resistant MCF-7 [99], a human breast cancer cell line, and inhibits apoptosis caused by adriamycin cytotoxicity [100]. CDDP (cis-diamminedichloroplatinum) is a first-line chemotherapeutic drug for a large number of malignant tumors; it is genotoxic and works by cross-linking DNA, resulting in cell-cycle arrest and ultimately triggering apoptosis. Nakamura *et al.* showed that CDDP-resistant subclones of Hela cells exhibit higher levels of Grx compared to parental cells [59]. Overexpression of Grx1 increases the resistance of MCF7 breast cancer cells to Doxorubicin, a widely used anti-cancer agent [101]. siRNA-mediated silencing of Grx2 dramatically sensitizes the cells to doxorubicin- and phenylarsine oxide-induced cell death [69]. Overexpression of both mitochondrial and cytosolic Grx2 decreases the susceptibility of HeLa cells to doxorubicin-induced apoptosis as well as the antimetabolite 2-deoxy-D-glucose by attenuation of cytochrome c release and caspase activation induced by both agents [70]. Their findings demonstrate a crucial role of Grx2 in regulating the mitochondrial redox status and cell death at the mitochondrial checkpoint. Notably, there is one report showing the pro-apoptotic function of Grx3 [102]. In this study, it was found that Grx3 depletion and overexpression of caspase-cleaved Grx3, normally induced by chemotherapy drugs, inhibited the activation of caspase-3 by chemotherapy drugs and accordingly apoptosis [102]. The seemingly paradoxical conclusions drawn by different studies may reflect the complexity of Grx functions, which require further investigation.

3.4. The Involment of Grxs in Drug Metabolism

Human Grxs are involved in the metabolism of chemotherapeutic drugs because they are the main contributors to the formation of the pharmacologically active metabolite of clopidogrel from its GSH conjugate in the human liver [103]. Selenium compounds are known to decrease cell proliferation, cause DNA fragmentation and induce apoptosis in tumor cells at high concentrations [104-105]. For this reason, selenium is a potential therapeutic agent in cancer treatment and exhibits cytotoxicity through ROS generation [104]. Wallengerg's group discovered that selenium compounds, including selenite, GS-Se-SG, Se-DL-cystine and DL-cystine, are substrates of Grx1; suggesting Grx1 is involved in selenium metabolism [106]. They also showed that suppression of Grx1 increased cell viability after selenium compounds treatment. This effect may be explained by diminished redox-cycling of Grx with these compounds, generating less mixed disulfides and ROS. The finding reported by Olm *et al.* also indicates that Grxs contribute to selenium cytotoxicity by the reduction of cystine to cysteine intracellularly, leading to a more efficient uptake and consequently higher cytotoxicity [107]. In contrast to TrxR, which protects cells from selenium cytotoxicity [108], Grx1 contributes to selenium toxicity [106]. It is noteworthy that the Grx system is inhibited by bis-(glutathionato) platinum (II) (GS-Platinum complex, GS-Pt), a major route for cellular elimination of CDDP [109]. This observation also explains why CDDP-resistant cancer cells show high levels of Grxs. The role of Grx in drug metabolism and activity is a novel theme in studying the mechanisms of redox-based cancer treatment.

4. Grxs as Potential Targets in Cancer Treatment

4.1. Killing Cancer Cells by Targeting Grxs

As mentioned earlier in this chapter, Grxs protect cancer cells from oxidative stress generated by cancer cells themselves (due to high metabolism) or therapeutic chemicals to support their uncontrolled proliferation and malignant invading behaviors. The idea of selectively killing cancer cells by exploiting their metabolic and oxidative traits makes Grxs valuable targets in anticancer treatment. Inhibition of Grxs in cancer cells may shift the balance between high oxidative stress and antagonizing antioxidant capacity, and further magnify their vulnerabilities to oxidative stress. The combination of chemotherapeutic drugs with Grxs inhibition (e.g., knockdown or inhibitors) may be more effective in killing cancer cells than chemotherapy alone and thus reduce the occurrence of drug resistance and the side-effects of chemotherapy. Alternatively, Grx inhibition in combination with ROS-inducing drugs such as elesclomol [110], a chemical that selectively transporting copper to mitochondria to induce oxidative stress [111], may overwhelm cancer cells with ROS and thus induce apoptosis. Recently, a phase III clinical trial of elesclomol in combination with paclitaxel in melanoma shows that patients with low and normal baseline levels of lactate dehydrogenase (LDH), a well-known indicator for hypoxia and poor prognosis in cancer, had an improvement in progression-free survival [112]. This suggests that ROS-generating agents may hold promise as novel anticancer therapies. Therefore, it is reasonable to speculate that Grxs blockade may also render cancer cells more sensitive to cytotoxic therapies.

4.2. Detection of Grxs in Serum as Biomarkers

Grx levels are found to be correlated with disease status. A study by Godoy *et al.* shows that Hela cells overexpressing Grx1-3 and 5 displayed higher survival/ proliferation rates and lower oxidative damage compared to control cells when subjected to hypoxia and reoxygenation [101]. As mentioned earlier, Trx and Grx can be detected in the serum from patients. More importantly, extracellular Trx and Grx levels are both capable of modulating the uptake of selenium by cancer cells, which is crucial to the specific selenite (a type of selenium compounds) cytotoxicity [107]. Detection of serum Trx1 showed diagnostic value in malignant diseases [113-114]; therefore, whether Grx levels in serum can serve as a diagnostic or recurrent marker for cancer patients is an issue worth investigating.

4.3. Detection of Mutations and Post-Translational Modifications

The mutations in the Grx family, which are related to functional changes, have been discovered in other species [115-117]. Whether these similar mutations involving the function of Grx can also be found in human cancers is waiting to be solved. Despite the fact that Grxs are major regulators in maintaining redox homeostasis, they are also substrates of redox-related modifications. Grx1 can be regulated by oxidative stress through modification of its cysteinyl residues and this modification is related to activity loss [118]. In contrast, modification of Grx2 actually leads to the activation of its function [118]. Tyrosine phosphorylation of Grx3 renders its translocation to the nucleus under oxidative stress [55]. The mutations or post-translational modifications of Grxs may not only reflect their physical function, but their disease-specific roles as well.

Conclusion

The importance of the Grx system in cancer is increasingly recognized. Emerging evidence has strongly suggested a critical role of Grxs in the process of tumorigenesis and treatment resistance, though there are several studies that show opposite results. Whether redox stress is a friend or foe is the debate of the century. Likewise, the role of Grxs in cancer cells is also intricate and complex. For example, high levels of Grxs can either promote or suppress EMT. To make matters worse, different Grx members may exert distinct effects on cell functions. The molecular mechanisms of Grx members involved in signaling pathways in cancer are worthy of attention. The comprehensive investigations on Grxs will provide better understanding of cancer biology and contribute to the development of clinical applications. It is hoped that this review generates substantial interests in the role of Grxs in cancer, and that further investigations will establish Grx members as biomarkers and therapeutic targets in cancer. The increasingly obvious complexity in the biology of ROS in cancer development creates a compelling reason to unravel the mechanisms underlying the function of Grx.

Acknowledgements

We thank the support of National Institutes of Health (CA151610 and UL1TR000124), the Avon Foundation (02-2010-068), and David Salomon Research Fund to Xiaojiang Cui, and the support of the Agricultural Research Service, US Department of Agriculture (Cooperation Agreement 6250-51000-055) to Ninghui Cheng.

References

[1] Holmgren A, Aslund F. Glutaredoxin. *Methods Enzymol.* 1995;252:283-92.

[2] Fernandes AP, Holmgren A. Glutaredoxins: glutathione-dependent redox enzymes with functions far beyond a simple thioredoxin backup system. *Antioxid Redox Signal.* 2004 Feb;6(1):63-74.

[3] Nikkola M, Gleason FK, Saarinen M, Joelson T, Bjornberg O, Eklund H. A putative glutathione-binding site in T4 glutaredoxin investigated by site-directed mutagenesis. *J Biol Chem.* 1991 Aug 25;266(24):16105-12.

[4] Holmgren A. Hydrogen donor system for Escherichia coli ribonucleoside-diphosphate reductase dependent upon glutathione. *Proc Natl Acad Sci U S A.* 1976 Jul;73(7):2275-9.

[5] Nordlund P, Reichard P. Ribonucleotide Reductases. *Annual Review of Biochemistry.* 2006;75(1):681-706.

[6] Holmgren A. Thioredoxin and glutaredoxin systems. *J Biol Chem.* 1989 Aug 25;264(24):13963-6.
[7] Bushweller JH, Aslund F, Wuthrich K, Holmgren A. Structural and functional characterization of the mutant Escherichia coli glutaredoxin (C14----S) and its mixed disulfide with glutathione. *Biochemistry.* 1992 Sep 29;31(38):9288-93.
[8] Shelton MD, Chock PB, Mieyal JJ. Glutaredoxin: role in reversible protein s-glutathionylation and regulation of redox signal transduction and protein translocation. *Antioxid Redox Signal.* 2005 Mar-Apr;7(3-4):348-66.
[9] Lillig CH, Berndt C, Holmgren A. Glutaredoxin systems. Biochim Biophys Acta. 2008 Nov;1780(11):1304-17.
[10] Meyer Y, Siala W, Bashandy T, Riondet C, Vignols F, Reichheld JP. Glutaredoxins and thioredoxins in plants. *Biochim Biophys Acta.* 2008 Apr;1783(4):589-600.
[11] Rodriguez-Manzaneque MT, Ros J, Cabiscol E, Sorribas A, Herrero E. Grx5 glutaredoxin plays a central role in protection against protein oxidative damage in Saccharomyces cerevisiae. *Mol Cell Biol.* 1999 Dec;19(12):8180-90.
[12] Rodriguez-Manzaneque MT, Tamarit J, Belli G, Ros J, Herrero E. Grx5 is a mitochondrial glutaredoxin required for the activity of iron/sulfur enzymes. *Mol Biol Cell.* 2002 Apr;13(4):1109-21.
[13] Ojeda L, Keller G, Muhlenhoff U, Rutherford JC, Lill R, Winge DR. Role of glutaredoxin-3 and glutaredoxin-4 in the iron regulation of the Aft1 transcriptional activator in Saccharomyces cerevisiae. *J Biol Chem.* 2006 Jun 30;281(26):17661-9.
[14] Pujol-Carrion N, Belli G, Herrero E, Nogues A, de la Torre-Ruiz MA. Glutaredoxins Grx3 and Grx4 regulate nuclear localisation of Aft1 and the oxidative stress response in Saccharomyces cerevisiae. *J Cell Sci.* 2006 Nov 1;119(Pt 21):4554-64.
[15] Muhlenhoff U, Molik S, Godoy JR, Uzarska MA, Richter N, Seubert A, et al. Cytosolic monothiol glutaredoxins function in intracellular iron sensing and trafficking via their bound iron-sulfur cluster. *Cell Metab.* 2010 Oct 6;12(4):373-85.
[16] Witte S, Villalba M, Bi K, Liu Y, Isakov N, Altman A. Inhibition of the c-Jun N-terminal kinase/AP-1 and NF-kappaB pathways by PICOT, a novel protein kinase C-interacting protein with a thioredoxin homology domain. *J Biol Chem.* 2000 Jan 21;275(3):1902-9.
[17] Rahlfs S, Fischer M, Becker K. Plasmodium falciparum possesses a classical glutaredoxin and a second, glutaredoxin-like protein with a PICOT homology domain. *J Biol Chem.* 2001 Oct 5;276(40):37133-40.
[18] Cheng NH, Hirschi KD. Cloning and characterization of CXIP1, a novel PICOT domain-containing Arabidopsis protein that associates with CAX1. *J Biol Chem.* 2003 Feb 21;278(8):6503-9.
[19] Wingert RA, Galloway JL, Barut B, Foott H, Fraenkel P, Axe JL, et al. Deficiency of glutaredoxin 5 reveals Fe-S clusters are required for vertebrate haem synthesis. *Nature.* 2005 Aug 18;436(7053):1035-39.
[20] Herrero E, Ros J, Tamarit J, Belli G. Glutaredoxins in fungi. *Photosynth Res.* 2006 Sep;89(2-3):127-40.
[21] Cheng NH, Liu JZ, Brock A, Nelson RS, Hirschi KD. AtGRXcp, an Arabidopsis chloroplastic glutaredoxin, is critical for protection against protein oxidative damage. *J Biol Chem.* 2006 Sep 8;281(36):26280-8.

[22] Gallogly MM, Mieyal JJ. Mechanisms of reversible protein glutathionylation in redox signaling and oxidative stress. *Curr Opin Pharmacol*. 2007 Aug;7(4):381-91.

[23] Shenton D, Perrone G, Quinn KA, Dawes IW, Grant CM. Regulation of protein S-thiolation by glutaredoxin 5 in the yeast Saccharomyces cerevisiae. *J Biol Chem*. 2002 May 10;277(19):16853-9.

[24] Tamarit J, Belli G, Cabiscol E, Herrero E, Ros J. Biochemical characterization of yeast mitochondrial Grx5 monothiol glutaredoxin. *J Biol Chem*. 2003 Jul 11;278(28):25745-51.

[25] Zaffagnini M, Bedhomme M, Marchand CH, Morisse S, Trost P, Lemaire SD. Redox regulation in photosynthetic organisms: focus on glutathionylation. *Antioxid Redox Signal*. 2012 Mar 15;16(6):567-86.

[26] Zaffagnini M, Michelet L, Massot V, Trost P, Lemaire SD. Biochemical characterization of glutaredoxins from Chlamydomonas reinhardtii reveals the unique properties of a chloroplastic CGFS-type glutaredoxin. *J Biol Chem*. 2008 Apr 4;283(14):8868-76.

[27] Fernandes AP, Fladvad M, Berndt C, Andresen C, Lillig CH, Neubauer P, et al. A novel monothiol glutaredoxin (Grx4) from Escherichia coli can serve as a substrate for thioredoxin reductase. *J Biol Chem*. 2005 Jul 1;280(26):24544-52.

[28] Lillig CH, Berndt C, Vergnolle O, Lonn ME, Hudemann C, Bill E, et al. Characterization of human glutaredoxin 2 as iron-sulfur protein: a possible role as redox sensor. *Proc Natl Acad Sci U S A*. 2005 Jun 7;102(23):8168-73.

[29] Feng Y, Zhong N, Rouhier N, Hase T, Kusunoki M, Jacquot JP, et al. Structural insight into poplar glutaredoxin C1 with a bridging iron-sulfur cluster at the active site. *Biochemistry*. 2006 Jul 4;45(26):7998-8008.

[30] Rouhier N, Unno H, Bandyopadhyay S, Masip L, Kim SK, Hirasawa M, et al. Functional, structural, and spectroscopic characterization of a glutathione-ligated [2Fe-2S] cluster in poplar glutaredoxin C1. *Proc Natl Acad Sci U S A*. 2007 May 1;104(18):7379-84.

[31] Holmgren A, Johansson C, Berndt C, Lonn ME, Hudemann C, Lillig CH. Thiol redox control via thioredoxin and glutaredoxin systems. *Biochem Soc Trans*. 2005 Dec;33(Pt 6):1375-7.

[32] Picciocchi A, Saguez C, Boussac A, Cassier-Chauvat C, Chauvat F. CGFS-type monothiol glutaredoxins from the cyanobacterium Synechocystis PCC6803 and other evolutionary distant model organisms possess a glutathione-ligated [2Fe-2S] cluster. *Biochemistry*. 2007 Dec 25;46(51):15018-26.

[33] Fladvad M, Bellanda M, Fernandes AP, Mammi S, Vlamis-Gardikas A, Holmgren A, et al. Molecular mapping of functionalities in the solution structure of reduced Grx4, a monothiol glutaredoxin from Escherichia coli. *J Biol Chem*. 2005 Jul 1;280(26):24553-61.

[34] Gibson LM, Dingra NN, Outten CE, Lebioda L. Structure of the thioredoxin-like domain of yeast glutaredoxin 3. *Acta Crystallogr D Biol Crystallogr*. 2008 Sep;64(Pt 9):927-32.

[35] Iwema T, Picciocchi A, Traore DA, Ferrer JL, Chauvat F, Jacquamet L. Structural basis for delivery of the intact [Fe2S2] cluster by monothiol glutaredoxin. *Biochemistry*. 2009 Jul 7;48(26):6041-3.

[36] Li L, Cheng N, Hirschi KD, Wang X. Structure of Arabidopsis chloroplastic monothiol glutaredoxin AtGRXcp. *Acta crystallographica Section D, Biological crystallography*. 2010 Jun;66(Pt 6):725-32.
[37] Johansson C, Roos AK, Montano SJ, Sengupta R, Filippakopoulos P, Guo K, et al. The crystal structure of human GLRX5: iron-sulfur cluster co-ordination, tetrameric assembly and monomer activity. *The Biochemical journal*. 2011 Jan 15;433(2):303-11.
[38] Couturier J, Koh CS, Zaffagnini M, Winger AM, Gualberto JM, Corbier C, et al. Structure-function relationship of the chloroplastic glutaredoxin S12 with an atypical WCSYS active site. *J Biol Chem*. 2009 Apr 3;284(14):9299-310.
[39] Mesecke N, Mittler S, Eckers E, Herrmann JM, Deponte M. Two novel monothiol glutaredoxins from Saccharomyces cerevisiae provide further insight into iron-sulfur cluster binding, oligomerization, and enzymatic activity of glutaredoxins. *Biochemistry*. 2008 Feb 5;47(5):1452-63.
[40] Frazzon J, Dean DR. Formation of iron-sulfur clusters in bacteria: an emerging field in bioinorganic chemistry. *Curr Opin Chem Biol*. 2003 Apr;7(2):166-73.
[41] Lill R, Muhlenhoff U. Iron-sulfur-protein biogenesis in eukaryotes. *Trends Biochem Sci*. 2005 Mar;30(3):133-41.
[42] Balk J, Pilon M. Ancient and essential: the assembly of iron-sulfur clusters in plants. *Trends Plant Sci*. 2011 Apr;16(4):218-26.
[43] Li H, Mapolelo DT, Dingra NN, Keller G, Riggs-Gelasco PJ, Winge DR, et al. Histidine 103 in Fra2 is an iron-sulfur cluster ligand in the [2Fe-2S] Fra2-Grx3 complex and is required for in vivo iron signaling in yeast. *J Biol Chem*. 2011 Jan 7;286(1):867-76.
[44] Robbins JB, Smith D, Belfort M. Redox-responsive zinc finger fidelity switch in homing endonuclease and intron promiscuity in oxidative stress. *Curr Biol*. 2011 Feb 8;21(3):243-8.
[45] Liu X, Liu S, Feng Y, Liu J-Z, Chen Y, Pham K, et al. Structural insights into the N-terminal GIY–YIG endonuclease activity of Arabidopsis glutaredoxin AtGRXS16 in chloroplasts. Proceedings of the National Academy of Sciences. 2013 June 4, 2013;110(23):9565-70.
[46] White MF, Dillingham MS. Iron–sulphur clusters in nucleic acid processing enzymes. *Current Opinion in Structural Biology*. [doi: 10.1016/j.sbi.2011.11.004]. 2012;22(1):94-100.
[47] Wu Y, Brosh RM. DNA helicase and helicase–nuclease enzymes with a conserved iron–sulfur cluster. *Nucleic Acids Research*. 2012 May 1, 2012;40(10):4247-60.
[48] Gari K, León Ortiz AM, Borel V, Flynn H, Skehel JM, Boulton SJ. MMS19 Links Cytoplasmic Iron-Sulfur Cluster Assembly to DNA Metabolism. *Science*. 2012 July 13, 2012;337(6091):243-5.
[49] Stehling O, Vashisht AA, Mascarenhas J, Jonsson ZO, Sharma T, Netz DJA, et al. MMS19 Assembles Iron-Sulfur Proteins Required for DNA Metabolism and Genomic Integrity. *Science*. 2012 July 13, 2012;337(6091):195-9.
[50] Kuper J, Kisker C. Damage recognition in nucleotide excision DNA repair. *Current Opinion in Structural Biology*. [doi: 10.1016/j.sbi.2011.12.002]. 2012;22(1):88-93.
[51] Fernando MR, Sumimoto H, Nanri H, Kawabata S, Iwanaga S, Minakami S, et al. Cloning and sequencing of the cDNA encoding human glutaredoxin. *Biochim Biophys Acta*. 1994 Jun 21;1218(2):229-31.

[52] Pai HV, Starke DW, Lesnefsky EJ, Hoppel CL, Mieyal JJ. What is the functional significance of the unique location of glutaredoxin 1 (GRx1) in the intermembrane space of mitochondria? *Antioxid Redox Signal*. 2007 Nov;9(11):2027-33.

[53] Shelton MD, Distler AM, Kern TS, Mieyal JJ. Glutaredoxin regulates autocrine and paracrine proinflammatory responses in retinal glial (muller) cells. *J Biol Chem*. 2009 Feb 20;284(8):4760-6.

[54] Lundberg M, Johansson C, Chandra J, Enoksson M, Jacobsson G, Ljung J, et al. Cloning and expression of a novel human glutaredoxin (Grx2) with mitochondrial and nuclear isoforms. *J Biol Chem*. 2001 Jul 13;276(28):26269-75.

[55] Babichev Y, Isakov N. Tyrosine phosphorylation of PICOT and its translocation to the nucleus in response of human T cells to oxidative stress. *Adv Exp Med Biol*. 2001;495:41-5.

[56] Berndt C, Hudemann C, Hanschmann EM, Axelsson R, Holmgren A, Lillig CH. How does iron-sulfur cluster coordination regulate the activity of human glutaredoxin 2? *Antioxid Redox Signal*. 2007 Jan;9(1):151-7.

[57] Haunhorst P, Berndt C, Eitner S, Godoy JR, Lillig CH. Characterization of the human monothiol glutaredoxin 3 (PICOT) as iron-sulfur protein. *Biochem Biophys Res Commun*. 2010 Apr 2;394(2):372-6.

[58] Kumar S, Holmgren A. Induction of thioredoxin, thioredoxin reductase and glutaredoxin activity in mouse skin by TPA, a calcium ionophore and other tumor promoters. *Carcinogenesis*. 1999 Sep;20(9):1761-7.

[59] Nakamura H, Bai J, Nishinaka Y, Ueda S, Sasada T, Ohshio G, et al. Expression of thioredoxin and glutaredoxin, redox-regulating proteins, in pancreatic cancer. *Cancer Detect Prev*. 2000;24(1):53-60.

[60] Welss T, Papoutsaki M, Michel G, Reifenberger J, Chimenti S, Ruzicka T, et al. Molecular basis of basal cell carcinoma: analysis of differential gene expression by differential display PCR and expression array. *Int J Cancer*. 2003 Mar 10;104(1):66-72.

[61] Fernandes AP, Capitanio A, Selenius M, Brodin O, Rundlof AK, Bjornstedt M. Expression profiles of thioredoxin family proteins in human lung cancer tissue: correlation with proliferation and differentiation. *Histopathology*. 2009 Sep;55(3):313-20.

[62] Cha MK, Kim IH. Preferential overexpression of glutaredoxin3 in human colon and lung carcinoma. *Cancer Epidemiol*. 2009 Oct;33(3-4):281-7.

[63] Ohayon A, Babichev Y, Pasvolsky R, Dong G, Sztarkier I, Benharroch D, et al. Hodgkin's lymphoma cells exhibit high expression levels of the PICOT protein. *J Immunotoxicol*. 2010 Mar;7(1):8-14.

[64] Qu Y, Wang J, Ray PS, Guo H, Huang J, Shin-Sim M, et al. Thioredoxin-like 2 regulates human cancer cell growth and metastasis via redox homeostasis and NF-kappaB signaling. *J Clin Invest*. 2011 Jan 4;121(1):212-25.

[65] Said K, Glaumann H, Bjornstedt M, Bergquist A. The value of thioredoxin family proteins and proliferation markers in dysplastic and malignant gallbladders in patients with primary sclerosing cholangitis. *Digestive diseases and sciences*. 2012 May;57(5):1163-70.

[66] Lonn ME, Hudemann C, Berndt C, Cherkasov V, Capani F, Holmgren A, et al. Expression pattern of human glutaredoxin 2 isoforms: identification and

characterization of two testis/cancer cell-specific isoforms. *Antioxid Redox Signal.* 2008 Mar;10(3):547-57.
[67] Ferri A, Fiorenzo P, Nencini M, Cozzolino M, Pesaresi MG, Valle C, et al. Glutaredoxin 2 prevents aggregation of mutant SOD1 in mitochondria and abolishes its toxicity. *Hum Mol Genet.* 2010 Nov 15;19(22):4529-42.
[68] Beer SM, Taylor ER, Brown SE, Dahm CC, Costa NJ, Runswick MJ, et al. Glutaredoxin 2 catalyzes the reversible oxidation and glutathionylation of mitochondrial membrane thiol proteins: implications for mitochondrial redox regulation and antioxidant DEFENSE. *J Biol Chem.* 2004 Nov 12;279(46):47939-51.
[69] Lillig CH, Lonn ME, Enoksson M, Fernandes AP, Holmgren A. Short interfering RNA-mediated silencing of glutaredoxin 2 increases the sensitivity of HeLa cells toward doxorubicin and phenylarsine oxide. *Proceedings of the National Academy of Sciences of the United States of America.* 2004 Sep 7;101(36):13227-32.
[70] Enoksson M, Fernandes AP, Prast S, Lillig CH, Holmgren A, Orrenius S. Overexpression of glutaredoxin 2 attenuates apoptosis by preventing cytochrome c release. *Biochemical and biophysical research communications.* 2005 Feb 18;327(3):774-9.
[71] Wu WS. The signaling mechanism of ROS in tumor progression. *Cancer Metastasis Rev.* 2006 Dec;25(4):695-705.
[72] Anathy V, Aesif SW, Guala AS, Havermans M, Reynaert NL, Ho YS, et al. Redox amplification of apoptosis by caspase-dependent cleavage of glutaredoxin 1 and S-glutathionylation of Fas. *J Cell Biol.* 2009 Jan 26;184(2):241-52.
[73] Linares GR, Xing W, Govoni KE, Chen ST, Mohan S. Glutaredoxin 5 regulates osteoblast apoptosis by protecting against oxidative stress. *Bone.* 2009 May;44(5):795-804.
[74] Du Y, Zhang H, Lu J, Holmgren A. Glutathione and glutaredoxin act as a backup of human thioredoxin reductase 1 to reduce thioredoxin 1 preventing cell death by aurothioglucose. *J Biol Chem.* 2012 Nov 2;287(45):38210-9.
[75] Cha H, Kim JM, Oh JG, Jeong MH, Park CS, Park J, et al. PICOT is a critical regulator of cardiac hypertrophy and cardiomyocyte contractility. *J Mol Cell Cardiol.* 2008 Dec;45(6):796-803.
[76] Kren L, Brazdil J, Hermanova M, Goncharuk VN, Kallakury BV, Kaur P, et al. Prognostic significance of anti-apoptosis proteins survivin and bcl-2 in non-small cell lung carcinomas: a clinicopathologic study of 102 cases. Appl Immunohistochem *Mol Morphol.* 2004 Mar;12(1):44-9.
[77] Cheng NH, Zhang W, Chen WQ, Jin J, Cui X, Butte NF, et al. A mammalian monothiol glutaredoxin, Grx3, is critical for cell cycle progression during embryogenesis. *FEBS J.* 2011 Jul;278(14):2525-39.
[78] Shelton MD, Kern TS, Mieyal JJ. Glutaredoxin regulates nuclear factor kappa-B and intercellular adhesion molecule in Muller cells: model of diabetic retinopathy. *J Biol Chem.* 2007 Apr 27;282(17):12467-74.
[79] Allen EM, Mieyal JJ. Protein-thiol oxidation and cell death: regulatory role of glutaredoxins. *Antioxidants & redox signaling.* 2012 Dec 15;17(12):1748-63.
[80] Adachi T, Pimentel DR, Heibeck T, Hou X, Lee YJ, Jiang B, et al. S-glutathiolation of Ras mediates redox-sensitive signaling by angiotensin II in vascular smooth muscle cells. *J Biol Chem.* 2004 Jul 9;279(28):29857-62.

[81] Murata H, Ihara Y, Nakamura H, Yodoi J, Sumikawa K, Kondo T. Glutaredoxin exerts an antiapoptotic effect by regulating the redox state of Akt. *J Biol Chem.* 2003 Dec 12;278(50):50226-33.

[82] Caito S, Rajendrasozhan S, Cook S, Chung S, Yao H, Friedman AE, et al. SIRT1 is a redox-sensitive deacetylase that is post-translationally modified by oxidants and carbonyl stress. *FASEB J.* 2010 Sep;24(9):3145-59.

[83] Kim Y, Chay KO, Kim I, Song YB, Kim TY, Han SJ, et al. Redox regulation of the tumor suppressor PTEN by glutaredoxin 5 and Ycp4. *Biochem Biophys Res Commun.* 2011 Apr 1;407(1):175-80.

[84] Qanungo S, Starke DW, Pai HV, Mieyal JJ, Nieminen AL. Glutathione supplementation potentiates hypoxic apoptosis by S-glutathionylation of p65-NFkappaB. *J Biol Chem.* 2007 Jun 22;282(25):18427-36.

[85] Martinez-Outschoorn UE, Balliet RM, Rivadeneira DB, Chiavarina B, Pavlides S, Wang C, et al. Oxidative stress in cancer associated fibroblasts drives tumor-stroma co-evolution: A new paradigm for understanding tumor metabolism, the field effect and genomic instability in cancer cells. *Cell Cycle.* 2010 Aug 15;9(16):3256-76.

[86] Weinberg RA. Coevolution in the tumor microenvironment. *Nat Genet.* 2008 May;40(5):494-5.

[87] Rubartelli A, Bonifaci N, Sitia R. High rates of thioredoxin secretion correlate with growth arrest in hepatoma cells. *Cancer Res.* 1995 Feb 1;55(3):675-80.

[88] Banerjee R. Redox outside the box: linking extracellular redox remodeling with intracellular redox metabolism. *J Biol Chem.* 2012 Feb 10;287(7):4397-402.

[89] Chaiswing L, Zhong W, Liang Y, Jones DP, Oberley TD. Regulation of prostate cancer cell invasion by modulation of extra- and intracellular redox balance. *Free Radic Biol Med.* 2012 Jan 15;52(2):452-61.

[90] Lundberg M, Fernandes AP, Kumar S, Holmgren A. Cellular and plasma levels of human glutaredoxin 1 and 2 detected by sensitive ELISA systems. *Biochemical and biophysical research communications.* 2004 Jul 2;319(3):801-9.

[91] Bjornstedt M, Xue J, Huang W, Akesson B, Holmgren A. The thioredoxin and glutaredoxin systems are efficient electron donors to human plasma glutathione peroxidase. *J Biol Chem.* 1994 Nov 25;269(47):29382-4.

[92] Peltoniemi MJ, Rytila PH, Harju TH, Soini YM, Salmenkivi KM, Ruddock LW, et al. Modulation of glutaredoxin in the lung and sputum of cigarette smokers and chronic obstructive pulmonary disease. *Respiratory research.* 2006;7:133.

[93] Giannoni E, Parri M, Chiarugi P. EMT and oxidative stress: a bidirectional interplay affecting tumor malignancy. *Antioxid Redox Signal.* 2012 Jun 1;16(11):1248-63.

[94] Maillet A, Pervaiz S. Redox regulation of p53, redox effectors regulated by p53: a subtle balance. *Antioxid Redox Signal.* 2012 Jun 1;16(11):1285-94.

[95] Cui X. Reactive oxygen species: the achilles' heel of cancer cells? *Antioxid Redox Signal.* 2012 Jun 1;16(11):1212-4.

[96] Reynaert NL, van der Vliet A, Guala AS, McGovern T, Hristova M, Pantano C, et al. Dynamic redox control of NF-kappaB through glutaredoxin-regulated S-glutathionylation of inhibitory kappaB kinase beta. *Proc Natl Acad Sci U S A.* 2006 Aug 29;103(35):13086-91.

[97] Trachootham D, Zhou Y, Zhang H, Demizu Y, Chen Z, Pelicano H, et al. Selective killing of oncogenically transformed cells through a ROS-mediated mechanism by beta-phenylethyl isothiocyanate. *Cancer Cell.* 2006 Sep;10(3):241-52.
[98] Gupta SC, Hevia D, Patchva S, Park B, Koh W, Aggarwal BB. Upsides and downsides of reactive oxygen species for cancer: the roles of reactive oxygen species in tumorigenesis, prevention, and therapy. *Antioxid Redox Signal.* 2012 Jun 1;16(11):1295-322.
[99] Wells WW, Rocque PA, Xu DP, Meyer EB, Charamella LJ, Dimitrov NV. Ascorbic acid and cell survival of adriamycin resistant and sensitive MCF-7 breast tumor cells. *Free Radic Biol Med.* 1995 Apr;18(4):699-708.
[100] Meyer EB, Wells WW. Thioltransferase overexpression increases resistance of MCF-7 cells to adriamycin. *Free radical biology & medicine.* 1999 Mar;26(5-6):770-6.
[101] Godoy JR, Oesteritz S, Hanschmann EM, Ockenga W, Ackermann W, Lillig CH. Segment-specific overexpression of redoxins after renal ischemia and reperfusion: protective roles of glutaredoxin 2, peroxiredoxin 3, and peroxiredoxin 6. *Free Radic Biol Med.* 2011 Jul 15;51(2):552-61.
[102] Yun N, Kim C, Cha H, Park WJ, Shibayama H, Park IS, et al. Caspase-3-mediated cleavage of PICOT in apoptosis. *Biochemical and biophysical research communications.* 2013 Mar 15;432(3):533-8.
[103] Hagihara K, Kazui M, Kurihara A, Ikeda T, Izumi T. Glutaredoxin is involved in the formation of the pharmacologically active metabolite of clopidogrel from its GSH conjugate. *Drug metabolism and disposition: the biological fate of chemicals.* 2012 Sep;40(9):1854-9.
[104] Nilsonne G, Sun X, Nystrom C, Rundlof AK, Potamitou Fernandes A, Bjornstedt M, et al. Selenite induces apoptosis in sarcomatoid malignant mesothelioma cells through oxidative stress. *Free Radic Biol Med.* 2006 Sep 15;41(6):874-85.
[105] Lopez-Lazaro M, Willmore E, Elliott SL, Austin CA. Selenite induces topoisomerase I and II-DNA complexes in K562 leukemia cells. *Int J Cancer.* 2008 Nov 1;123(9):2217-21.
[106] Wallenberg M, Olm E, Hebert C, Bjornstedt M, Fernandes AP. Selenium compounds are substrates for glutaredoxins: a novel pathway for selenium metabolism and a potential mechanism for selenium-mediated cytotoxicity. *The Biochemical journal.* 2010 Jul 1;429(1):85-93.
[107] Olm E, Fernandes AP, Hebert C, Rundlof AK, Larsen EH, Danielsson O, et al. Extracellular thiol-assisted selenium uptake dependent on the x(c)- cystine transporter explains the cancer-specific cytotoxicity of selenite. *Proc Natl Acad Sci U S A.* 2009 Jul 7;106(27):11400-5.
[108] Madeja Z, Sroka J, Nystrom C, Bjorkhem-Bergman L, Nordman T, Damdimopoulos A, et al. The role of thioredoxin reductase activity in selenium-induced cytotoxicity. *Biochem Pharmacol.* 2005 Jun 15;69(12):1765-72.
[109] Arner ES, Nakamura H, Sasada T, Yodoi J, Holmgren A, Spyrou G. Analysis of the inhibition of mammalian thioredoxin, thioredoxin reductase, and glutaredoxin by cis-diamminedichloroplatinum (II) and its major metabolite, the glutathione-platinum complex. *Free Radic Biol Med.* 2001 Nov 15;31(10):1170-8.

[110] Qu Y, Wang J, Sim MS, Liu B, Giuliano A, Barsoum J, et al. Elesclomol, counteracted by Akt survival signaling, enhances the apoptotic effect of chemotherapy drugs in breast cancer cells. *Breast Cancer Res Treat.* 2010 Jun;121(2):311-21.

[111] Nagai M, Vo NH, Shin Ogawa L, Chimmanamada D, Inoue T, Chu J, et al. The oncology drug elesclomol selectively transports copper to the mitochondria to induce oxidative stress in cancer cells. *Free Radic Biol Med.* 2012 May 15;52(10):2142-50.

[112] O'Day SJ, Eggermont AM, Chiarion-Sileni V, Kefford R, Grob JJ, Mortier L, et al. Final results of phase III SYMMETRY study: randomized, double-blind trial of elesclomol plus paclitaxel versus paclitaxel alone as treatment for chemotherapy-naive patients with advanced melanoma. *J Clin Oncol.* 2013 Mar 20;31(9):1211-8.

[113] Tabata C, Terada T, Tabata R, Yamada S, Eguchi R, Fujimori Y, et al. Serum thioredoxin-1 as a diagnostic marker for malignant peritoneal mesothelioma. *J Clin Gastroenterol.* 2013 Jan;47(1):e7-11.

[114] Berghella AM, Pellegrini P, Del Beato T, Ciccone F, Contasta I. The potential role of thioredoxin 1 and CD30 systems as multiple pathway targets and biomarkers in tumor therapy. *Cancer Immunol Immunother.* 2011 Oct;60(10):1373-81.

[115] Odeh H, Hunker KL, Belyantseva IA, Azaiez H, Avenarius MR, Zheng L, et al. Mutations in Grxcr1 are the basis for inner ear dysfunction in the pirouette mouse. *Am J Hum Genet.* 2010 Feb 12;86(2):148-60.

[116] Hakansson KO, Ostergaard H, Winther JR. Crystallization of mutant forms of glutaredoxin Grx1p from yeast. A*cta Crystallogr Sect F Struct Biol Cryst Commun.* 2006 Sep 1;62(Pt 9):920-2.

[117] Porras P, Padilla CA, Krayl M, Voos W, Barcena JA. One single in-frame AUG codon is responsible for a diversity of subcellular localizations of glutaredoxin 2 in Saccharomyces cerevisiae. *J Biol Chem.* 2006 Jun 16;281(24):16551-62.

[118] Hashemy SI, Johansson C, Berndt C, Lillig CH, Holmgren A. Oxidation and S-nitrosylation of cysteines in human cytosolic and mitochondrial glutaredoxins: cffects on structure and activity. *J Biol Chem.* 2007 May 11;282(19):14428-36.

[119] Camaschella C, Campanella A, De Falco L, Boschetto L, Merlini R, Silvestri L, et al. The human counterpart of zebrafish shiraz shows sideroblastic-like microcytic anemia and iron overload. *Blood.* 2007 Aug 15;110(4):1353-8.

[120] Ye H, Jeong SY, Ghosh MC, Kovtunovych G, Silvestri L, Ortillo D, et al. Glutaredoxin 5 deficiency causes sideroblastic anemia by specifically impairing heme biosynthesis and depleting cytosolic iron in human erythroblasts. *J Clin Invest.* 2010 May;120(5):1749-61.

[121] Zhou Q, Chipperfield H, Melton DA, Wong WH. A gene regulatory network in mouse embryonic stem cells. *Proc Natl Acad Sci U S A. 2007* Oct 16;104(42):16438-43.

[122] Jeong D, Kim JM, Cha H, Oh JG, Park J, Yun SH, et al. PICOT attenuates cardiac hypertrophy by disrupting calcineurin-NFAT signaling. *Circ Res.* 2008 Mar 28;102(6):711-9.

[123] Jeong D, Cha H, Kim E, Kang M, Yang DK, Kim JM, et al. PICOT inhibits cardiac hypertrophy and enhances ventricular function and cardiomyocyte contractility. *Circ Res.* 2006 Aug 4;99(3):307-14.

[124] Reinbothe TM, Ivarsson R, Li DQ, Niazi O, Jing X, Zhang E, et al. Glutaredoxin-1 mediates NADPH-dependent stimulation of calcium-dependent insulin secretion. *Mol Endocrinol.* 2009 Jun;23(6):893-900.

[125] Ivarsson R, Quintens R, Dejonghe S, Tsukamoto K, in 't Veld P, Renstrom E, et al. Redox control of exocytosis: regulatory role of NADPH, thioredoxin, and glutaredoxin. *Diabetes*. 2005 Jul;54(7):2132-42.

In: Free Radicals
Editor: Bill Stone
ISBN: 978-1-63117-177-2

Chapter V

Pharmacological Ascorbate: Oxidative Stress and the Treatment of Pancreatic Cancer

John A. Cieslak, M.D., Ph.D. and Joseph J. Cullen, M.D. *

Free Radical and Radiation Biology Program, Departments of Surgery and Radiation Oncology, Holden Comprehensive Cancer Center, University of Iowa Hospitals and Clinics and the University of Iowa College of Medicine, Iowa City, IA, US

Abstract

Adenocarcinoma of the pancreas remains the 4th leading cause of cancer related deaths in the United States and is steadily increasing in incidence. Whereas notable advances have been made in the treatment of other cancers, new therapies in the treatment of pancreatic cancer have been lacking, and the prognosis remains dismal. However, recent studies have demonstrated that high dose intravenous, pharmacological ascorbate (ascorbic acid, vitamin C) induces cytotoxicity and oxidative stress selectively in pancreatic cancer cells vs. normal cells, suggesting a promising new role of ascorbate as a therapeutic agent. At physiologic concentrations, ascorbate functions as a reducing agent and antioxidant. However, in the presence of catalytic metal ions and at pharmacological levels, ascorbate can induce oxidative stress through the generation of hydrogen peroxide (H_2O_2). Ascorbate absorption and excretion is a tightly regulated process, resulting in micromolar concentrations when ascorbate is taken orally. However, when pharmacological ascorbate is given intravenously, millimolar levels are achieved. This knowledge rekindled interest into the clinical potential of pharmacological ascorbate in the treatment of cancer and several new studies into its efficacy and mechanisms of action were launched. Recent *in vitro* and *in vivo* studies have demonstrated ascorbate oxidation occurs extracellularly, generating H_2O_2 flux into cells resulting in oxidative stress. Pancreatic cancer cells have increased sensitivity to ascorbate-induced cytotoxicity compared to normal cells, which may be due to the lower levels of antioxidant enzymes

* Corresponding Author Address: Department of Surgery, 1528 JCP, University of Iowa College of Medicine, Iowa City, IA 52242; Email: joseph-cullen@uiowa.edu

and higher endogenous levels of reactive oxygen species that occur in cancer cells. Pharmacologic ascorbate also inhibits the growth of pancreatic tumor xenografts and displays synergistic cytotoxic effects when combined with gemcitabine in pancreatic cancer. Phase I trials of pharmacological ascorbate in pancreatic cancer patients have demonstrated safety and potential efficacy. In this chapter we will review the mechanism of ascorbate-induced cytotoxicity, examine the use of pharmacological ascorbate in treatment and assess the current data supporting its efficacy as an adjuvant in pancreatic cancer.

Keywords: ascorbate, oxidative stress, hydrogen peroxide, pancreatic cancer, cancer therapy

Abbreviations

hydrogen peroxide (H_2O_2)
5-fluorouracil (5-FU)
oxaliplatin, irinotecan, fluorouracil, and leucovorin (FOLFIRINOX)
ascorbate radical ($Asc^{\bullet-}$)
dehydroascorbic acid (DHA)
glucose transporters (GLUTs)
ascorbate anion ($AscH^-$)
hydroxyl radicals ($HO^\bullet$)
alkoxyl radicals ($RO^\bullet$)
peroxyl radicals ($LOO^\bullet$)
thiol radicals ($GS^\bullet$)
superoxide radical ($O_2^{\bullet-}$)
L-Ascorbate 2-phosphate (A2P)
superoxide dismutase (SOD)
1,3 *bis* (2-chloroethyl)-1-nitrosurea (BCNU)
2-deoxy-D-glucose (2DG)
glutathione disulfide reductase (GR)
glucose-6-phosphate dehydrogenase (G6PD)
Quality of Life (QOL)
Clinical Global Impression of Change (CGIC)
dose-limiting toxicity (DLT)
maximum tolerated dose (MTD)

Introduction and Background

Pancreatic Cancer

The commonly used term "pancreatic cancer" typically refers to ductal adenocarcinoma of the pancreas. Derived from the exocrine pancreas, these tumors represent 85% of all pancreatic neoplasms. Adenocarcinoma of the pancreas is the fourth leading cause of cancer related death in the United States and second only to colorectal cancer as a cause of digestive cancer-related death. Furthermore its incidence is steadily increasing [1]. Current National Cancer Institute SEER (Surveillance Epidemiology and End Results) data estimates that 45,220 men and women (22,740 men, 22,480 women) will be diagnosed with pancreatic cancer in calendar year 2013 (age-adjusted incidence rate of 12.2 per 100,000 men and women per year) [2]. The median age at diagnosis for cancer of the pancreas is 71 years of age. The prognosis is dismal, with an overall 5-year relative survival rate of only 6%, and median age at death of 73 (age-adjusted death rate of 10.9 per 100,000 men and women per year) [2-4]. Indeed, the challenge in treating such an aggressive and deadly cancer was reflected in a recent NCI cancer bulletin article on pancreatic cancer, "the slow but steady march toward more individualized care in cancer medicine has left pancreatic cancer behind. Patients diagnosed with this disease live no longer today than patients diagnosed two decades ago, despite more than a dozen large clinical trials. Even as many patients with other cancers have benefited from targeted drugs, pancreatic cancer remains as deadly as ever" [5].

One of the primary difficulties in treating this disease is its late presentation. Presenting symptoms vary based on tumor location within the pancreas, with the most commonly reported symptoms being abdominal/epigastric pain, jaundice, and anorexia/weight loss, and these symptoms are most commonly associated with cancers located within the head of the pancreas (60-70% of pancreatic cancers) [6]. Currently, surgical resection via pancreaticoduodenectomy is the only potentially curative treatment, but unfortunately only 15-20% of patients have surgically resectable disease at the time of presentation, with 40% of patients presenting with metastatic disease and the remaining patients presenting with locally advanced tumors.

Even with complete resection, prognosis is poor, with expected 5-year survival rates of approximately 25% [7-10]. For locally advanced and metastatic disease, median survival is approximately 10 and 6 months, respectively [11]. For the majority of patients with pancreatic cancer, adjuvant chemotherapy (and in certain cases combination radiotherapy) remains the only treatment option with the goal of palliating symptoms and improving quality of life [12]. During the 1990's several studies investigated the use of gemcitabine as a new chemotherapeutic in the treatment of pancreatic cancer as an alternative to the previously established therapy, 5-fluorouracil (5-FU). A clear improvement of the one-year median survival rate in patients treated with gemcitabine over those who received 5-FU was observed (18 vs. 2%, p=0.0001), as well as a reduction in pain intensity and daily analgesic consumption, and an improvement in performance status (p=0.002) [13]. For many years since that time, gemcitabine was the standard of care in the adjuvant chemotherapeutic treatment for advance pancreatic cancer patients. However, a recent multi-site randomized control trial of a chemotherapy regimen consisting of oxaliplatin, irinotecan, fluorouracil, and leucovorin (FOLFIRINOX), showed 4.3 months increased survival compared to patients treated with gemcitabine, as well as prolonged progression-free survival [14]. However, while FOLFIRINOX showed a survival benefit, it was associated with more severe adverse events and added toxicity, which were not well tolerated by many patients. Despite this, FOLFIRINOX is now considered the first line standard of care treatment for advanced pancreatic cancer. Even with the modest improvement in survival time attained with FOLFIRINOX, several clinical trials of multiple new therapies have been performed, and no drug or combination of drugs has significantly improved the overall prognosis [12-15].

Ascorbate (Ascorbic Acid, Vitamin C)

Ascorbate (ascorbic acid, Vitamin C) is an essential nutrient for humans and plays a role in several important biochemical functions. Ascorbic acid is a water-soluble ketolactone with two ionizable hydroxyl groups, making it an excellent reducing agent and anti-oxidant at physiologic concentrations. Indeed, it readily undergoes two consecutive, one electron oxidations to form ascorbate radical ($Asc^{\bullet -}$) and dehydroascorbic acid (DHA), though the ascorbate radical is relatively unreactive due to resonance stabilization of the unpaired electron [16]. Though ascorbate oxidizes readily, its rate of oxidation is pH dependent and can be further accelerated by the presence of catalytic metal ions [17]. At physiological pH, the autoxidation of ascorbate is fairly slow, with a rate constant of approximately 300 M^{-1} s^{-1}[18].

Biologically, ascorbate functions across a various range of cell and organ systems as an anti-oxidant. In general, intracellular ascorbate concentrations are higher than extracellular fluids, reaching millimolar concentrations in circulating neutrophils, lymphocytes, monocytes, and platelets [19, 20]. The exception to this finding seems to be erythrocytes, which have intracellular ascorbate levels similar to extracellular plasma [21, 22]. High levels of intracellular ascorbate are hypothesized to help maintain an intracellular reducing environment, but it has also been demonstrated that ascorbate can help quench extracellular oxidants by transferring electrons across the plasma membrane, or through efflux of ascorbate itself (as observed in astrocyte transfer of ascorbate to nearby neurons) [23, 24]. Furthermore, millimolar levels of ascorbate are found in the cornea and lens of the eye, which may help protect them from solar radiation damage [25, 26].

Besides its role as an antioxidant, ascorbate functions as a co-factor in various enzymatic pathways. In humans, the highest concentration of ascorbate is found in the adrenal and pituitary glands, where it acts as a physiologic reductant in the conversion of dopamine to norepinephrine, and as a co-factor for peptidyl glycine α-amidating monooxygenase [26-29]. It is also a known cofactor for Fe^{2+}-2-oxoglutarate dioxygenases, where it is necessary for maintaining iron in the ferrous state – required for the full activity of these enzymes [30, 31]. Fe^{2+}-2-oxoglutarate dioxygenases serve several biologically important functions, including: the promotion of collagen synthesis, and its proper assembly [32, 33]; regulation of hypoxia-inducible transcription factor (HIF) – with over 800 target genes, yielding more than 60 gene products involved in angiogenesis, cell survival, glucose uptake, glycolysis and iron homeostasis [34-37]; and a cofactor in histone demethylation [38-41], to name a few.

Ascorbate can be synthesized from glucose in plants and most animals. Humans and other primates, however, lack functional L-gulonolactone oxidase; the enzyme required for the last step of ascorbate synthesis, and are dependent on dietary intake to maintain essential stores [43]. Both ascorbate and dehydroascorbic acid (DHA) are absorbed via the enterocytes of the small intestine. Ascorbate absorption is mediated by Na^+-dependent vitamin C transporters (SVCTs), whereas DHA is absorbed by Na^+-independent facilitative glucose transporters (GLUTs) [43-46]. Because plasma glucose concentrations are much higher than plasma DHA concentrations (mM vs. μM respectively), the majority of intracellular ascorbate is due to absorption via SVCTs, rather than indirectly through DHA absorption via GLUTs [47, 48]. Besides the brush border of enterocytes, SVCTs are also found within the renal tubular cells. Furthermore, plasma ascorbate concentrations are tightly regulated; both by the limited affinity of SVCT for ascorbate, as well as by a negative feedback loop in which high intracellular ascorbate concentrations leads to down-regulation of SVCT present on the enterocyte membranes [49-51]. Pharmacokinetic modeling has shown that it is a combination of saturable intestinal absorption, tissue accumulation, and renal re-absorption and excretion that determines the bioavailability of ascorbate [16, 52, 53]. Thus, the bioavailability of orally administered ascorbate is much lower than when administered intravenously because of this tight regulation of absorption by the gut. Indeed, fasting plasma concentrations of ascorbic acid achievable through oral vs. i.v. administration of the drug result in micromolar vs. millimolar levels, respectively [53].

At physiologic concentrations and pH, ascorbate anion ($AscH^-$) functions primarily as a reducing agent and antioxidant, readily donating an electron to potentially damaging free radicals such as hydroxyl radicals ($HO^•$), alkoxyl radicals ($RO^•$), peroxyl radicals ($LOO^•$), and thiol radicals ($GS^•$), as well playing a pivotal role in the prevention of LDL and lipid peroxidation synergistically with vitamin E [16, 54-57]. The oxidation of ascorbate anion produces ascorbate radical ($Asc^{•-}$), which is relatively unreactive and is reduced back to ascorbate by NADH/NADPH reductases [58]. Interestingly, in the presence of catalytic metal ions, ascorbate can also function as a pro-oxidant and induce oxidative stress [17, 59, 60]. Ascorbate reduces ferric iron to ferrous iron, which is then free to react with oxygen, producing superoxide radical ($O_2^{•-}$). Superoxide radical then dismutates into hydrogen peroxide (H_2O_2), which in turn reacts with ferrous iron through the Fenton reaction, resulting in a cascade of reactive oxygen species (ROS). This process also occurs in the absence of catalytic metals through autoxidation of ascorbate, albeit at a slower rate.

Ascorbate as a Cancer Therapeutic Agent

As early as the 1950's, it was suggested that ascorbate may limit the spread of cancer [61]. It was hypothesized that ascorbate inhibited hyaluronidases, preventing the breakdown of the extracellular matrix and therefore cancer cell migration [62, 63]. Parenteral ascorbate first demonstrated clinical benefit in the treatment of cancer in the early trials of Cameron, Pauling, and Campbell in the 1970s, with treatment correlating with decreased tumor growth, tumor regression, and increased survival time [64-67]. Cameron and Campbell published case reports of 50 patients treated with high-dose ascorbate, with some report of benefit [64]. Cameron and Pauling then published a follow up study of 100 patients with terminal cancer who were given intravenous ascorbate that showed that patients who received ascorbate survived 300 days longer than retrospective control patients with similar disease [67]. However, two randomized, double-blinded clinical trials performed at the Mayo Clinic between 1979 and 1985 utilizing *orally* administered ascorbate (10 g per day) showed no difference in symptoms or survival between treatment groups and placebo controls, and ascorbate was dismissed as a potential chemotherapeutic agent in the treatment of cancer by the research and medical communities [68, 69].

It was only later realized after pharmacokinetic studies that the bioavailability of orally administered ascorbate is much lower than when administered intravenously [19, 70]. Oral doses of ascorbate ranging from 30 to 100 mg daily produced average fasting plasma concentrations of only 60 μM. Even doses of 1000 mg daily produced average fasting plasma concentrations of only 75-80 μM. There were minimal further increases in plasma concentrations when daily doses were increased to 2500 mg [19, 53, 70]. As discussed above, the tight regulation of plasma ascorbate concentration is a result of the combination of saturable intestinal absorption, tissue accumulation, and renal re-absorption and excretion [16, 52, 53]. Riordan and associates found that intravenous administration of ascorbate produced peak plasma concentrations approximately 25-fold higher than that attained by the same dose given orally [71]. Thus, potentially therapeutic doses are attainable only through parenteral administration [72]. Rodent studies using intraperitoneal dosing of ascorbate (mimicking intravenous infusions in humans), confirmed that only parenteral injection could produce pharmacologic ascorbate concentrations similar to those obtained by i.v. infusion in humans [73-74] These data suggest that the lack of efficacy of ascorbate as a cancer treatment as determined by the Mayo Clinic studies may have been due to the fact that patients were receiving sub-therapeutic doses throughout the trials. This knowledge rekindled interest into the clinical potential of pharmacological ascorbate in the treatment of cancer and several new studies into its efficacy and mechanisms of action were launched.

Ascorbate Induced Cytotoxicity in Pancreatic Cancer

In Vitro Studies

Selective cytotoxicity of pharmacologic ascorbate on cancer cells was first demonstrated *in vitro* by Chen *et al.* in 2005 [76]. In their study, cell death in 10 cancer cell lines and 4 normal cell types was measured after one-hour exposure to up to 20 mM ascorbate. Cancer cell lines studied included one human lymphoma and one human colon cell line, three human breast cancer cell lines, and lung, kidney, colon, and melanoma cell lines from mice. Normal cells were unaffected by 20 mM ascorbate, where as all but one cancer cell line showed decreased survival with ascorbate exposure; 5 of which had EC_{50} doses < 4 mM. Interestingly, cell death was suggested to be dependent upon H_2O_2 formation. Shortly after, the same laboratory expanded their study to 43 cancer cell lines [73]. Again, the results were impressive, with EC_{50} doses of ascorbate less than 10 mM for 34 of the 43 cell lines investigated (75%), and with normal cells insensitive to concentrations of ascorbate exceeding 20 mM. This study did include one pancreatic cancer cell line (Pan02), which was exceedingly sensitive to ascorbate ($EC_{50} \approx$ 1mM). Furthermore, the addition of catalase to the medium ameliorated death of ovarian carcinoma (Ovcar5), pancreatic carcinoma (Pan02), and glioblastoma (9L) cells exposed to 10 mM ascorbate (1 h), supporting their earlier finding that cytotoxicity was mediated by H_2O_2. These studies demonstrated that pharmacological doses of ascorbate achievable by parenteral administration of the drug have selective toxicity against cancer cells vs. normal cells, and paved the way for additional studies on the efficacy of pharmacologic ascorbate and mechanism of action in additional cancer cell lines.

In a the first study specific to pancreatic cancer cell susceptibility to ascorbate, Du et al. demonstrated selective sensitivity of three pancreatic cancer cell lines (MIA PaCa-2, AsPC-1, and BxPC-3) vs. a normal immortalized pancreatic ductal epithelial cell line (H6c7) to 1 hour treatment with both 5 and 10 mM ascorbate [77]. All of the pancreatic cancer cell lines demonstrated decreased cell metabolic viability as well as decreased clonogenic survival when treated with ascorbate [78, 79]. This study demonstrated a time and dose-dependent increase in measured H_2O_2 production with increased concentrations of ascorbate leading to the hypothesis that ascorbate associated H_2O_2 production induced oxidative stress within cancer cells, leading to caspase-independent cell death consistent with autophagy. Indeed, when cells were treated with scavengers of H_2O_2, ascorbate-associated decreases in clonogenic survival could be reversed. It was suggested that the difference in sensitivity observed in cancer cells vs. normal cells toward ascorbate might be explained by the low levels of antioxidant enzymes and high levels of endogenous ROS in cancer cells [16, 80-82].

In Vivo Studies

Before studies of cancer cell cytotoxicity could be performed *in vivo*, it first had to be demonstrated that animals exhibit the same relationship between oral and parenteral ascorbate, as do humans. Rodent studies using intraperitoneal dosing of ascorbate confirmed that only parenteral injection could produce pharmacologic ascorbate concentrations similar to those obtained by i.v. infusion in humans [73-75]. One study in mice showed that a bolus intravenous injection of ascorbate at a dose of 1g kg^{-1} resulted in plasma concentration of 15 mM, whereas supplementation of the drinking water with the same dose only increased plasma concentration to 50 μM [75]. Once confirmed that pharmacologic concentrations of ascorbate can only be attained via parenteral administration in animals, studies were designed to test for ascorbate-induced cytotoxicity *in vivo*.

In 2008, Chen *et al.* published the first *in vivo* study of pharmacologic ascorbate on tumors xenografts in mice [73]. In mice bearing glioblastoma xenografts, a single pharmacologic dose of ascorbate produced sustained concentrations of both ascorbate radical and hydrogen peroxide within the interstitial fluids of the tumor. In contrast, the same pharmacologic ascorbate concentrations in whole blood generated little detectable ascorbate radical and no detectable H_2O_2. Using a microdialysis technique, the authors were able to show that the putative metallocatalyst for the generation of ascorbate radical and H_2O_2 was present within extracellular fluids, including tumor interstitial space [83]. However, the lack of ascorbate radical and peroxide in the blood suggested that erythrocytes were acting as a sink, actively recycling $Asc^{\bullet-}$ and H_2O_2 through more efficient and redundant H_2O_2 catabolic pathways relative to the extracellular fluid, including high levels of associated catalase, glutathione peroxidase and membrane associated ascorbate radical reductase [84-89]. Therefore, pharmacologic ascorbate may serve as a pro-drug for H_2O_2 delivery to the extracellular milieu, without accumulation in blood. This may also help explain why ascorbate is selectively cytotoxic to cancer cells rather than normal tissues.

In the extracellular space and interstitial fluid of the tumor, it was proposed that the catalytic activity needed for the generation of $Asc^{\bullet-}$ and H_2O_2 was provided by metal ions associated with protein collected there [76]. It is known that tumor vessels have much higher permeability compared to normal endothelium and this permits the accumulation of macromolecules such as proteins in the interstitial fluid [90-91]. Furthermore, iron, copper, and other catalytic metals are known to associate with damaged protein within the extracellular fluid [92-94]. These data suggest an explanation as to why ascorbate radical and hydrogen peroxide were found in sustainable concentrations in the interstitial fluids of the tumor after a single dose of pharmacologic ascorbate. Furthermore, the H_2O_2 generated by ascorbate oxidation in the extracellular space could accumulate to concentrations greater than found intracellularly, resulting in a net diffusion across the cell membrane, resulting in greater toxicity to tumor cells [16, 83] (Figure 1).

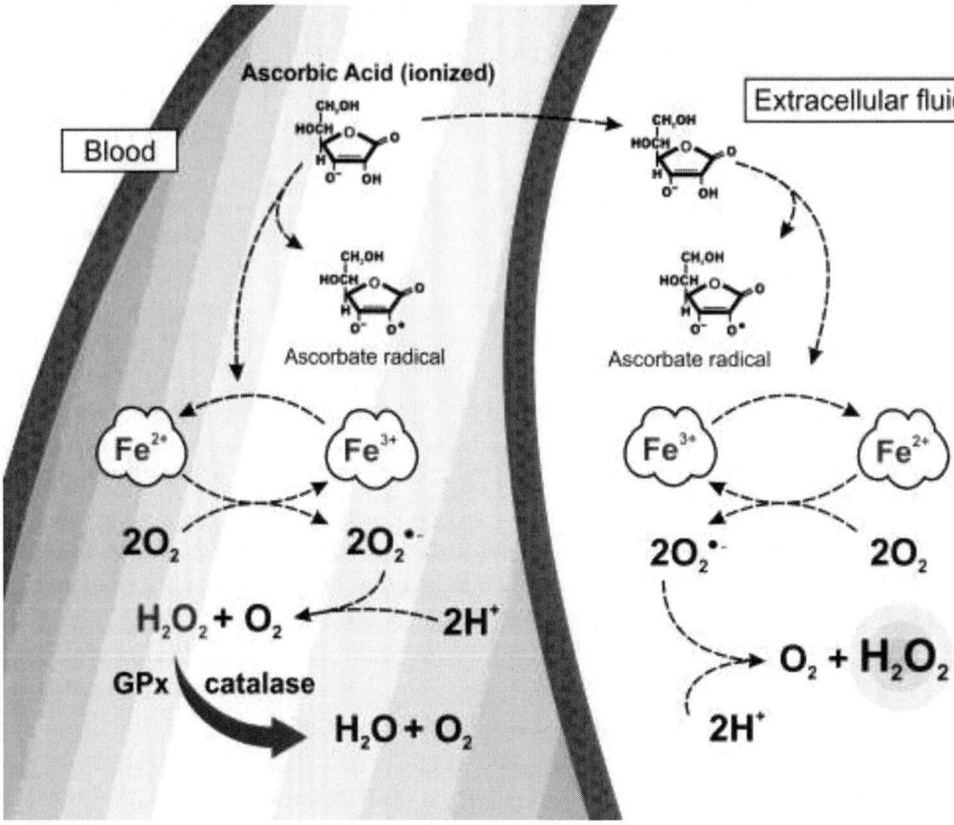

Figure 1. Possible mechanism of ascorbate oxidation generating H_2O_2 in extracellular fluid. Ascorbate undergoes oxidation with metal catalysts forming H_2O_2. In blood H_2O_2 is converted to water and oxygen due to the abundance of catalase and glutathione peroxidase so that H_2O_2 is not detectable and without evidence of systemic oxidative stress. However, in the extracellular fluid, pharmacologic ascorbate reacts with metal ion catalysts subsequently forming H_2O_2. This production of extracellular H_2O_2 diffuses into cells causing cell death. Thus, pharmacological ascorbate is a pro-drug for delivery of H_2O_2 *in vitro* and *in vivo*.

In the same study, Chen *et al.* investigated the efficacy of pharmacologic ascorbate administration on the growth of ovarian (Ovcar5), pancreatic (Pan02), and glioblastoma (9L) tumors in nude mice. A treatment dose of 4 g ascorbate/kg body weight, administered intraperitoneally twice daily (once daily for Pan02 tumors) commenced after tumors reached a palpable size of 5–7 mm in diameter. Treatment was continued for 30, 12, and 13 days, respectively. Parenteral ascorbate as the only treatment significantly decreased both tumor growth rates and overall weight by 41–53% (P=0.04–0.001) for Ovcar5, Pan02, and 9L tumors [73].

In 2010, Du *et al.* published a complimentary study focusing on pancreatic tumor xenografts [77]. MIA PaCa-2 tumor cells were injected into the flank region of nude mice and tumors were allowed to grow to between 3 and 4 mm in dimension before treatment was initiated. The treatment group received 4 g/kg ascorbate intraperitoneally, twice daily for 14 days. Animals were sacrificed once tumors reached a predetermined size of 1,000 mm^3. Animals that received ascorbate had significantly slower tumor growth when compared with animals that received saline ($P < 0.001$). Furthermore, there was a greater than 3-fold decrease in tumor size in animals receiving ascorbate when compared to those treated with saline ($P < 0.001$). On day 21 of the experiment, the control group had a mean tumor volume of 472 mm^3, whereas the ascorbate group had a mean tumor volume of 138 mm^3. Log-rank analyses of survival showed that the animals that received ascorbate had increased survival compared with controls (68 days versus 78 days, $P < 0.0001$). All mice completed the treatment period, with none of the animals having to be sacrificed for continued weight loss or cachexia, further supporting the hypothesis that pharmacologic ascorbate is non-toxic to normal, healthy cells and tissues. In combination, the *in vitro and in vivo* studies of Chen *et al.* and Du *et al.*, strongly suggested that pharmacologic doses of ascorbate achievable in humans might have potential for therapy in pancreatic cancer.

Mechanism of Ascorbate Induced Cytotoxicity in Pancreatic Cancer

As noted above, the administration of pharmacologic ascorbate is associated with the formation of hydrogen peroxide in the extracellular fluid surrounding a tumor [17, 59. 60. 73, 76, 77, 83, 95]. In the presence of catalytic metal ions, ascorbate functions as a pro-oxidant and induces oxidative stress, but even in the absence of metals the autoxidation of ascorbate generates significant amounts of H_2O_2 when ascorbate is at millimolar concentrations [17, 59, 60]. Because ascorbate readily oxidizes to produce H_2O_2, pharmacologic ascorbate has been proposed as a pro-drug for the delivery of peroxide to tumors [16, 73, 76, 77, 83]. H_2O_2 generation is dependent on ascorbate concentration and incubation time, and has a linear relationship with ascorbate radical formation [83]. Peroxide can affect both extracellular and intracellular targets, as it is permeable across lipid membranes [96, 97]. Extracellular H_2O_2 may attack membrane lipids forming lipid hydroperoxides and causing leaky membranes. Intracellularly, oxidative stress and DNA damage promotes cell death, possibly via autophagy. This mechanism has been substantiated both *in vitro* and *in vivo* by the studies of Chen *et al.*, and Du *et al.* (see above) [73, 76, 77, 83].

Furthermore, it has been demonstrated that increasing intracellular levels of ascorbate does not enhance cytotoxicity. L-Ascorbate 2-phosphate (A2P) is a form of ascorbate that is protected from oxidation by the presence of a phosphate moiety. A2P binds to cell membranes where the phosphate group is hydrolyzed by cell membrane associated esterases, resulting in the transport of ascorbate into cells [98-100]. The addition of A2P to cell culture media will increase intracellular ascorbate to millimolar levels [101]. However, Olney *et al.* showed that the addition of A2P to treatment with pharmacological ascorbate does not enhance cytotoxicity in MIA PaCa-2 cells [102]. Indeed, cells treated with A2P showed no changes in clonogenic survival when compared to controls, while cells treated with ascorbate had significant decreases in clonogenic survival. Additionally, clonogenic survival was similar in cells treated with the combination of A2P and ascorbate when compared to ascorbate alone, suggesting that increases in intracellular ascorbate are not responsible for the ascorbate-induced cytotoxicity observed when ascorbate is added to the extracellular medium. These data support the hypothesis that ascorbate-induced cytotoxicity is due to the formation of extracellular H_2O_2, which then diffuses into the cell and causes cytotoxicity as opposed to intracellular ascorbate oxidation.

Further evidence supporting the importance of H_2O_2 production in selective cancer cell cytotoxicity is offered by experiments that have investigated the neutralization of peroxide by endogenous and exogenous catalase. Klingelhoeffer *et al.* demonstrated differential sensitivity to ascorbate and H_2O_2 by pretreatment with extracellular exogenous catalase, which they also correlated with endogenous intracellular catalase production in 11 cancer cell lines [103]. Sensitivity of three pancreatic cancer cell lines (MIA PaCa-2, AsPC-1, and BxPC-3) to pharmacologic ascorbate was reversed both by the pretreatment of cells with exogenous catalase (extracellular), as well as by overexpression of intracellular catalase by transfecting cells using adenovirus containing catalase cDNA [77]. Additionally, ascorbate toxicity has been enhanced in Ehrlich ascites carcinoma cells *in vitro* by treatment with the catalase inhibitor aminotriazole [104]. Taken together, these studies suggest that extracellular pharmacologic ascorbate mediates cancer cell death by H_2O_2 formation [53].

The role of catalytic metal ions in the formation of H_2O_2 via pharmacologic ascorbate cannot be understated. In the presence of iron, ascorbate is oxidized rapidly as it reduces Fe^{3+} to Fe^{2+}, which is then free to react with oxygen, producing superoxide radical ($Fe^{2+} + O_2 \rightarrow Fe^{3+} + O_2^{\bullet-}$). Superoxide radical then dismutates into hydrogen peroxide ($O_2^{\bullet-} + O_2^{\bullet-} + 2H^+ \rightarrow H_2O_2 + O_2$), which in turn reacts with ferrous iron through the Fenton reaction producing hydroxyl radical ($Fe^{2+} + H_2O_2 \rightarrow Fe^{3+} + HO^\bullet$). The presence of ascorbate can allow the recycling of Fe^{3+} to Fe^{2+}, which in turn will catalyze the formation of highly reactive oxidants from H_2O_2[16].

The quantity and availability of catalytic metal ions available to induce the pro-oxidant effects of ascorbate may play a significant role in the amount of resulting cytotoxicity. Normally, iron is not free in solution but is sequestered by iron binding proteins such as transferrin and ferritin [105, 106]. Transferrin is the major iron transport protein, moving iron absorbed in the diet from enterocytes to the cell surface where it binds to transferrin receptor, promoting endocytosis and internalization of the protein. Once intracellular, the iron is released from transferrin where it is bound to ferritin, the iron storage protein.

In pathological states, such as thalassemia and hemochromatosis, free iron is found in the plasma and extracellular fluid. Chronic inflammatory diseases are also associated with increased oxidative stress and levels of catalytic metal ions in tissues. For example, decreased levels of ascorbate and increased deposition of iron protein has been demonstrated in the synovial membranes in patients with rheumatoid arthritis [107, 108]. Additionally, septic patients have been found to have increased catalytic iron levels with decreased ascorbate concentrations [109]. In these situations the administration of ascorbate without an iron chelator could potentially lead to extensive oxidative tissue damage, similar to what is observed in ischemia/reperfusion injury [17, 110, 111].

In this same light, it has been shown that patients with various malignancies have elevated serum levels of ferritin [112-114]. It is known that in cancer, tumor vessels have increased permeability compared to normal endothelium, permitting the accumulation of macromolecules such as protein into the interstitial fluid [90, 91]. As discussed above, the presence of extracellular metal-containing proteins is thought to be essential for the pro-oxidant effects of ascorbate [59, 83]. Given the increase in ferritin in cancer, and the potential for its extracellular accumulation, it has been proposed that iron-saturated ferritin may be the source of catalytic iron required for the selective ascorbate-induced cytotoxicity observed in pancreatic and other cancers [16]. Indeed, ferritin staining was detected in the stroma surrounding the neoplastic cells of breast cancer tissue [115], and serum ferritin levels have been shown to correlate to the tumor stage and volume in cervical cancer [116]. Furthermore, it is known that iron can be released from ferritin by biological reductants, including ascorbate [67]. Therefore, increased ferritin may provide a continuous source of catalytic iron required for pharmacologic ascorbate-mediated H_2O_2 production and cytotoxicity.

As to why ascorbate seems to have selective toxicity against tumor cells vs. normal cells, a few hypotheses have already been discussed: 1) the difference in sensitivity observed in cancer cells vs. normal cells toward ascorbate may be explained by the low levels of antioxidant enzymes and high levels of endogenous ROS in cancer cells [16, 80-82]. 2) Erythrocytes act as a sink for $Asc^{\bullet-}$ and especially H_2O_2 due to redundant H_2O_2 catabolic pathways relative to the extracellular fluid, preventing peroxide buildup in the blood and delivery to healthy tissues, while ensuring H_2O_2 delivery to the extracellular milieu (Figure 1).

Enhancement of Ascorbate-Induced Cytotoxicity in Pancreatic Cancer

Because catalytic metals are known to increase the rate of ascorbate-induced peroxide formation and therefore oxidative stress-mediated cytotoxicity, the question has been raised if redox-active metals can also be provided exogenously. Porphyrin-based superoxide dismutase (SOD) mimetics contain a catalytic redox-active metal (Mn, Fe, or Cu) coordinated within a stable porphyrin ring. In the presence of a reducing agent such as ascorbate, manganese porphyrins function as superoxide reductases rather than dismutases, with Mn(III) reduced to Mn(II) by ascorbate, allowing Mn(II) to react with O_2 forming superoxide, which can then form peroxide [16]. Several studies have demonstrated enhanced ascorbate oxidation using manganese porphyrins *in vitro*, with synergistic killing of prostatic, pancreatic, and hepatic cancer cell lines vs. pharmacologic ascorbate alone [117, 118]. It is also advantageous that manganese porphyrins have already been tested alone *in vivo* and have low toxicities at micromolar concentrations [119]. Therefore, there is great potential for the use of these porphyrins as adjuvants to enhance the efficacy of pharmacologic ascorbate in the treatment of pancreatic cancer in the future.

In this same regard, oxidative stress has been shown to increase the levels of catalytic iron in tissues; ionizing radiation and some chemotherapeutic drugs have been shown to do the same [120-122]. Therefore, it is entirely feasible that combination therapies, such as chemotherapy plus pharmacologic ascorbate, and radiation therapy plus pharmacologic ascorbate would act synergistically to potentiate ascorbate-induced cytotoxicity *in vivo*. This is an important consideration because in the mouse studies performed by Du *et al.* (discussed above), pharmacologic ascorbate as a single agent was cytostatic rather than cytotoxic, i.e., high dose i.v. ascorbate did not completely eliminate pancreatic cancer tumors from the mice but rather slowed their growth rate, resulting in decreased tumor volume – the treatment was not curative.

To test for synergism between chemotherapy and ascorbate, Espey *et al.,* studied pharmacologic ascorbate in combination with gemcitabine, the standard of care chemotherapeutic in pancreatic cancer at the time, both *in vitro* and *in vivo* [123]. Pharmacologic ascorbate was found to enhance gemcitabine cytotoxicity in eight pancreatic cell lines (7 human, 1 murine). Furthermore, as the ratio of ascorbate to gemcitabine was increased, cell death elicited per unit gemcitabine increased, suggesting that when used in combination, a lower gemcitabine dose could be used to obtain the same antitumor activity (as indicated by a dose reduction index > 1) [53]. Indeed, gemcitabine doses could be decreased 2 to 6 logs when combined with pharmacologic concentrations of ascorbate. To determine whether pancreatic cancer cell growth rate dictated sensitivity to gemcitabine and ascorbate, *in vitro* doubling times were analyzed. The authors found no correlation between growth rate and ascorbate sensitivity, but a positive correlation between growth rate and sensitivity to both gemcitabine alone and combination therapy. To further examine these results *in vivo,* PAN-02 and PANC-1 cell line xenografts were placed into mice as representative gemcitabine-sensitive and gemcitabine-resistant pancreatic carcinomas, respectively. In both cases, combination of gemcitabine-ascorbate therapy resulted in significantly larger decreases in tumor volume compared to gemcitabine alone. The effect was quite striking in the PANC-1 gemcitabine resistant tumors in which tumor volume decreased 52% with combined gemcitabine/ascorbate therapy compared with a decrease of only 4% when treated with gemcitabine alone ($P = 0.002$) [123]. These findings are promising and demonstrate that combining clinically achievable concentrations of pharmacologic ascorbate with gemcitabine increases the chemosensitivity of pancreatic cancer cells *in vitro* and *in vivo*, and that pharmacologic ascorbate synergizes with gemcitabine to improve therapeutic efficacy.

As previously discussed, the cytotoxicity of pharmacologic ascorbate is directly related to the production of H_2O_2 in the extracellular space, and its flux into cancer cells, resulting in oxidative stress, DNA damage, and ultimately cell death. In a recent study, Olney *et al.* proposed that inhibiting intracellular hydroperoxide removal during the administration of pharmacologic ascorbate would increase the cytotoxicity observed in pancreatic cancer cells [102]. Human pancreatic cancer cells were treated with ascorbate alone or in combination with intracellular inhibitors of H_2O_2 removal including the glutathione disulfide reductase inhibitor 1,3 *bis* (2-chloroethyl)-1-nitrosurea (BCNU), siRNA targeted to glutathione disulfide reductase (siGR), and an inhibitor of glucose metabolism, 2-deoxy-D-glucose (2DG). Also, endogenous catalase (removal of H_2O_2 via reduction to water) activity was inhibited using aminotriazole so that ascorbate-induced changes in intracellular H_2O_2 could be determined.

BCNU is a clinically used chemotherapeutic agent that causes DNA alkylation but is also known to inhibit glutathione disulfide reductase (GR). With GR inhibited, cells have reduced ability to remove H_2O_2 via the glutathione peroxidase system. 2DG is a glucose analog and a competitive inhibitor for uptake via the glucose transporters. Competition between 2DG and glucose is thought to cause inhibition of glucose metabolism, thereby creating a chemically induced state of glucose deprivation resulting in inhibition of hydroperoxide detoxification [79]. Likewise, knockdown of endogenous GR protein levels using siRNA could also prevent H_2O_2 via the glutathione peroxidase system.

The authors found that inhibitors of peroxide metabolism increased ascorbate induced cytotoxicity, as well as intracellular H_2O_2 concentrations. Pancreatic cancer cells treated with BCNU alone had no effect on clonogenic survival or viability, whereas with the combination of BCNU and ascorbate, clonogenic survival dramatically decreased. Similarly, utilizing siGR to decrease endogenous GR levels by >50%, the authors demonstrated significant decreases in clonogenic survival in cells treated with siGR + ascorbate, vs. siGR or ascorbate alone ($P < 0.001$). Finally, using the glucose analog 2DG, experiments demonstrated that combination treatment with 2DG and ascorbate enhanced cytotoxicity with decreased clonogenic survival and cell viability in pancreatic cancer cell lines [102]. When endogenous catalase activity was inhibited using aminotriazole, the authors were also able to demonstrate significantly increased intracellular H_2O_2 concentrations using all three methodologies of inhibiting hydroperoxide removal discussed above. Taken collectively, these data demonstrate that inhibitors of H_2O_2 removal enhance the increase in the intracellular steady-state concentration of H_2O_2 induced by treatment with pharmacological ascorbate, and therefore cytotoxicity to pancreatic cancer cells. Thus, treatments consisting of a combination of ascorbate and inhibitors of the removal of H_2O_2 may potentially be an effective therapy for pancreatic adenocarcinoma.

Phase I Clinical Trials of Ascorbate in Pancreatic Cancer

Intravenous Ascorbate in Patients with Advanced Cancers to Investigate Dose Tolerance, Pharmacokinetics, Plasma Concentrations and Safety

Since ascorbate had demonstrated few adverse events in case reports of human trials, it was expected that i.v. ascorbate therapy would be safe in most patients. However, there were reasons to be cautious. Because ascorbate acts as a pro-drug for the delivery of H_2O_2, high dose ascorbate can induce intravascular hemolysis in patients with glucose-6-phosphate dehydrogenase (G6PD) deficiency that cannot efficiently regenerate glutathione, a scavenger of peroxide in the blood [124-126]. In patients with pre-existing renal insufficiency or past medical history of kidney stones, there is also a risk of forming calcium oxalate crystals within the urinary space, as oxalic acid is one of the end products of ascorbate oxidation[127]. Additionally, because of the rapid oxidation of ascorbate into H_2O_2 by catalytic metals, administration of pharmacologic ascorbate to individuals with iron overload (hemochromatosis, thalassemia, and other conditions requiring multiple transfusions) is likely contraindicated [71, 128]. Finally, in the early trials of Cameron and Campbell, there have been rare cases of massive tumor hemorrhage reported after administration of high-dose i.v. ascorbate in patients with advanced cancers [64, 129]. At this time, several phase I clinical trials of intravenous ascorbate in patients with advanced cancers have been performed [74, 130-133]. The main focus of these initial trials has been pharmacokinetics, dosing, resulting ascorbate plasma concentrations, and most importantly safety. In addition, some trials have also examined the clinical consequences of the pharmacologic ascorbate therapy.

In 2004, Riordan *et al.* published case reports of patients with renal cell carcinoma, breast cancer, pancreatic cancer and lymphoma in which i.v. ascorbate was administered in doses of 10 to 100 grams/day, up to three times per week, with improved patient well being, and in some cases reduced tumor size, with minimal toxicity [134]. Based on these reports Riordan and colleagues performed a phase I clinical trial the following year in which 24 late stage terminal cancer patients were given continuous infusions of ascorbate at doses of 150 to 710 mg/kg/day for up to eight weeks [131]. During therapy, serum ascorbate concentrations ranged from 0.28 to 3.8 mM, with a mean of 1.1 mM. The most commonly reported adverse events reported during the study were minor and included nausea, dry mouth, dry skin and minor edema. Two Grade 3 adverse events were reported as 'possibly related' to the ascorbate, including one patient who developed a kidney stone (but who had prior history of kidney stones) and another patient who developed hypokalemia after six weeks of treatment. Blood creatinine, blood urea nitrogen, glucose, and uric acid concentrations where monitored during the duration of therapy and either decreased or remained stable in all patients demonstrating that high-dose intravenous ascorbate does not adversely affect renal function at the doses studied, and was well-tolerated provided that the patient did not have a prior history of kidney stones.

In 2008, Hoffer *et al.* performed a phase I dose-escalating and pharmacokinetic study of i.v. ascorbate in patients with advanced malignancies with the primary objective of determining a recommended dosage for phase II trials, and secondary objectives of determining any adverse effects, any anti-tumor effects, and patient quality of life during treatment [74]. Ascorbate was administered three times per week at fixed doses of 0.4, 0.6, 0.9, and 1.5 g/kg. During therapy, serum ascorbate concentrations ranged from 2.4 to 26 mM. At the highest dosage (1.5 g/kg), pharmacokinetic studies determined that plasma ascorbate concentrations exceeding 10 mM were achievable for approximately 4.5 hours, levels that are known to induce cytotoxicity in a variety of cancer cells [73, 76, 77]. Adverse effects were mild and included nausea, headache, abdominal cramping, diarrhea, flushing and vomiting. Virtually all the side effects that occurred were consistent with the side effects expected from the rapid infusion of any high osmolarity solution. The symptoms were preventable by encouraging patients to drink fluids before and during the infusion. No unusual biochemical or hematologic abnormalities were observed during the study. The authors reported that patients whose ascorbate dose was $\geq$ 0.6 g/kg maintained their physical quality of life throughout the trial, whereas those at the lowest dose did not. None of the patients were found to have objective tumor responses to the treatment, and all patients eventually experienced disease progression. In the end, the study concluded that 1.5 g/kg ascorbic acid infused three times weekly is essentially free of risk and major side effects. The authors recommended 1.5 g/kg as the starting dose for future phase II trials, but noted that this is not the absolute maximal tolerated dose, as the potential for larger or more frequent dosing might also be tolerated [74]. Furthermore, they concluded that ascorbate might need to be combined with cytotoxic or other redox-active molecules to be an efficacious treatment.

In 2012, a phase I clinical trial was performed by Takahashi *et al.* that exclusively examined the impact of pharmacologic ascorbate therapy on the quality of life in patients with cancer [133]. In this prospective, observational study, 60 patients with various newly diagnosed malignant cancers receiving adjuvant intravenous ascorbate were asked to fill out a Quality of Life (QOL) questionnaire developed by the European Organization of Research and Treatment of Cancer (EORTC) before initiating treatment, and then after 2 and 4 weeks of therapy [135, 136]. The questionnaire addressed global health status as a function of "Functional Scales," including physical, role, emotional, cognitive and social functioning, as well as "Symptom Scales," including fatigue, nausea/vomiting, pain, dyspnea, insomnia, appetite loss, constipation, diarrhea and financial difficulties. In addition, attending physicians who were treating the patients were asked to fill out a Clinical Global Impression of Change (CGIC) survey at 2 and 4 weeks post i.v. ascorbate therapy [137].

Patients received pharmacologic ascorbate with biweekly infusions and target blood ascorbate concentrations of 350-400 mg/dL immediately following infusion [138]. The study did not address peak plasma ascorbate levels or clinical disease progression. Interestingly, the QOL scores significantly improved at both 2 weeks ($p < 0.05$) and 4 weeks ($p < 0.01$) of treatment, compared to initial scores. In the "Functional Scales," patients showed significant increases in physical, role, emotional, cognitive and social functioning after 4 weeks of intravenous ascorbate therapy. Furthermore, patients showed significant relief of fatigue, pain, insomnia, constipation and financial difficulties scores in the "Symptoms Scales." According to the CGIC, attending physicians demonstrated that 47% of their patients at two weeks and 60% of their patients at four weeks had minimally, to much improved quality of life. At the conclusion of their study, the authors proposed that pharmacologic ascorbate therapy can safely improve the quality of life of cancer patients, and suggest further use of i.v. ascorbate as a palliative care procedure, focusing on improving QOL, and in particular relief from fatigue.

Most recently, Stephenson *et al.,* performed an additional phase I clinical trial to evaluate the safety, tolerability, and pharmacokinetics of high dose pharmacologic ascorbate as a monotherapy in patients with advanced cancers which were refractory to standard therapy [132]. The authors proposed that the relatively poor anticancer response observed in the prior phase I studies with ascorbate was either due to inadequate concentrations of ascorbate achieved within the systemic compartment, or failure to achieve the adequate duration of elevated concentration necessary for cytotoxicity. Their goal was to obtain higher blood levels, longer exposure times, and higher dose intensity to better assess both toxicity and potential for antitumor efficacy.

In the study, five cohorts of three patients received i.v. ascorbate for 4 consecutive days per week, for 4 weeks. The ascorbate was administered at 1 g/min starting at a total dose of 30 g/m^2 in the first cohort. Subsequent cohorts would have the dose increased by 20 g/m^2 until a maximum tolerated dose was found. To do this, the authors monitored for a dose-limiting toxicity (DLT), defined as any reversible adverse event $\geq$ grade 3. If a DLT was observed in $\geq$ 2 patients, then the maximum tolerated dose (MTD) would be defined as the dose just below the dose at which the DLT was observed. Data were obtained for cohorts treated with 30, 50, 70, 90, and 110 g/m^2.

Pharmacokinetics showed that ascorbate was eliminated by simple first-order kinetics and did not accumulate to any significant level during consecutive daily administrations. The half life (2.0 ± 0.6 h) and clearance rate values (21 ± 5 dL/h m^2) of ascorbate were similar for all patients across all the cohorts. The maximum plasma concentration (C_{max}) and area under the curve (AUC – the time spent at a given plasma concentration, i.e., bioavailability), increased proportionately with increasing ascorbate doses before maxing out at 70 g/m^2. A C_{max} value of 49 mM was obtained for the 70 and 90 g/m^2 doses, whereas the 110 g/m^2 dose produced a C_{max} value of 37 mM. Each of the three highest doses maintained plasma ascorbate levels between 10-20 mM for 5-6 hours. Even at the higher doses intravenous ascorbate was well tolerated, again with the most common side effects being headache and nausea. Other reported adverse events included hypertension, insomnia, loss of appetite, fatigue, chills, and hyperglycemia. Unfortunately, none of the patients in the study experienced any objective tumor response from the treatments, with 3 patients having stable disease and the rest with tumor progression. Because a C_{max} of 49 mM was obtained with 70 g/m^2 without further increase at higher doses, a treatment dose of 70-80 g/m^2 is recommended for future studies of pharmacologic ascorbate to provide patients with the highest possible drug exposure benefits without subjecting them to unnecessarily higher doses and infusion times.

Collectively, the studies discussed above have demonstrated that i.v. ascorbate is safe and well tolerated. The relatively mild side effects related to its administration are thought to be due to its high osmolality and include nausea, vomiting, headache, dry mouth, flushing, diarrhea and minor edema [74, 130-132]. These symptoms were widely preventable by encouraging patients to drink fluids before and during the infusion [74]. Additionally, Takahashi *et al.* suggest that pharmacologic ascorbate therapy can improve patients QOL and relieve certain symptoms related to cancer burden, including fatigue [133]. The one major side effect directly attributable to pharmacologic ascorbate seems to be the risk of subsequent kidney stone formation in patients with prior history of stones [131]. Importantly, Stephenson *et al.,* have now demonstrated plasma ascorbate concentrations up to 49 mM are attainable and levels of 10-20 mM are sustainable for 5-6 hours.

Pharmacological Ascorbate in the Treatment of Pancreatic Cancer: Clinical Trials

In 2012, Monti *et al.* published the results of a phase I clinical trial specifically aimed at examining the safety and efficacy of intravenous ascorbate in the treatment of patients with metastatic stage IV pancreatic ductal adenocarcinoma [130]. Fourteen patients were enrolled to receive intravenous ascorbate at either 50, 75, or 100 grams per infusion over 90-120 minutes, three times per week for 8 weeks, combined with the standard of care chemotherapy gemcitabine and erlotinib (an epidermal growth factor receptor inhibitor). Gemcitabine was administered intravenously at a dose of 1000 mg/m^2 over 30 minutes on day 1, once weekly for 7 weeks followed by a 1 week of rest. Erlotinib was given orally in a single daily dose of 100 mg per day for 8 weeks. The primary aim of the trial was assessing safety with a secondary aim of assessing response to treatment. Out of 14 patients who enrolled in the study, 9 patients completed the treatment (3 per dosage group). Of the 5 patients who did not complete the study, two subjects chose to discontinue the study because it was too difficult for them to come into the hospital for treatments, and three subjects died from rapid disease progression before completing therapy. At the beginning and end of the treatment cycle, patients received a CT scan that was evaluated by an expert radiologist who was blinded to the treatment group.

Overall, for the total cohort of 14 patients, 23 adverse events were reported, with the most common being nausea and mild lightheadedness. Of the 23 adverse events, 8 were considered serious and were attributed to progression of disease and/or concomitant treatment with gemcitabine and erlotinib. In patients receiving 100 grams of ascorbate, peak plasma levels of between 25 to 32 mM were reported. At the end of the study, 8 out of 9 patients who completed 8 weeks of treatments had reduction in the size of their primary tumor, and 1 patient's tumor was stable in size. By RECIST criteria, 7 patients had stable disease and 2 patients had progressive disease [139]. Progression-free survival time was similar to previously reported data from patients treated with gemcitabine/erlotinib alone.

Most importantly, Monti *et al.* demonstrated that there was no increased toxicity when pharmacologic ascorbate was added to gemcitabine and erlotinib treatments in patients with metastatic pancreatic cancer. With promising results, the combination therapy decreased primary tumor size in eight out of the nine subjects studied. The lack of improvement in progression-free survival with the addition of ascorbate might be explained by the fact that the duration of treatment may not have been sufficient.

More recently in 2013, Welsh *et al.* published the results of a phase I clinical trial performed at the University of Iowa examining the toxicity and efficacy of pharmacological ascorbate combined with gemcitabine in patients with stage IV pancreatic adenocarcinoma [140]. Fourteen subjects were enrolled to receive 15-125 g of ascorbate per infusion, twice weekly for 4 week cycles. The dose of ascorbate escalated each week and was tailored to each patient to achieve plasma ascorbate concentrations of ≥ 20 mM, In addition, each patient received 1000 mg/m^2 intravenous gemcitabine once weekly for 3 weeks followed by one week of rest. Ascorbate treatments cycles continued until a patient experienced a ≥ grade 3 dose limiting toxicity or until disease progression, as defined by the RECIST criteria [139]. CT imaging was obtained at baseline and then after completing every 2 cycles of therapy to assess for tumor progression. Disease burden, weight, performance status, hematologic and metabolic laboratories, time to progression and overall survival were monitored.

Nine subjects completed at least two cycles of treatment. No dose limiting toxicities or serious adverse effects attributable to intravenous ascorbate occurred during the study. The most common side effects reported were nausea, diarrhea and dry mouth. Pharmacologically, plasma ascorbate levels ranged from 20 to 25 mM in the first hour post-infusion, and mean trough levels remained significantly elevated compared to baseline levels in all subjects. Ascorbate radical was measured in pre and post-infusion blood samples, and was only detectable during pharmacological levels of ascorbate, consistent with a greatly increased rate of ascorbate oxidation [141]. Additionally, F_2-isoprostane levels were measured before and after ascorbate infusions as a marker of systemic oxidative stress [142]. In all patients, F_2-isoprostane levels were decreased after ascorbate infusions suggesting that ascorbate does not induce systemic oxidative stress, but rather acts as a tissue protectant and antioxidant systemically, while inducing pro-oxidant and cytotoxic effects that are localized to the tumor bed.

By the end of the study, six out of nine patients improved their overall performance status. Compared to the trial reported by Monti and colleagues, which only treated patients for 8 weeks, the average treatment duration in the Welsh *et al.* trial was 6 months. Additionally, no subjects were lost to follow-up. Encouraging to investigators, the mean time to disease progression was 26 ± 7 weeks, while mean overall survival was 13 ± 2 months, a significant improvement compared to trials of gemcitabine alone for advanced pancreatic cancer (mean progression free survival and mean overall survival of 9 weeks and 6 months, respectively) [13]. This study again demonstrated that the use of pharmacological ascorbate in combination with gemcitabine is safe and well tolerated. Combined, these studies provide a strong justification for the establishment of a phase II clinical trial sufficiently powered to determine the efficacy of pharmacological ascorbate combined with gemcitabine; the next step in the validation of this new and exciting therapy for the treatment of pancreatic cancer.

Future Directions

Pharmacological Ascorbate as an Adjuvant to Radiotherapy

For the majority of patients with pancreatic cancer, adjuvant chemotherapy and radiotherapy remain the only treatment option with the goal of palliating symptoms and improving quality of life [12]. Ionizing radiation has been shown to increase the levels of catalytic iron in tissues, which increases the rate of ascorbate-induced peroxide formation and cytotoxicity [17, 121]. Therefore, investigation into whether pharmacologic ascorbate acts synergistically with radiation therapy as a radio-sensitizer to increase radiation-induced pancreatic cancer cell death is of interest. Studies have shown that the sensitivity of glioblastoma multiforme cells to radiation was enhanced by exposure to pharmacological ascorbate [143]. Combination treatment was shown to increase the number of double stranded DNA breaks relative to that produced by radiation alone. Similar findings were demonstrated in the human leukemia cell line, HL60 [144].

Perspectives

Unfortunately, adenocarcinoma of the pancreas remains the 4th leading cause of cancer related deaths in the United States and continues to rise in incidence. The only chance of complete cure is offered by a major surgical resection of the tumor that often necessitates removal of surrounding structures, including the duodenum, the common bile duct, the gallbladder and a the portion of the pancreas itself. This procedure, technically known as a pancreaticoduodenectomy is also commonly known at the "Whipple procedure." Such a major procedure carries a high morbidity and mortality of ~5% across the United States as a whole. Even with complete resection, prognosis is poor, with expected 5-year survival rates of approximately 25%. Indeed, one of the primary difficulties in treating this disease is its late presentation with only 15-20% of patients have surgically resectable disease at the time of presentation, with 40% of patients presenting with metastatic disease and the remaining patients presenting with locally advanced tumors.

For the majority of patients with pancreatic cancer, adjuvant chemotherapy (and in certain cases combination radiotherapy) remains the only treatment option but survival remains poor. Current chemotherapeutic regimens can have significant toxicities and adverse events including febrile neutropenia, neutropenia, thrombocytopenia, sensory neuropathy and cardiac toxicity.

Pharmacologic ascorbate offers a new and exciting option in the treatment of pancreatic cancer. Although as a single agent it appears to be cytostatic rather than cytotoxic, ascorbate has been shown to work synergistically with chemotherapy and even radiation to enhance cytotoxicity and tumor cell death. Two phase I clinical trials have already demonstrated great promise in its efficacy. Importantly, parenteral ascorbate is extremely well tolerated with a mild side effect profile, and selective tumor cytotoxicity, even at millimolar plasma concentrations. With continued research and further trials, pharmacological ascorbate promises to be an effective therapy in the future battle against pancreatic cancer.

Summary

It has been over fifty years since ascorbate was described as a potential therapy for cancer. Parenteral ascorbate first demonstrated clinical benefit in the treatment of cancer in the early trials of Cameron, Pauling, and Campbell in the 1970s. Later Moertel conducted two randomized, double-blinded clinical trials at the Mayo Clinic between 1979 and 1985 utilizing orally administered ascorbate; neither study showed any benefit and ascorbate was dismissed as a potential chemotherapeutic agent in the treatment of cancer by the research and medical communities. It wasn't until relatively recently that studies showed that oral and i.v. ascorbate have strikingly different pharmacokinetic properties and that the bioavailability of orally administered ascorbate is much lower than when administered intravenously. Clinical data show that when ascorbate is given orally, fasting plasma concentrations are tightly controlled at <100 μmol/L. However, we now know that intravenous doses of ~ 80 g/m^2 are able to achieve plasma concentrations of up to 49 mmol! Thus, interest into the clinical potential of pharmacological ascorbate in the treatment of cancer was rekindled. Interestingly, at pharmacologic concentrations and in the presence of catalytic metal ions, ascorbate functions as a pro-oxidant and can induce oxidative stress via the generation of extracellular hydroperoxide (H_2O_2).

The selective cytotoxicity of pharmacologic ascorbate to tumor cells has been confirmed in several cancer cell lines in both *in* vitro and in *vivo* models in several laboratories. Several phase I trials have demonstrated that i.v. ascorbate is safe and well tolerated, with mild side effects and possible improvement in quality of life during treatment. Two recent phase I clinical trials investigating the safety and efficacy of pharmacologic ascorbate in combination with gemcitabine chemotherapy in the treatment of stage IV pancreatic adenocarcinoma were performed demonstrating safety without increased toxicity, with promising and possible efficacy.

This is an exciting time in the field of free radical and redox biology, specifically in the treatment of pancreatic cancer. Whereas notable advances have been made in the treatment of other cancers, new therapies in the treatment of pancreatic cancer have been lacking. However, encouraging studies thus far show promise for pharmacologic ascorbate as an adjuvant to existing chemotherapeutic and radiation therapies in pancreatic cancer.

References

[1] Siegel R, Naishadham D, Jemal A, Naishadham D. (2013) Cancer statistics, 2013. *CA Cancer J Clin*. 63:11-30.

[2] Howlader N NA, Krapacho M, Garshell J, Neyman N, Altekruse SF, Kosary CL, Yu M, Ruhl J, Tatalovich Z, Cho H, Mariotto A, Lewis DR, Chen HS, Feuer EJ, Cronin KA. SEER Cancer Statistics Review, 1975-2010. National Cancer Institute. Bethesda, MD, *http://seer.cancer.gov/csr/1975_2010/*, based on November 2012 SEER data submission, posted to the SEER web site, April 2013.

[3] Bramhall SR, Allum WH, Jones AG, Allwood A, Cummins C, Neoptolemos JP. Treatment and survival in 13,560 patients with pancreatic cancer, and incidence of the

disease, in the West Midlands: an epidemiological study. *The British journal of surgery.* 1995 Jan;82(1):111-5. PubMed PMID: 7881926.

[4] Yeo CJ, Cameron JL. Pancreatic cancer. *Current problems in surgery.* 1999 Feb;36(2):59-152. PubMed PMID: 10021685.

[5] Winstead E. Pancreatic Cancer Report Urges Changes in Clinical Trials: National Cancer Institute. Bethesda, MD; November, 1999. Volume 6 / Number 21:[Available from: *http://www.cancer.gov/ncicancerbulletin/archive/2009/110309/page2.*

[6] Porta M, Fabregat X, Malats N, Guarner L, Carrato A, de Miguel A, et al. Exocrine pancreatic cancer: symptoms at presentation and their relation to tumour site and stage. *Clinical & translational oncology : official publication of the Federation of Spanish Oncology Societies and of the National Cancer Institute of Mexico.* 2005 Jun;7(5):189-97. PubMed PMID: 15960930.

[7] Bakkevold KE, Kambestad B. Long-term survival following radical and palliative treatment of patients with carcinoma of the pancreas and papilla of Vater--the prognostic factors influencing the long-term results. A prospective multicentre study. *European journal of surgical oncology : the journal of the European Society of Surgical Oncology and the British Association of Surgical Oncology.* 1993 Apr;19(2):147-61. PubMed PMID: 7684003.

[8] Geer RJ, Brennan MF. Prognostic indicators for survival after resection of pancreatic adenocarcinoma. *American journal of surgery.* 1993 Jan;165(1):68-72; discussion -3. PubMed PMID: 8380315.

[9] Trede M, Schwall G, Saeger HD. Survival after pancreatoduodenectomy. 118 consecutive resections without an operative mortality. *Annals of surgery.* 1990 Apr;211(4):447-58. PubMed PMID: 2322039. Pubmed Central PMCID: 1358031.

[10] Yeo CJ, Cameron JL, Lillemoe KD, Sitzmann JV, Hruban RH, Goodman SN, et al. Pancreaticoduodenectomy for cancer of the head of the pancreas. 201 patients. *Annals of surgery.* 1995 Jun;221(6):721-31; discussion 31-3. PubMed PMID: 7794076. Pubmed Central PMCID: 1234702.

[11] Ghaneh P, Costello E, Neoptolemos JP. Biology and management of pancreatic cancer. *Gut.* 2007 Aug;56(8):1134-52. PubMed PMID: WOS:000247968700022. English.

[12] Di Marco M, Di Cicilia R, Macchini M, Nobili E, Vecchiarelli S, Brandi G, et al. Metastatic pancreatic cancer: is gemcitabine still the best standard treatment? (Review). *Oncology reports.* 2010 May;23(5):1183-92. PubMed PMID: 20372829.

[13] Burris HA, 3rd, Moore MJ, Andersen J, Green MR, Rothenberg ML, Modiano MR, et al. Improvements in survival and clinical benefit with gemcitabine as first-line therapy for patients with advanced pancreas cancer: a randomized trial. *Journal of clinical oncology : official journal of the American Society of Clinical Oncology.* 1997 Jun;15(6):2403-13. PubMed PMID: 9196156.

[14] Conroy T, Desseigne F, Ychou M, Bouche O, Guimbaud R, Becouarn Y, et al. FOLFIRINOX versus gemcitabine for metastatic pancreatic cancer. *The New England journal of medicine.* 2011 May 12;364(19):1817-25. PubMed PMID: 21561347.

[15] Ghaneh P, Neoptolemos J. Adjuvant chemotherapy - the standard after resection for pancreatic cancer. *American journal of surgery.* 2007 Oct;194(4A):S131-S7. PubMed PMID: WOS:000250084000027. English.

[16] Du J, Cullen JJ, Buettner GR. Ascorbic acid: chemistry, biology and the treatment of cancer. *Biochimica et biophysica acta.* 2012 Dec;1826(2):443-57. PubMed PMID: 22728050. Pubmed Central PMCID: 3608474.

[17] Buettner GR, Jurkiewicz BA. Catalytic metals, ascorbate and free radicals: combinations to avoid. *Radiation research.* 1996 May;145(5):532-41. PubMed PMID: 8619018.

[18] Williams NH, Yandell JK. Outer-Sphere Electron-Transfer Reactions of Ascorbate Anions. *Aust J Chem.* 1982;35(6):1133-44. PubMed PMID: WOS:A1982NU72100007. English.

[19] Levine M, Wang Y, Padayatty SJ, Morrow J. A new recommended dietary allowance of vitamin C for healthy young women. *Proceedings of the National Academy of Sciences of the United States of America.* 2001 Aug 14;98(17):9842-6. PubMed PMID: 11504949. Pubmed Central PMCID: 55540.

[20] Lloyd JV, Davis PS, Emery H, Lander H. Platelet ascorbic acid levels in normal subjects and in disease. *Journal of clinical pathology.* 1972 Jun;25(6):478-83. PubMed PMID: 4504974. Pubmed Central PMCID: 477361.

[21] Evans RM, Currie L, Campbell A. The distribution of ascorbic acid between various cellular components of blood, in normal individuals, and its relation to the plasma concentration. *The British journal of nutrition.* 1982 May;47(3):473-82. PubMed PMID: 7082619.

[22] Li H, Tu H, Wang Y, Levine M. Vitamin C in mouse and human red blood cells: an HPLC assay. *Analytical biochemistry.* 2012 Jul 15;426(2):109-17. PubMed PMID: 22522059.

[23] Lane DJ, Lawen A. Ascorbate and plasma membrane electron transport--enzymes vs efflux. *Free radical biology & medicine.* 2009 Sep 1;47(5):485-95. PubMed PMID: 19501649.

[24] Wilson JX. Antioxidant defense of the brain: a role for astrocytes. *Canadian journal of physiology and pharmacology.* 1997 Oct-Nov;75(10-11):1149-63. PubMed PMID: 9431439.

[25] Brubaker RF, Bourne WM, Bachman LA, McLaren JW. Ascorbic acid content of human corneal epithelium. *Investigative ophthalmology & visual science.* 2000 Jun;41(7):1681-3. PubMed PMID: 10845585.

[26] Kern HL, Zolot SL. Transport of vitamin C in the lens. *Current eye research.* 1987 Jul;6(7):885-96. PubMed PMID: 3621982.

[27] Hornig D. Distribution of ascorbic acid, metabolites and analogues in man and animals. *Annals of the New York Academy of Sciences.* 1975 Sep 30;258:103-18. PubMed PMID: 1106295.

[28] Rumsey SC, Levine M. Absorption, transport, and disposition of ascorbic acid in humans. *J Nutr Biochem.* 1998 Mar;9(3):116-30. PubMed PMID: WOS:000072679500001. English.

[29] Streeter ML, Rosso P. Transport mechanisms for ascorbic acid in the human placenta. *The American journal of clinical nutrition.* 1981 Sep;34(9):1706-11. PubMed PMID: 7282597.

[30] Ozer A, Bruick RK. Non-heme dioxygenases: cellular sensors and regulators jelly rolled into one? *Nature chemical biology.* 2007 Mar;3(3):144-53. PubMed PMID: 17301803.

[31] Englard S, Seifter S. The biochemical functions of ascorbic acid. *Annual review of nutrition.* 1986;6:365-406. PubMed PMID: 3015170.

[32] Kivirikko KI, Prockop DJ. Enzymatic hydroxylation of proline and lysine in protocollagen. *Proceedings of the National Academy of Sciences of the United States of America.* 1967 Mar;57(3):782-9. PubMed PMID: 16591531. Pubmed Central PMCID: 335576.

[33] Myllyharju J, Kivirikko KI. Collagens, modifying enzymes and their mutations in humans, flies and worms. *Trends in genetics : TIG.* 2004 Jan;20(1):33-43. PubMed PMID: 14698617.

[34] Bruick RK, McKnight SL. A conserved family of prolyl-4-hydroxylases that modify HIF. *Science.* 2001 Nov 9;294(5545):1337-40. PubMed PMID: 11598268.

[35] Mole DR, Blancher C, Copley RR, Pollard PJ, Gleadle JM, Ragoussis J, et al. Genome-wide association of hypoxia-inducible factor (HIF)-1alpha and HIF-2alpha DNA binding with expression profiling of hypoxia-inducible transcripts. *The Journal of biological chemistry.* 2009 Jun 19;284(25):16767-75. PubMed PMID: 19386601. Pubmed Central PMCID: 2719312.

[36] Semenza GL. Targeting HIF-1 for cancer therapy. *Nature reviews Cancer.* 2003 Oct;3(10):721-32. PubMed PMID: 13130303.

[37] Semenza GL. Hypoxia-inducible factors: mediators of cancer progression and targets for cancer therapy. *Trends in pharmacological sciences.* 2012 Apr;33(4):207-14. PubMed PMID: 22398146. Pubmed Central PMCID: 3437546.

[38] Chung TL, Brena RM, Kolle G, Grimmond SM, Berman BP, Laird PW, et al. Vitamin C promotes widespread yet specific DNA demethylation of the epigenome in human embryonic stem cells. *Stem cells.* 2010 Oct;28(10):1848-55. PubMed PMID: 20687155.

[39] Cloos PA, Christensen J, Agger K, Helin K. Erasing the methyl mark: histone demethylases at the center of cellular differentiation and disease. *Genes & development.* 2008 May 1;22(9):1115-40. PubMed PMID: 18451103. Pubmed Central PMCID: 2732404.

[40] Cyr AR, Domann FE. The redox basis of epigenetic modifications: from mechanisms to functional consequences. *Antioxidants & redox signaling.* 2011 Jul 15;15(2):551-89. PubMed PMID: 20919933. Pubmed Central PMCID: 3118659.

[41] Esteban MA, Pei D. Vitamin C improves the quality of somatic cell reprogramming. *Nature genetics.* 2012 Apr;44(4):366-7. PubMed PMID: 22456737.

[42] Nishikimi M, Fukuyama R, Minoshima S, Shimizu N, Yagi K. Cloning and chromosomal mapping of the human nonfunctional gene for L-gulono-gamma-lactone oxidase, the enzyme for L-ascorbic acid biosynthesis missing in man. *The Journal of biological chemistry.* 1994 May 6;269(18):13685-8. PubMed PMID: 8175804.

[43] Diliberto EJ, Jr., Heckman GD, Daniels AJ. Characterization of ascorbic acid transport by adrenomedullary chromaffin cells. Evidence for Na+-dependent co-transport. *The Journal of biological chemistry.* 1983 Nov 10;258(21):12886-94. PubMed PMID: 6630211.

[44] Savini I, Rossi A, Pierro C, Avigliano L, Catani MV. SVCT1 and SVCT2: key proteins for vitamin C uptake. *Amino acids.* 2008 Apr;34(3):347-55. PubMed PMID: 17541511.

[45] Vera JC, Rivas CI, Velasquez FV, Zhang RH, Concha, II, Golde DW. Resolution of the facilitated transport of dehydroascorbic acid from its intracellular accumulation as

ascorbic acid. *The Journal of biological chemistry.* 1995 Oct 6;270(40):23706-12. PubMed PMID: 7559541.

[46] Welch RW, Bergsten P, Butler JD, Levine M. Ascorbic acid accumulation and transport in human fibroblasts. *The Biochemical journal.* 1993 Sep 1;294 (Pt 2):505-10. PubMed PMID: 8373364. Pubmed Central PMCID: 1134483.

[47] Corpe CP, Tu H, Eck P, Wang J, Faulhaber-Walter R, Schnermann J, et al. Vitamin C transporter Slc23a1 links renal reabsorption, vitamin C tissue accumulation, and perinatal survival in mice. *The Journal of clinical investigation.* 2010 Apr;120(4):1069-83. PubMed PMID: 20200446. Pubmed Central PMCID: 2847422.

[48] Tsukaguchi H, Tokui T, Mackenzie B, Berger UV, Chen XZ, Wang Y, et al. A family of mammalian Na+-dependent L-ascorbic acid transporters. *Nature.* 1999 May 6;399(6731):70-5. PubMed PMID: 10331392.

[49] MacDonald L, Thumser AE, Sharp P. Decreased expression of the vitamin C transporter SVCT1 by ascorbic acid in a human intestinal epithelial cell line. *The British journal of nutrition.* 2002 Feb;87(2):97-100. PubMed PMID: 11895172.

[50] Padayatty SJ, Sun H, Wang Y, Riordan HD, Hewitt SM, Katz A, et al. Vitamin C pharmacokinetics: implications for oral and intravenous use. *Annals of internal medicine.* 2004 Apr 6;140(7):533-7. PubMed PMID: 15068981.

[51] Savini I, Catani MV, Arnone R, Rossi A, Frega G, Del Principe D, et al. Translational control of the ascorbic acid transporter SVCT2 in human platelets. *Free radical biology & medicine.* 2007 Mar 1;42(5):608-16. PubMed PMID: 17291984.

[52] Graumlich JF, Ludden TM, Conry-Cantilena C, Cantilena LR, Jr., Wang Y, Levine M. Pharmacokinetic model of ascorbic acid in healthy male volunteers during depletion and repletion. *Pharmaceutical research.* 1997 Sep;14(9):1133-9. PubMed PMID: 9327438.

[53] Parrow NL, Leshin JA, Levine M. Parenteral Ascorbate As a Cancer Therapeutic: A Reassessment Based on Pharmacokinetics. *Antioxidants & redox signaling.* 2013 Jun 19. PubMed PMID: 23621620.

[54] Buettner GR. The pecking order of free radicals and antioxidants: lipid peroxidation, alpha-tocopherol, and ascorbate. *Archives of biochemistry and biophysics.* 1993 Feb 1;300(2):535-43. PubMed PMID: 8434935.

[55] Burton GW, Ingold KU. Vitamin-E - Application of the Principles of Physical Organic-Chemistry to the Exploration of Its Structure and Function. *Accounts Chem Res.* 1986 Jul;19(7):194-201. PubMed PMID: WOS:A1986D981100001. English.

[56] Golumbic C, Mattill, H.A. Antioxidants and the autoxidation of fats. XIII. The antioxygenic action of ascorbic acid in association with tocopherols, hydroquinones and related compounds. *J Am Chem Soc.* 1941;63:1279-80.

[57] Suh J, Zhu BZ, Frei B. Ascorbate does not act as a pro-oxidant towards lipids and proteins in human plasma exposed to redox-active transition metal ions and hydrogen peroxide. *Free Radical Bio Med.* 2003 May 15;34(10):1306-14. PubMed PMID: WOS:000182573500010. English.

[58] Linster CL, Van Schaftingen E. Vitamin C. Biosynthesis, recycling and degradation in mammals. *The FEBS journal.* 2007 Jan;274(1):1-22. PubMed PMID: 17222174.

[59] Frei B, Lawson S. Vitamin C and cancer revisited. *Proceedings of the National Academy of Sciences of the United States of America.* 2008 Aug 12;105(32):11037-8. PubMed PMID: 18682554. Pubmed Central PMCID: 2516245.

[60] Halliwell B. Vitamin C: poison, prophylactic or panacea? *Trends in biochemical sciences*. 1999 Jul;24(7):255-9. PubMed PMID: 10390611.

[61] Mc CW. Cancer: a collagen disease, secondary to a nutritional deficiency. *Archives of pediatrics.* 1959 Apr;76(4):166-71. PubMed PMID: 13638066.

[62] Cameron E, Pauling L. Ascorbic acid and the glycosaminoglycans. An orthomolecular approach to cancer and other diseases. *Oncology*. 1973;27(2):181-92. PubMed PMID: 4267127.

[63] Cameron E, Rotman D. Ascorbic acid, cell proliferation, and cancer. *Lancet*. 1972 Mar 4;1(7749):542. PubMed PMID: 4110043.

[64] Cameron E, Campbell A. The orthomolecular treatment of cancer. II. Clinical trial of high-dose ascorbic acid supplements in advanced human cancer. *Chemico-biological interactions.* 1974 Oct;9(4):285-315. PubMed PMID: 4430016.

[65] Cameron E, Campbell A, Jack T. The orthomolecular treatment of cancer. III. Reticulum cell sarcoma: double complete regression induced by high-dose ascorbic acid therapy. *Chemico-biological interactions.* 1975 Nov;11(5):387-93. PubMed PMID: 1104207.

[66] Cameron E, Pauling L. Supplemental ascorbate in the supportive treatment of cancer: Prolongation of survival times in terminal human cancer. *Proceedings of the National Academy of Sciences of the United States of America.* 1976 Oct;73(10):3685-9. PubMed PMID: 1068480. Pubmed Central PMCID: 431183.

[67] Cameron E, Pauling L. Supplemental ascorbate in the supportive treatment of cancer: reevaluation of prolongation of survival times in terminal human cancer. *Proceedings of the National Academy of Sciences of the United States of America.* 1978 Sep;75(9):4538-42. PubMed PMID: 279931. Pubmed Central PMCID: 336151.

[68] Creagan ET, Moertel CG, O'Fallon JR, Schutt AJ, O'Connell MJ, Rubin J, et al. Failure of high-dose vitamin C (ascorbic acid) therapy to benefit patients with advanced cancer. A controlled trial. *The New England journal of medicine*. 1979 Sep 27;301(13):687-90. PubMed PMID: 384241.

[69] Moertel CG, Fleming TR, Creagan ET, Rubin J, O'Connell MJ, Ames MM. High-dose vitamin C versus placebo in the treatment of patients with advanced cancer who have had no prior chemotherapy. A randomized double-blind comparison. *The New England journal of medicine.* 1985 Jan 17;312(3):137-41. PubMed PMID: 3880867.

[70] Levine M, Conry-Cantilena C, Wang Y, Welch RW, Washko PW, Dhariwal KR, et al. Vitamin C pharmacokinetics in healthy volunteers: evidence for a recommended dietary allowance. *Proceedings of the National Academy of Sciences of the United States of America.* 1996 Apr 16;93(8):3704-9. PubMed PMID: 8623000. Pubmed Central PMCID: 39676.

[71] Padayatty SJ, Riordan HD, Hewitt SM, Katz A, Hoffer LJ, Levine M. Intravenously administered vitamin C as cancer therapy: three cases. *CMAJ : Canadian Medical Association journal = journal de l'Association medicale canadienne.* 2006 Mar 28;174(7):937-42. PubMed PMID: 16567755. Pubmed Central PMCID: 1405876.

[72] Padayatty SJ, Levine M. New insights into the physiology and pharmacology of vitamin C. CMAJ : *Canadian Medical Association journal = journal de l'Association medicale canadienne.* 2001 Feb 6;164(3):353-5. PubMed PMID: 11232136. Pubmed Central PMCID: 80729.

[73] Chen Q, Espey MG, Sun AY, Pooput C, Kirk KL, Krishna MC, et al. Pharmacologic doses of ascorbate act as a pro-oxidant and decrease growth of aggressive tumor xenografts in mice. *Proceedings of the National Academy of Sciences of the United States of America.* 2008 Aug 12;105(32):11105-9. PubMed PMID: 18678913. Pubmed Central PMCID: 2516281.

[74] Hoffer LJ, Levine M, Assouline S, Melnychuk D, Padayatty SJ, Rosadiuk K, et al. Phase I clinical trial of i.v. ascorbic acid in advanced malignancy. *Annals of oncology : official journal of the European Society for Medical Oncology / ESMO.* 2008 Nov;19(11):1969-74. PubMed PMID: 18544557.

[75] Verrax J, Calderon PB. Pharmacologic concentrations of ascorbate are achieved by parenteral administration and exhibit antitumoral effects. *Free radical biology & medicine.* 2009 Jul 1;47(1):32-40. PubMed PMID: 19254759.

[76] Chen Q, Espey MG, Krishna MC, Mitchell JB, Corpe CP, Buettner GR, et al. Pharmacologic ascorbic acid concentrations selectively kill cancer cells: action as a pro-drug to deliver hydrogen peroxide to tissues. *Proceedings of the National Academy of Sciences of the United States of America.* 2005 Sep 20;102(38):13604-9. PubMed PMID: 16157892. Pubmed Central PMCID: 1224653.

[77] Du J, Martin SM, Levine M, Wagner BA, Buettner GR, Wang SH, et al. Mechanisms of ascorbate-induced cytotoxicity in pancreatic cancer. *Clinical cancer research : an official journal of the American Association for Cancer Research.* 2010 Jan 15;16(2):509-20. PubMed PMID: 20068072. Pubmed Central PMCID: 2807999.

[78] Heeg K, Reimann J, Kabelitz D, Hardt C, Wagner H. A rapid colorimetric assay for the determination of IL-2-producing helper T cell frequencies. *Journal of immunological methods.* 1985 Mar 18;77(2):237-46. PubMed PMID: 3156935.

[79] Coleman MC, Asbury CR, Daniels D, Du J, Aykin-Burns N, Smith BJ, et al. 2-deoxy-D-glucose causes cytotoxicity, oxidative stress, and radiosensitization in pancreatic cancer. *Free radical biology & medicine.* 2008 Feb 1;44(3):322-31. PubMed PMID: 18215740.

[80] Liu J, Hinkhouse MM, Sun W, Weydert CJ, Ritchie JM, Oberley LW, et al. Redox regulation of pancreatic cancer cell growth: role of glutathione peroxidase in the suppression of the malignant phenotype. *Human gene therapy.* 2004 Mar;15(3):239-50. PubMed PMID: 15018733.

[81] Oberley LW. Mechanism of the tumor suppressive effect of MnSOD overexpression. *Biomedicine & pharmacotherapy = Biomedecine & pharmacotherapie.* 2005 May;59(4):143-8. PubMed PMID: 15862707.

[82] Schafer FQ, Buettner GR. Redox environment of the cell as viewed through the redox state of the glutathione disulfide/glutathione couple. *Free radical biology & medicine.* 2001 Jun 1;30(11):1191-212. PubMed PMID: 11368918.

[83] Chen Q, Espey MG, Sun AY, Lee JH, Krishna MC, Shacter E, et al. Ascorbate in pharmacologic concentrations selectively generates ascorbate radical and hydrogen peroxide in extracellular fluid in vivo. *Proceedings of the National Academy of Sciences of the United States of America.* 2007 May 22;104(21):8749-54. PubMed PMID: 17502596. Pubmed Central PMCID: 1885574.

[84] Brown JM, Grosso MA, Terada LS, Beehler CJ, Toth KM, Whitman GJ, et al. Erythrocytes decrease myocardial hydrogen peroxide levels and reperfusion injury. *The*

American journal of physiology. 1989 Feb;256(2 Pt 2):H584-8. PubMed PMID: 2916691.

[85] Chance B, Sies H, Boveris A. Hydroperoxide metabolism in mammalian organs. *Physiological reviews.* 1979 Jul;59(3):527-605. PubMed PMID: 37532.

[86] Guemouri L, Artur Y, Herbeth B, Jeandel C, Cuny G, Siest G. Biological variability of superoxide dismutase, glutathione peroxidase, and catalase in blood. *Clinical chemistry.* 1991 Nov;37(11):1932-7. PubMed PMID: 1934468.

[87] Motoyama S, Saito S, Inaba H, Kitamura M, Minamiya Y, Suzuki H, et al. Red blood cells attenuate sinusoidal endothelial cell injury by scavenging xanthine oxidase-dependent hydrogen peroxide in hyperoxic perfused rat liver. *Liver.* 2000 Jun;20(3):200-8. PubMed PMID: 10902969.

[88] Low FM, Hampton MB, Winterbourn CC. Peroxiredoxin 2 and peroxide metabolism in the erythrocyte. *Antioxidants & redox signaling.* 2008 Sep;10(9):1621-30. PubMed PMID: 18479207.

[89] May JM, Qu Z, Cobb CE. Recycling of the ascorbate free radical by human erythrocyte membranes. *Free radical biology & medicine.* 2001 Jul 1;31(1):117-24. PubMed PMID: 11425497.

[90] Baronzio G, Schwartz L, Kiselevsky M, Guais A, Sanders E, Milanesi G, et al. Tumor interstitial fluid as modulator of cancer inflammation, thrombosis, immunity and angiogenesis. *Anticancer research.* 2012 Feb;32(2):405-14. PubMed PMID: 22287726.

[91] Casciari JJ, Riordan NH, Schmidt TL, Meng XL, Jackson JA, Riordan HD. Cytotoxicity of ascorbate, lipoic acid, and other antioxidants in hollow fibre in vitro tumours. *British journal of cancer.* 2001 Jun 1;84(11):1544-50. PubMed PMID: 11384106. Pubmed Central PMCID: 2363673.

[92] Halliwell B. Oxygen radicals, nitric oxide and human inflammatory joint disease. *Annals of the rheumatic diseases.* 1995 Jun;54(6):505-10. PubMed PMID: 7632097. Pubmed Central PMCID: 1009913.

[93] Klockars M, Weber T, Tanner P, Hellstrom PE, Pettersson T. Pleural fluid ferritin concentrations in human disease. *Journal of clinical pathology.* 1985 Jul;38(7):818-24. PubMed PMID: 4019803. Pubmed Central PMCID: 499311.

[94] Weinberger A, Simkin PA. Plasma proteins in synovial fluids of normal human joints. *Seminars in arthritis and rheumatism.* 1989 Aug;19(1):66-76. PubMed PMID: 2672342.

[95] Du J, Nelson ES, Simons AL, Olney KE, Moser JC, Schrock HE, et al. Regulation of pancreatic cancer growth by superoxide. *Molecular carcinogenesis.* 2012 Mar 5. PubMed PMID: 22392697. Pubmed Central PMCID: 3375391.

[96] Antunes F, Cadenas E. Estimation of H2O2 gradients across biomembranes. *Febs Lett.* 2000 Jun 16;475(2):121-6. PubMed PMID: WOS:000087772900011. English.

[97] Wang XY, Liu JK, Yokoi I, Kohno M, Mori A. Direct Detection of Circulating Free-Radicals in the Rat Using Electron-Spin-Resonance Spectrometry. *Free Radical Bio Med.* 1992;12(2):121-6. PubMed PMID: WOS:A1992HE05800004. English.

[98] Chepda T, Cadau M, Girin P, Frey J, Chamson A. Monitoring of ascorbate at a constant rate in cell culture: effect on cell growth. *In vitro cellular & developmental biology Animal.* 2001 Jan;37(1):26-30. PubMed PMID: 11249202.

[99] Frikke-Schmidt H, Lykkesfeldt J. Keeping the intracellular vitamin C at a physiologically relevant level in endothelial cell culture. *Analytical biochemistry.* 2010 Feb 1;397(1):135-7. PubMed PMID: 19782654.

[100] Fujiwara M, Nagao N, Monden K, Misumi M, Kageyama K, Yamamoto K, et al. Enhanced protection against peroxidation-induced mortality of aortic endothelial cells by ascorbic acid-2-O-phosphate abundantly accumulated in the cell as the dephosphorylated form. *Free radical research.* 1997 Jul;27(1):97-104. PubMed PMID: 9269584.

[101] Vislisel JM, Schafer FQ, Buettner GR. A simple and sensitive assay for ascorbate using a plate reader. *Analytical biochemistry.* 2007 Jun 1;365(1):31-9. PubMed PMID: 17433246. Pubmed Central PMCID: 2129083.

[102] Olney KE, Du J, van 't Erve TJ, Witmer JR, Sibenaller ZA, Wagner BA, et al. Inhibitors of hydroperoxide metabolism enhance ascorbate-induced cytotoxicity. *Free radical research.* 2013 Mar;47(3):154-63. PubMed PMID: 23205739. Pubmed Central PMCID: 3674878.

[103] Klingelhoeffer C, Kammerer U, Koospal M, Muhling B, Schneider M, Kapp M, et al. Natural resistance to ascorbic acid induced oxidative stress is mainly mediated by catalase activity in human cancer cells and catalase-silencing sensitizes to oxidative stress. *BMC complementary and alternative medicine.* 2012;12:61. PubMed PMID: 22551313. Pubmed Central PMCID: 3404974.

[104] Benade L, Howard T, Burk D. Synergistic killing of Ehrlich ascites carcinoma cells by ascorbate and 3-amino-1,2,4,-triazole. *Oncology.* 1969;23(1):33-43. PubMed PMID: 5774953.

[105] Richardson DR, Ponka P. The molecular mechanisms of the metabolism and transport of iron in normal and neoplastic cells. *Biochimica et biophysica acta.* 1997 Mar 14;1331(1):1-40. PubMed PMID: 9325434.

[106] Wang W, Knovich MA, Coffman LG, Torti FM, Torti SV. Serum ferritin: Past, present and future. *Biochimica et biophysica acta.* 2010 Aug;1800(8):760-9. PubMed PMID: 20304033. Pubmed Central PMCID: 2893236.

[107] Buettner GR, Chamulitrat W. The catalytic activity of iron in synovial fluid as monitored by the ascorbate free radical. *Free radical biology & medicine.* 1990;8(1):55-6. PubMed PMID: 2157634.

[108] Dabbagh AJ, Trenam CW, Morris CJ, Blake DR. Iron in joint inflammation. *Annals of the rheumatic diseases.* 1993 Jan;52(1):67-73. PubMed PMID: 8427520. Pubmed Central PMCID: 1004961.

[109] Galley HF, Davies MJ, Webster NR. Ascorbyl radical formation in patients with sepsis: effect of ascorbate loading. *Free radical biology & medicine.* 1996;20(1):139-43. PubMed PMID: 8903690.

[110] Coudray C, Pucheu S, Boucher F, Arnaud J, de Leiris J, Favier A. Effect of ischemia/reperfusion sequence on cytosolic iron status and its release in the coronary effluent in isolated rat hearts. *Biological trace element research.* 1994 Apr-May;41(1-2):69-75. PubMed PMID: 7946910.

[111] Spencer KT, Lindower PD, Buettner GR, Kerber RE. Transition metal chelators reduce directly measured myocardial free radical production during reperfusion. *Journal of cardiovascular pharmacology.* 1998 Sep;32(3):343-8. PubMed PMID: 9733345.

[112] Basso D, Fabris C, Del Favero G, Meggiato T, Panozzo MP, Vianello D, et al. Hepatic changes and serum ferritin in pancreatic cancer and other gastrointestinal diseases: the role of cholestasis. *Annals of clinical biochemistry.* 1991 Jan;28 (Pt 1):34-8. PubMed PMID: 2024931.

[113] Guner G, Kirkali G, Yenisey C, Tore IR. Cytosol and serum ferritin in breast carcinoma. *Cancer letters.* 1992 Dec 24;67(2-3):103-12. PubMed PMID: 1483258.

[114] Miyata Y, Koga S, Nishikido M, Hayashi T, Kanetake H. Relationship between serum ferritin levels and tumour status in patients with renal cell carcinoma. *BJU international.* 2001 Dec;88(9):974-7. PubMed PMID: 11851623.

[115] Rossiello R, Carriero MV, Giordano GG. Distribution of ferritin, transferrin and lactoferrin in breast carcinoma tissue. *Journal of clinical pathology.* 1984 Jan;37(1):51-5. PubMed PMID: 6323544. Pubmed Central PMCID: 498617.

[116] Jacobs A. Serum ferritin and malignant tumours. *Medical oncology and tumor pharmacotherapy.* 1984;1(3):149-56. PubMed PMID: 6085815.

[117] Tian J, Peehl DM, Knox SJ. Metalloporphyrin synergizes with ascorbic acid to inhibit cancer cell growth through fenton chemistry. *Cancer biotherapy & radiopharmaceuticals.* 2010 Aug;25(4):439-48. PubMed PMID: 20735206.

[118] Zhong W, Yan T, Webber MM, Oberley TD. Alteration of cellular phenotype and responses to oxidative stress by manganese superoxide dismutase and a superoxide dismutase mimic in RWPE-2 human prostate adenocarcinoma cells. *Antioxidants & redox signaling.* 2004 Jun;6(3):513-22. PubMed PMID: 15130278.

[119] Batinic-Haberle I, Reboucas JS, Spasojevic I. Superoxide dismutase mimics: chemistry, pharmacology, and therapeutic potential. *Antioxidants & redox signaling.* 2010 Sep 15;13(6):877-918. PubMed PMID: 20095865. Pubmed Central PMCID: 2935339.

[120] Carmine TC, Evans P, Bruchelt G, Evans R, Handgretinger R, Niethammer D, et al. Presence of iron catalytic for free radical reactions in patients undergoing chemotherapy: implications for therapeutic management. *Cancer letters.* 1995 Aug 1;94(2):219-26. PubMed PMID: 7543367.

[121] Persson HL. Radiation-induced lysosomal iron reactivity: implications for radioprotective therapy. *IUBMB life.* 2006 Jul;58(7):395-401. PubMed PMID: 16801214.

[122] Reif DW. Ferritin as a source of iron for oxidative damage. *Free radical biology & medicine.* 1992;12(5):417-27. PubMed PMID: 1317328.

[123] Espey MG, Chen P, Chalmers B, Drisko J, Sun AY, Levine M, et al. Pharmacologic ascorbate synergizes with gemcitabine in preclinical models of pancreatic cancer. *Free radical biology & medicine.* 2011 Jun 1;50(11):1610-9. PubMed PMID: 21402145. Pubmed Central PMCID: 3482496.

[124] Campbell GD, Jr., Steinberg MH, Bower JD. Letter: Ascorbic acid-induced hemolysis in G-6-PD deficiency. *Annals of internal medicine.* 1975 Jun;82(6):810. PubMed PMID: 1138591.

[125] Mehta JB, Singhal SB, Mehta BC. Ascorbic-acid-induced haemolysis in G-6-PD deficiency. *Lancet.* 1990 Oct 13;336(8720):944. PubMed PMID: 1976956.

[126] Rees DC, Kelsey H, Richards JD. Acute haemolysis induced by high dose ascorbic acid in glucose-6-phosphate dehydrogenase deficiency. *Bmj.* 1993 Mar 27;306(6881):841-2. PubMed PMID: 8490379. Pubmed Central PMCID: 1677333.

[127] Wong K, Thomson C, Bailey RR, McDiarmid S, Gardner J. Acute oxalate nephropathy after a massive intravenous dose of vitamin C. *Australian and New Zealand journal of medicine*. 1994 Aug;24(4):410-1. PubMed PMID: 7980244.

[128] Fleming RE, Ponka P. Iron overload in human disease. *The New England journal of medicine*. 2012 Jan 26;366(4):348-59. PubMed PMID: 22276824.

[129] Campbell A, Jack T. Acute reactions to mega ascorbic acid therapy in malignant disease. *Scottish medical journal*. 1979 Apr;24(2):151-3. PubMed PMID: 227054.

[130] Monti DA, Mitchell E, Bazzan AJ, Littman S, Zabrecky G, Yeo CJ, et al. Phase I evaluation of intravenous ascorbic acid in combination with gemcitabine and erlotinib in patients with metastatic pancreatic cancer. *PloS one*. 2012;7(1):e29794. PubMed PMID: 22272248. Pubmed Central PMCID: 3260161.

[131] Riordan HD, Casciari JJ, Gonzalez MJ, Riordan NH, Miranda-Massari JR, Taylor P, et al. A pilot clinical study of continuous intravenous ascorbate in terminal cancer patients. *Puerto Rico health sciences journal*. 2005 Dec;24(4):269-76. PubMed PMID: 16570523.

[132] Stephenson CM, Levin RD, Spector T, Lis CG. Phase I clinical trial to evaluate the safety, tolerability, and pharmacokinetics of high-dose intravenous ascorbic acid in patients with advanced cancer. *Cancer chemotherapy and pharmacology*. 2013 Jul;72(1):139-46. PubMed PMID: 23670640. Pubmed Central PMCID: 3691494.

[133] Tahahashi HM, H.; Yanagisawa, A. High-dose intravenous vitamin C improves quality of life in cancer patients. *Personalized Medicine Universe*. 2012;1(1):49-53.

[134] Riordan HD, Riordan NH, Jackson JA, Casciari JJ, Hunninghake R, Gonzalez MJ, et al. Intravenous vitamin C as a chemotherapy agent: a report on clinical cases. *Puerto Rico health sciences journal*. 2004 Jun;23(2):115-8. PubMed PMID: 15377059.

[135] Kato J, Nagahara A, Iijima K, Yoshimura M, Osada T, Yoshizawa T, et al. Evaluation of EORTC QLQ-C30 questionnaire in patients undergoing in-hospital chemotherapy for gastrointestinal cancer in Japan. *Journal of gastroenterology and hepatology*. 2008 Dec;23 Suppl 2:S268-72. PubMed PMID: 19120910.

[136] Kobayashi K, Takeda F, Teramukai S, Gotoh I, Sakai H, Yoneda S, et al. A cross-validation of the European Organization for Research and Treatment of Cancer QLQ-C30 (EORTC QLQ-C30) for Japanese with lung cancer. *European journal of cancer*. 1998 May;34(6):810-5. PubMed PMID: 9797690.

[137] Farrar JT, Young JP, Jr., LaMoreaux L, Werth JL, Poole RM. Clinical importance of changes in chronic pain intensity measured on an 11-point numerical pain rating scale. *Pain*. 2001 Nov;94(2):149-58. PubMed PMID: 11690728.

[138] Riordan HD, Hunninghake RB, Riordan NH, Jackson JJ, Meng X, Taylor P, et al. Intravenous ascorbic acid: protocol for its application and use. *Puerto Rico health sciences journal*. 2003 Sep;22(3):287-90. PubMed PMID: 14619456.

[139] Eisenhauer EA, Therasse P, Bogaerts J, Schwartz LH, Sargent D, Ford R, et al. New response evaluation criteria in solid tumours: revised RECIST guideline (version 1.1). *European journal of cancer*. 2009 Jan;45(2):228-47. PubMed PMID: 19097774.

[140] Welsh JL, Wagner BA, van't Erve TJ, Zehr PS, Berg DJ, Halfdanarson TR, et al. Pharmacological ascorbate with gemcitabine for the control of metastatic and node-positive pancreatic cancer (PACMAN): results from a phase I clinical trial. *Cancer chemotherapy and pharmacology*. 2013 Mar;71(3):765-75. PubMed PMID: 23381814. Pubmed Central PMCID: 3587047.

[141] Buettner GR, Jurkiewicz BA. Ascorbate free radical as a marker of oxidative stress: an EPR study. *Free radical biology & medicine*. 1993 Jan;14(1):49-55. PubMed PMID: 8384150.

[142] Morrow JD, Hill KE, Burk RF, Nammour TM, Badr KF, Roberts LJ, 2nd. A series of prostaglandin F2-like compounds are produced in vivo in humans by a non-cyclooxygenase, free radical-catalyzed mechanism. *Proceedings of the National Academy of Sciences of the United States of America.* 1990 Dec;87(23):9383-7. PubMed PMID: 2123555. Pubmed Central PMCID: 55169.

[143] Herst PM, Broadley KW, Harper JL, McConnell MJ. Pharmacological concentrations of ascorbate radiosensitize glioblastoma multiforme primary cells by increasing oxidative DNA damage and inhibiting G2/M arrest. *Free radical biology & medicine.* 2012 Apr 15;52(8):1486-93. PubMed PMID: 22342518.

[144] Shinozaki K, Hosokawa Y, Hazawa M, Kashiwakura I, Okumura K, Kaku T, et al. Ascorbic acid enhances radiation-induced apoptosis in an HL60 human leukemia cell line. *Journal of radiation research.* 2011;52(2):229-37. PubMed PMID: 21343676.

In: Free Radicals
Editor: Bill Stone
ISBN: 978-1-63117-177-2

Chapter VI

The Design, Synthesis and *In Vitro* Evaluation of a Novel Pro-Oxidant Anticancer Prodrug Substrate Targeted to Acylamino-Acid-Releasing Enzyme

William L. Stone[1*], Yu Lin Jiang[2], Christopher McGoldrick[1], Marianne Brannon[1] and Koymangalath Krishnan[3]

[1]Department of Pediatrics, James H. Quillen College of Medicine, East Tennessee State University, Johnson City, TN, US

[2]Chemistry Department, [3]Department of Internal Medicine, Division of Hematology/Oncology, James H. Quillen College of Medicine, East Tennessee State University, Johnson City, TN, US

Abstract

Cancer cells often exhibit a high level of intrinsic oxidative stress due to an increased formation of reactive oxygen species and a decreased expression of enzymatic antioxidants. Prodrugs inducing additional oxidative stress can selectively induce apoptosis in cancer cells already having a high level of intrinsic oxidative stress. This study focused on the rational design and *in vitro* evaluation of a novel prodrug ester, (4-[(nitrooxy)methyl]phenyl-N-acetyl-L-alaninate or NPAA) activated by acylamino-acid-releasing enzyme (AARE, EC 3.4.19.1) to yield a quinone methide (QM) intermediate capable of depleting glutathione (GSH), a key intracellular antioxidant. NPAA shares structural features with both nitric oxide donating aspirin (NO-ASA), a well-characterized QM releasing anticancer prodrug, and N-acetyl-L-alanine-4-nitroanailide (AANA), a known specific substrate for AARE. AARE is a serine peptidase that is overexpressed in some tumors and cancer cell lines. The overall approach was to first predict the 3-dimensional structure of both rat (rAARE) and human AARE (hAARE) and then use the resulting low-resolution models to determine if NPAA was a plausible

* Department of Pediatrics, James H. Quillen College of Medicine, East Tennessee State University, Johnson City, TN, 37614 USA. Email: stone@etsu.edu.

prodrug by estimating its affinity to hAARE and rAARE in comparison to AANA. The AARE models were constructed using a bioinformatic-based protein structure prediction webserver (I-TASSER) followed by energy minimization and refinement. The resulting models were subjected to a variety of structural quality assessments. The optimal models of hAARE and rAARE were found to have similar three-dimensional structures with a β-propeller domain and an α/β-hydrolase domain containing an exopeptidase catalytic site with active site residue distances typically found in serine peptidases. Protein-ligand docking studies showed that both AANA and NPAA could bind to the exopeptidase catalytic site of the hAARE and rAARE models with reasonable affinities and in a region with a highly druggable pocket. In order to validate the *in silico* results, NPAA was synthesized, purified, physically characterized and evaluated for its *in vitro* ability to deplete GSH in the presence of rAARE. As anticipated, NPAA was found to deplete GSH and this effect was completely blocked by diisopropylfluorophosphate (DFP), an irreversible inhibitor of serine proteases, including rAARE. These studies support further efforts to optimize the design of QM releasing anticancer prodrugs targeted to AARE. Moreover, the molecular models presented here could be useful for the rational design of AARE inhibitors, which could also be exploited as potential anticancer agents.

Keywords: glutathione, cancer, bioinformatics, prodrug, acylamino-acid-releasing enzyme, chemotherapy

Abbreviations

NPAA	4-[(nitrooxy)methyl]phenyl-N-acetyl-L-alaninate
AARE	acylamino-acid-releasing enzyme
GSH	glutathione
NO-ASA	nitric oxide donating aspirin
QM	quinone methide
ROS	reactive oxygen species
APH	acyl-peptide hydrolase
AAP	acylaminoacyl peptidase
OPH	oxidized protein hydrolase
DTNB	5,5'-dithiobis-2-nitrobenzoic acid
DFP	diisopropylfluorophosphat
TBM	template-based modeling
POP	prolyl oligopeptidase
AANA	N-acetyl-L-alanine-4-nitroanilide
HR-ESI-TOF	high resolution-electrospray ionization-time-of-flight-mass spectra

Introduction

Oxidative Stress and Cancer

Oxidative stress induced apoptosis has been termed the "Achilles heel" of cancer [1]. As recently pointed out by Dr. Jim Watson, most agents that kill cancer cells do so by inducing reactive oxygen species (ROS) that block key steps in the cell cycle [2]. Numerous observations support the view that cancer cells often exhibit a high level of intrinsic oxidative stress, that is not just a metabolic quirk, but is required for an aggressive cancer phenotype and to escape apoptosis [1,3-6]. This high level of intrinsic oxidative stress makes cancer cells particularly susceptible to apoptosis induced by chemotherapeutic agents causing additional oxidative stress.

Akt Activation, Glutathione (GSH) and Oxidative Stress in Cancer Cells

The heightened oxidative stress in cancer cells has been attributed to the activation of the Akt kinase signaling cascade, which increases cellular reactive oxygen species (ROS), impairs enzymatic ROS detoxifying mechanisms and increases cellular susceptibility to ROS induced apoptosis [1,4]. Akt is a serine/threonine kinase that plays a cardinal node for a diverse set of signaling cascades important for regulating cell survival, cell growth, glucose metabolism, cell motility and angiogenesis [7]. The activation of Akt (caused by its phosphorylation) in cancer cells normally inhibits apoptosis caused by a variety of apoptotic stimuli but this is not the case for ROS-induced apoptosis, i.e., Akt activation plays a pro-apoptotic role in ROS-induced apoptosis [8]. Chemotherapeutic agents that induce oxidative stress therefore hold the potential for being selective at inducing apoptosis in cancer cells compared to normal cells [1].

Glutathione (L-γ-glutamyl-L-cysteinylglycine or GSH) is the primary intracellular antioxidant and this tripeptide plays a key role modulating tumor cell proliferation and the resistance of tumors to chemotherapeutic drugs [9]. GSH depletion has been found to cause a growth inhibition in many types of cancers including pancreatic cancer [10]. In an animal model, GSH depletion was found to sensitize melanoma cancer cells to combination chemotherapy and eliminate metastatic disease [11].

Acylamino-acid-releasing Enzyme (AARE) as an Anticancer Drug Target

Acylamino-acid-releasing enzyme (AARE, EC3.4.19.1) has recently been proposed as a potential target for the development of anticancer drugs [12]. Histological data in the Human Protein Atlas shows that AARE can be strongly expressed in cases of colorectal, breast, prostate, ovarian, endometrial and liver cancers [13]. AARE has well-documented substrate specificity towards N-acetylated-L-alaninate esters [14]. The studies presented here focus on the on the rational design and organic synthesis of a potential chemotherapeutic nitrooxy N-acetyl-L-alaninate prodrug that could be activated by the hydrolase activity of AARE and subsequently deplete intracellular GSH causing oxidative stress induced apoptosis (see Figure 1).

The Known Functions of AARE

AARE, also called acyl-peptide hydrolase (APH), acylaminoacyl peptidase (AAP) or, oxidized protein hydrolase (OPH), is a serine protease and a member of the prolyl oligopeptidase (POP) family. There are three known functions associated with AARE: (1) an exopeptidase activity that unblocks N-acetyl peptides with a preference for N-acetyl alanyl peptides [15]; (2) an endopeptidase activity towards oxidized and glycated proteins [16-20] and; (3) an ability to associate with aggresomes, which are pericentrosomal accumulations of misfolded or oxidized protein [19]. Moreover, work by Shimizu *et al.* [19] suggests that the proteasome and AARE work coordinately to clear cells of oxidized (carbonylated) proteins. A comprehensive physiological understanding of AARE remains elusive. Nevertheless, the acetylation of the N-terminal α-amine group of proteins is the most common post-translational modification in eukaryotic proteins yet, little is known about the biological role of N-alpha-terminal acetylation, and even less is known about the role of enzymes (like AARE) that catalyze the hydrolysis of an N-terminally acetylated peptide to release an N-acetylamino acid.

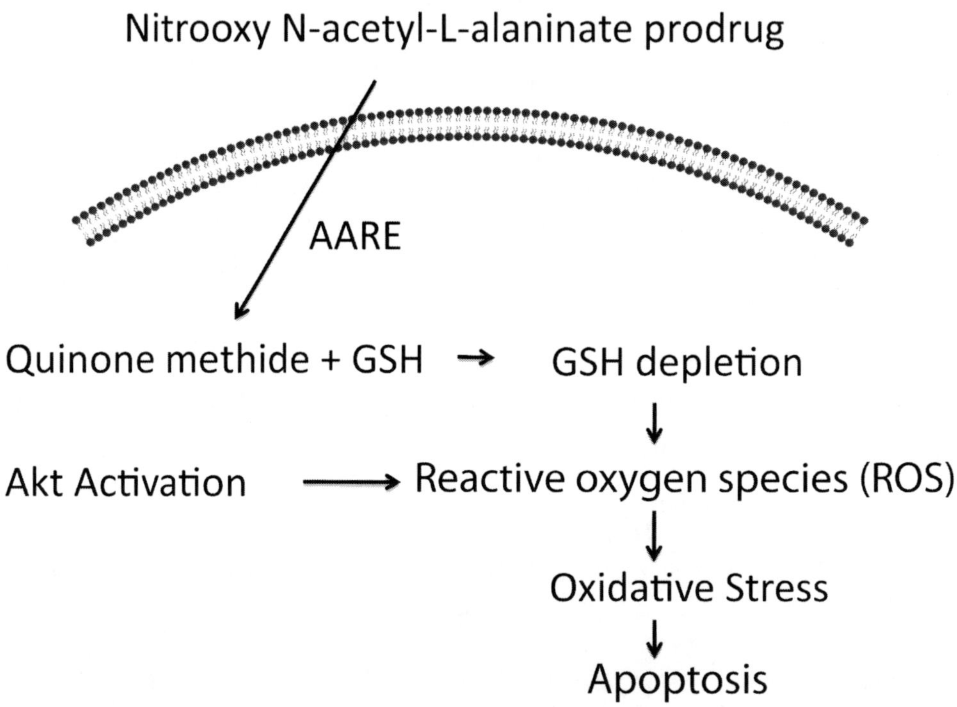

Figure 1. Oxidative stress induced apoptosis in cancer cells. We hypothesize that the novel prodrug, 4-[(nitrooxy)methyl]phenyl-N-acetyl-L-alaninate (NPAA), can exert an anticancer effect by being activated by the hydrolase activity of acylamino-acid-releasing enzyme (AARE) to yield a quinone methide (QM) intermediate that can deplete glutathione (GSH), an intracellular antioxidant. Depletion of GSH can cause oxidative stress-induced apoptosis by activation of the intrinsic death pathway. Cancer cells with activated Akt kinase would be particularly susceptible oxidative stress-induced apoptosis due to a high level of intrinsic oxidative stress.

Nitric oxide Generating Prodrugs and Oxidative Stress Induced Apoptosis in Cancer Cells

We previously described a novel synthetic route to nitric oxide (NO) donating acetylsalicylic acid (NO-ASA or NCX 4040) [21]. Both extensive *in vitro* and *in vivo* data suggest that NO-ASA (also called nitric oxide-donating aspirin) has potential as an anticancer prodrug and also has a toxicology profile superior to that of aspirin [22-29]. NO-ASA is thought to exert its anticancer effects by promoting oxidative stress induced apoptosis caused by the hydrolytic release of an electrophile quinone methide (QM) intermediate that selectively reacts with and depletes intracellular GSH (see Figure 2)[24,30]. Although a matter of some controversy [31], it is unlikely that the "NO-releasing" moiety of NO-ASA is a contributing factor for its anticancer effects [30,32]. This cannot, however, be completely ruled out in an *in vivo* situation [31].

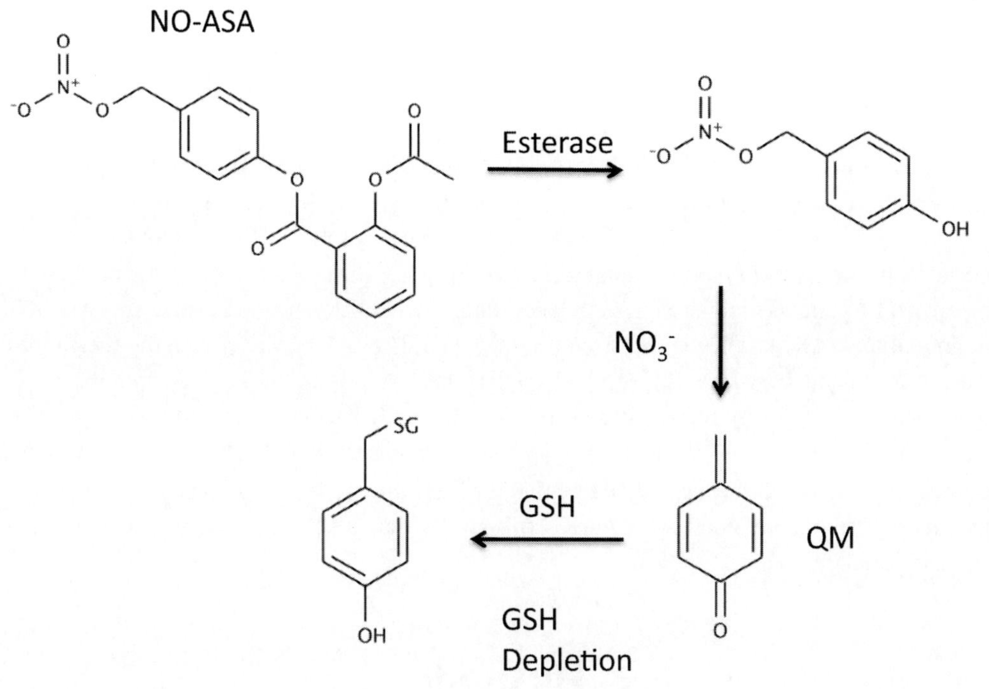

Figure 2. The anticancer effects of nitric oxide donating aspirin (NO-ASA). The anticancer effect of NO-ASA has been attributed to an esterase-catalyzed release of an electrophilic quinone methide (QM) intermediate that covalently reacts with and depletes glutathione (GSH), a key intracellular antioxidant. Depletion of intracellular GSH results in oxidative stress induced apoptosis. Cancer cells often have a high level of intrinsic oxidative stress, which renders them sensitive to prodrugs that induce additional oxidative stress.

The Rational Design and *In Vitro* Evaluation of a Novel Prodrug Ester, (4-[(nitrooxy) Phenyl-N-acetyl-L-alaninate or NPAA) Activated by Acylamino-acid-releasing Enzyme

The objectives of the work presented here are to: (1) use openly available protein modeling webservers to construct complete three-dimensional (3D) models of human (hAARE) and rat AARE (rAARE); (2) use *in silico* protein-docking software to determine if the optimal AARE models (the receptors) have a reasonable affinity for a prototype nitrooxy N-acetyl-L-alaninate QM releasing prodrug ester (the ligand); (3) validate any positive *in silico* results by synthesizing and physically characterizing the proposed novel prodrug ester and evaluating its *in vitro* ability to deplete GSH in the presence of rAARE which has a 92% sequence identity with hAARE (using the Basic Local Alignment Search Tool (BLAST) with a compositional matrix adjustment http://blast.ncbi.nlm.nih.gov)). This work will lay the foundation for future efforts aimed at optimizing AARE targeted prodrugs as well as preclinical cancer studies with cell and animal models.

There Are No Reported Structures for Any Mammalian AARE

There are no reported X-ray or NMR structures for any mammalian AAREs. Feese *et al.* [33] were, however, able to crystallize human erythrocyte AARE and obtain preliminary X-ray data. Similarly, Wright *et al.* [34] have crystallized porcine AARE (pAARE) and have reported a preliminary crystallographic analysis showing that pAARE has four molecules in the asymmetric unit, which is consistent with the known homotetrameric quaternary structure of mammalian AAREs. The crystal structure of AARE (PDB ID 1VE6) from the thermophilic archaeon *Aeropyrum pernix* K1 (apAARE) has been reported to 2.1 A^o and has a 29% sequence identity (55% sequence similarity) with hAARE but has a homodimeric quaternary structure [35]. The apAARE structure has two domains: a β-propeller domain in the N-terminus and an α/β-hydrolase domain in the C-terminus [35]. More recently, the crystal structure of *Pyrococcus horikoshii* AARE (pkAARE) has also been determined but it has a hexameric quaternary structure [36].

Methods

Protein-Structure Modeling

The FASTA format amino acid sequence of hAARE (P13798, ACPH_HUMAN) and rAARE (P13676, ACPH_RAT) were obtained from the Universal Protein Resource (UniProt) athttp://www.uniprot.org/uniprot/P13798). Highly conserved amino acids residues were identified using the POLYVIEW-3D server (http://polyview.cchmc.org/polyview3d.html) and protein sequence identity and similarity calculated using the UVa FAST server (http://fasta.bioch.virginia.edu/). The 3-D structures of hAARE were initially modeled from the amino acid sequence using three different protein structure prediction webservers, i.e., I-TASSER [37-39] (http://zhanglab.ccmb.med.umich.edu/I-TASSER/), Phyre2 [40] (http://www. sbg.bio.ic.ac.uk/phyre2/html/) , and M4T[41-43] (http://manaslu.aecom.yu.edu/ M4T/). For rAARE, only the I-TASSER was employed since this server gave the overall best results with hAARE. All the webservers employed in this research are freely available for academic use.

Energy Minimization and Refinement of Initial AARE Models

The models produced by all three servers were further refined using the YASARA energy minimization server (http://www.yasara.org/minimizationserver.htm).The YASARA server runs molecular dynamics simulations with explicit solvent using a knowledge-based, all atom force field derived from Amber [44]. In particular, the YASARA Amber force field parameters were modified to keep untoward damage to protein crystal structures to a minimum [44].

Structural Quality of AARE Models before and after Energy Minimization

The models, both before and after YASARA minimization, were initially screened for structural quality using: (1) the RAMPAGE Ramachandran Plot server [45] (http://mordred.bioc.cam.ac.uk/~rapper/rampage.php); (2) the ProSA web service https://prosa.services.came.sbg.ac.at/prosa.php) for the recognition of errors in the 3D structures of proteins [46]; (3) deviations from the expected α-carbon (CA) distances for the residues forming the catalytic Asp-His-Ser triad, as well as potential disruptions in the spatial arrangement of the highly conserved residues caused by YASARA energy minimization protocol.

Selected 3D models were then further evaluated for using the MolProbity structure-validation web service (http://molprobity.biochem.duke.edu/) which provides the MolProbity Score (MPscore), a single score combining the clash score, rotamer, and Ramachandran evaluations into a single score that is normalized to be on the same scale as protein structures obtained at X-ray resolution [47].

Protein-ligand Docking and Drug Binding Sites in AARE

Protein-ligand docking for the optimal structural models was performed using the PyRx 0.8 software for computational drug discovery (http://pyrx.sourceforge.net/),which is available under an open source license. A locally installed version of Autodock Vina was the docking protocol (http://vina.scripps.edu/) selected for use by PyRx [48]. Open Babel was used for importing the ligand SDF files and for initial ligand energy minimization. PyBabel was used calculating the ligand partial charges (i.e., PDBQT files) as described on the PyRx webpage (http://pyrx.sourceforge.net/). The ligands were considered flexible but the sidc chains on the protein models considered as rigid. The ligand-binding grid (or search space) for all docking calculations was set (automatically) at the maximum. This setting provided a grid with x, y z dimensions of 72 Å, 76 Å, 67 Å, respectively, that enclosed the entire protein.

This approach does not assume a particular location for the ligand-binding site, i.e., blind docking. The Vina exhaustiveness parameter was set to a value of 40.

Potential ligand binding sites/pockets for hAARE were also identified and characterized using the DoGSiteScorer (http://dogsite.zbh.uni-hamburg.de/) and the CAVER plugin for PyMol (http://caver.cz/). The DogSiteScorer is an automated pocket detection and analysis tool that provides a "druggability" estimation of the detected pockets, i.e., an estimate of how useful the pocket could be as drug target. [49]. The CAVER PyMol plugin provides a fully automated calculation of tunnels and channels in protein structures.

Organic Synthesis of the Novel 4-[(nitrooxy)phenyl-N-acetyl-L-alaninate (NPAA) Prodrug

The N-acetyl-L-alaninate quinone methide donor, 4-[(nitrooxy)phenyl-N-acetyl-L-alaninate was synthesized as outline in Figure 3. All chemicals were purchased from Sigma-Aldrich (St. Louis, MO), TCI (Portland, OR), Acros Organics (Thermo Fisher Scientific, New Jersey) and Lancaster (Ward Hill, MA) and used without further purification. Flash chromatography was performed with 70 to 230-mesh silica (Silicycle Inc., Quebec, Canada) and monitored by thin layer chromatography (TLC) with silica plates (Merck, Kieselgel 60 F254). The melting points were determined using MEL-TEMP, infrared spectroscopy (IR) spectra were recorded with a Genesis II FT-IRTM spectrometer and the ^{1}H and ^{13}C NMR spectra measured with a 400 MHz Varian instrument. The spectra were recorded in hexa-deuterocacetone (acetone-d_6), tetra-deuteromethanol (methanol-d_4) or hexa-deuterodimethylsulfoxide (DMSO-d_6). The chemical shifts of protons are given in ppm with tetramethylsilane as an internal standard. The chemical shifts of carbons were obtained in ppm with solvent peaks used as internal standards.

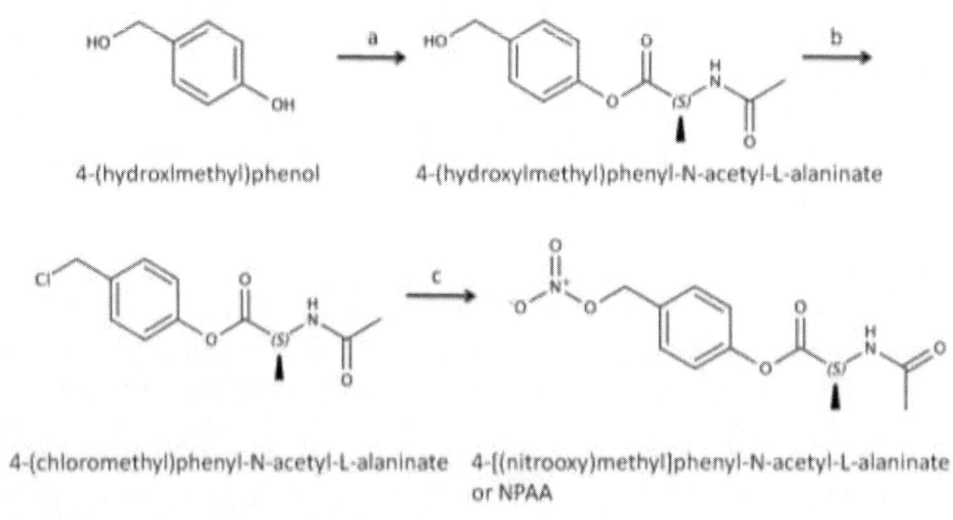

Figure 3. Organic Synthesis of a novel 4-[(nitrooxy)methyl]phenyl-N-acetyl-L-alaninate (NPAA) prodrug. The synthetic steps are steps: (a) N-acetyl-L-alanine, N,N'-dicyclohexylcarbodiimide, 4-dimethylaminopyridine, acetonitrile, 70%; (b) PCl_5, dichloromethane, 0 °C, 77%; (c) $AgNO_3$, acetonitrile, room temperature, 65%. The (S)- label in the above structures refers to the configuration of the chiral center using the R-S-system.

4-(Hydroxylmethyl)phenyl N-acetyl-L-alaninate was first synthesized (step a in Figure 3) by adding L-N-acetylalanine (0.26 g, 2.0 mmol), 4-(hydroxymethyl)phenol (0.496 g, 4.0 mmol) and 4-dimethylaminopyridine (2.4 mg, 0.02 mmol) to a one-neck round bottom flask containing 4 mL of acetonitrile. The mixture was stirred, heated to dissolve the solids and then cooled to room temperature. N,N'-dicyclohexylcarbodiimide (0.496 g, 2.4 mmol) was added to this solution followed by overnight stirring at room temperature. The resulting mixture was filtered, concentrated and subjected to silica gel column chromatography using a mixed solvent as the eluant (0-4.5% of methanol in dichloromethane by volume) to afford 4-(hydroxylmethyl)phenyl-N-acetyl-L-alaninate (0.33 g, 70%) as a colorless oil which showed one spot by TLC with a R_f value of 0.19 using 4% methanol in dichloromethane IR (neat, cm-1): 812, 885, 1014, 1040, 1136, 1165, 1188, 1375, 1456, 1506, 1541, 1651, 1755, 3272. ^{1}H NMR (400 MHz, DMSO-d_6, ppm) δ 1.43 (d, 3 H, J = 7.2 Hz, CH_3), 1.88 (s, 3 H, CH_3), 4.43 (m, 1 H, CH), 4.50 (d, 2 H, J = 5.6 Hz, CH_2), 5.27 (t, 1 H, J = 6.0 Hz, OH), 7.05 (d, 2 H, J = 8.4 Hz, phenyl); 7.36 (d, 2 H, J = 8.4 Hz, phenyl); 8.52 (d, 1 H, J = 6.4 Hz, NH); ^{13}C NMR (100 MHz, DMSO-d_6, ppm) δ 17.24, 22.72, 48.55, 62.89, 121.70, 128.07, 140.77, 149.69, 170.08, 172.45; high resolution-electrospray ionization-time-of-flight-mass spectra (HR-ESI-TOF) calculated for $C_{12}H_{16}NO_4^+$ (M + H^+) 238.107, found 238.108.

4-(Chloromethyl)phenyl N-acetyl-L-alaninate was next synthesized (step b in Figure 3) by adding 4-(hydroxylmethyl)phenyl-N-acetyl-L-alaninate (0.30 g, 1.27 mmol) to a one-neck round bottom flask with 4 mL dichloromethane. The mixture was stirred, cooled in an ice-water bath and PCl_5 (0.31 g, 1.48 mmol) was added followed by stirring for 15 minutes at (0°C). 4-(Chloromethyl)phenyl N-acetyl-L-alaninate (0.25 g, 77%) was purified as white solid from the resulting mixture by silica gel column chromatography using 2.0% (by volume) methanol in dichloromethane as the eluant. TLC showed one spot with a Rf value 0.19 using 2% methanol in dichloromethane. M.P. 139-140°C. IR (neat, cm-1): 667, 893, 1018, 1068, 1101, 1142, 1167, 1188, 1213, 1271, 1337, 1369, 1452, 1510, 1549, 1651, 1753, 3287. ^{1}H NMR (400 MHz, acetone-d_6, ppm) δ 1.50 (d, 3 H, J = 7.2 Hz, CH_3), 1.93 (s, 3 H, CH_3), 4.56 (m, 1 H, CH), 4.72 (s, 2 H, CH_2), 7.14 (d, 2 H, J = 8.4 Hz, phenyl); 7.50 (d, 2 H, J = 8.8 Hz, phenyl); 7.68 (s, 1 H, NH); ^{13}C NMR (100 MHz, acetone-d_6, ppm) δ 16.60, 21.70, 45.39, 48.47, 121.97, 130.02, 135.75, 151.05, 169.49, 171.61; HR-ESI-TOF calculated for $C_{12}H_{15}NO_3Cl^+$(M + H^+) 256.074, found 256.073.

Finally, 4-[(nitrooxy)methyl]phenyl N-acetyl-L-alaninate (NPAA) was synthesized (step c in Figure 3) by adding 4-(chloromethyl)phenyl N-acetyl-L-alaninate (0.25 g, 0.98 mmol) and acetonitrile (7 mL) to a one-neck round bottom flask followed by the addition of solid AgNO3 (0.332 g, 1.95 mmol). After stirring at room temperature for 48 h, the resulting mixture was subjected to column chromatography purification, using 25% of acetone in hexane (by volume) as the eluant, to give 4-[(nitrooxy)methyl]phenyl N-acetyl-L-alaninate as a white solid (0.18 g, 65%). TLC showed one spot with a Rf value of 0.14 with 25% acetone in hexane. M.p. 111-113 °C. IR (neat, cm-1): 678, 756, 837, 860, 889, 974, 1109, 1138, 1169, 1188, 1279, 1339, 1371, 1452, 1508, 1543, 1626, 1753, 3283. ^{1}H NMR (400 MHz, DMSO-d_6, ppm) δ 1.43 (d, 3 H, J = 6.8 Hz, CH_3), 1.88 (s, 3 H, CH_3), 4.42 (m, 1 H, CH), 5.58 (s, 2 H, CH2), 7.17 (d, 2 H, J = 8.4 Hz, phenyl); 7.55 (d, 2 H, J = 8.4 Hz, phenyl); 8.54 (d, 1 H, J = 6.2 Hz, NH); ^{13}C NMR (100 MHz, DMSO-d_6, ppm) δ 17.15, 22.68, 48.60, 75.07, 122.49, 130.50, 131.45, 151.68, 170.11, 172.26; HR-ESI-TOF calculated for $C_{12}H_{15}N_2O_6^+$ (M + H+) 283.092, found 283.093.

Rat Liver AARE (rAARE)

rAARE was semi-purified from rat liver (100 g) using the method described by Tsunasawa *et al.* [50] with the following modifications. After eluting samples from the DEAE-cellulose column, the AARE fractions were combined and subjected to gel filtration on a Superose 12 (10/300 GL) column (GE Healthcare, Pittsburgh, PA) using a Biologic Duo Flow Protein Purification System (Bio-Rad, Hercules, CA). Fractions were eluted with 50 mM pH 7 sodium phosphate buffer containing 1.0 mM EDTA and 0.2 M NaCl at a rate of 0.5 mL/min in 0.5 mL fractions. Fractions containing rAARE activity, which eluted as one peak, were combined (2 ml total volume, 0.12 mg protein/ml) and analyzed by reverse phase nanospray-spray liquid chromatography with tandem mass spectrometry (RP nano-LC-MS/MS).

For RP nano-LC-MS/MS, in-solution tryptic digests were prepared with the In-Gel tryptic Digestion kit (Pierce, Rockford, IL) using a 10 μL aliquot of the purified rAARE. Disulfide bonds were reduced, unmodified thiol groups alkylated, and proteins digested with trypsin overnight according to the manufacturer's instructions.

After digestion, samples were dried using a DNA Speed Vac Concentrator (Thermo Fisher Scientific, NC), the peptides rehydrated with 0.1% formic acid and further purified using zip tips (ZipTipU-C18, Millipore Corp., Billerica, MA) according to manufacturer's instructions. Peptides eluted from zip tips were transferred to vial inserts, dried and rehydrated in 4 μl of formic acid/acetonitrile/water (0.1:20:79.9, v/v/v) and 2 μl injected into a C18 picofrit column (New Objective, Inc., MA). The column was first equilibrated in solvent A (0.1% formic acid in water/acetonitrile (98:2, v/v)) and then eluted with a gradient of 2 – 40% of solvent B containing 0.1% formic acid in acetonitrile over 60 min at a flow rate of 200 nL/min. The eluted peptides were analyzed by nanospray ionization using a LTQ-XL ion trap MS (Thermo Scientific, Waltham, MA). MS data were acquired using data-dependent acquisition with a series of one full scan followed by a zoom scan and then a MS/MS scan of the ions. The dynamic exclusion duration was 30 ms. Proteins were identified using Bioworks (v3.3.1) software (Thermo Scientific, Waltham, MA).

In Vitro Glutathione (GSH) Depletion Assay

GSH depletion catalyzed by rAARE was monitored using Ellman's reagent, i.e., 5,5'-dithiobis-2-nitrobenzoic acid (DTNB). GSH and DTNB were obtained from Sigma Chemical Co. (St. Louis, MO). A 180 μl aliquot of freshly prepared solution containing 65 μM GSH and 160 μM of NPAA in 50mM pH 6.5 phosphate buffer was added to each well of a 96-well plate. A 20 μL aliquot of rAARE (0.12 mg protein/ml) in 50 mM pH 6.5 phosphate buffer was added to three wells immediately followed by a 50 μl aliquot of 1.25 mM DTNB (in pH 7.4 PBS buffer) for the zero time point and the absorbance at 412 nm was measured with a SpectraMax Plus 384 plate reader (Molecular Devices, Sunnyvale, CA). For each additional time point, the process was repeated using three wells per time point. A parallel series of measurements were made in which rAARE was pretreated with the serine protease inhibitor diisopropylfluorophosphate (DFP).

Results and Discussion

Predicted Protein Structures, Refinement and Structural Evaluation Analyses

The structural quality of the initial models returned from the three protein structure prediction webservers was initially evaluated (see Table 1) using the RAMPAGE Ramachandran Plot server [45] and the ProSA server [46]. The Z-score provided by the ProSA web server is an overall measure of protein model quality and values outside the range for known structures suggest a poor model [46]. For proteins with 732 residues (AARE), the known X-ray structures have a Z-score range between -5 and -15 but most X-ray structures are clustered around a Z-score between -7 and -12.

Table 1. Ramachandran plot assessment and ProSA Z-Scores for predicted models of human (h) and rat (r) acylamino-acid-releasing enzyme (AARE)

Model Server	% Residues in Ramachandran Regions			Z-Score**
	Favored	Allowed	Outliers	
Initial values from the protein structure prediction webservers				
h-I-TASSER*	80.0	11.6	8.4	-6.51
r-I-TASSER	79.7	11.4	8.9	-6.43
h-Phyre2	84.4	8.5	7.1	-2.79
h-M4T	87.8	8.2	4.0	-5.01
After YASARA energy minimization				
h-I-TASSER	86.6	10.3	3.2	-7.11
r-I-TASSER	84.4	11.9	3.7	-7.36
h-Phyre2	85.8	11.1	3.2	-5.72
h-M4T	84.2	11.5	4.2	-6.30

*This column specifies whether the predicted model is for human (h) or rat (r) AARE as well as the webserver (I-TASSER, Phyre2, etc.) used to obtain the predicted model.

** For a protein with 732 residues, most X-ray structures have a Z-score between -5 and -15 but most X-ray structures are clustered around a Z-score of -7 to -12.

I-TASSER (IT) is ranked as the number one server for protein structure prediction by the Protein Structure Prediction Center in the CASP7, CASP8 and CASP9 experiments [51,52]. This webserver uses a combination of *ab initio* folding, evolutionary and knowledge-based information (collectively termed "free-modeling" or FM) and template-based modeling (TBM) [53]. The I-TASSER webserver provides both structural and function predictions, e.g., the location amino acid residues involved in ligand binding sites. Although the I-TASSER server produced a model with the most plausible ProSA Z-scores, the percentage of outliers in the Ramachandran plots (i.e., the distribution of backbone dihedral angles) was high (see Table 1). The Z-score for the model returned by the Phyre2 server, which uses TBM methods, was unacceptably high and out of the range for native structures with 732 residues. The 3D model obtained by the M4T server, which uses a combination of TBM and iterative optimization of alternative alignments, had the best Ramachandran plot but a Z-value that was just plausible.

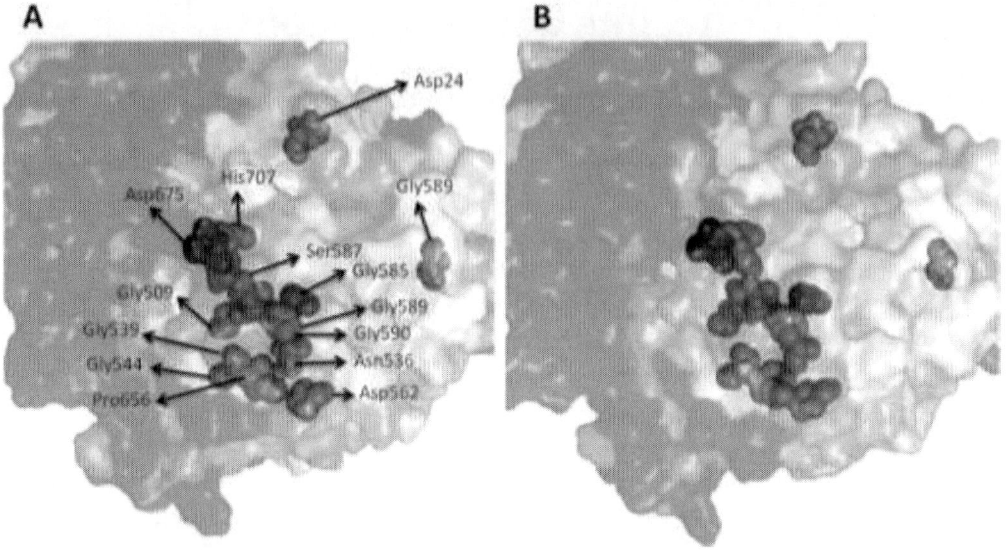

Figure 4. The spatial arrangement of the highly conserved residues in hAARE is not altered by YASARA energy minimization. Panel A shows the highly conserved residues for the I-TASSER human (h) AARE model before YASARA (Y) energy minimization (IT-hAARE) and panel B show the same residues after YASARA energy minimization (ITY-hAARE). Ser587, Asp675 and His707 comprise the exopeptidase catalytic triad characteristic of serine peptidases. These views were generated by the POLYVIEW-3D web-based tool for macromolecular structure visualization and analysis (http://polyview.cchmc.org/polyview3d.html).

The initial 3D models produced by all three modeling servers were subjected to refinement using the YASARA (Y) energy minimization server for improving physical realism in predicted models and the results are also provided in Table 1. After YASARA energy minimization, the Ramachandran plot quality, as well as the ProSA Z-scores, were all markedly improved, with the I-TASSER model producing the best overall quality for hAARE (see Table 1). The ProSA web service, in addition to calculating Z-scores, also provides a plot showing local model quality as a function of amino acid sequence position. For ITY-hAARE, the region with least local quality lies between residues 60 and 210, which does not contain any highly conserved residues. The residues with a high conservation scores include 24, 508, 509, 529, 536, 539, 544, 562, 585, 587, 589, 590, 656, 675 and 707, for a total of 15 residues. As indicated in Figure 4, most of the conserved residues were spatially clustered at the active site of the AARE models.

The Active Site of AARE as Compared to other Serine Proteases: An Additional Measure of AARE Structural Quality

Multiple sources of evidence [35,54,54,55] support the role of a charge relay system [56] formed by Ser587, Asp675 and His707 at the active exopeptidase site of AARE. Given the importance of the catalytic Asp-His-Ser triad, we next examined the α-carbon (CA) distances between these residues before and after YASARA energy minimization. For trypsin like serine proteases the CA-CA distances between Asp-His, Asp-Ser and His-Ser are known to be well conserved and close to 6.4 Å, 10.2 Å and 8.3 Å, respectively [57]. These distances can, however, vary by as much as 2 Å between different families of serine proteinases. The catalytic triad CA distances are a key measure of protein structural quality for serine peptidases, such as AARE, since any distances outside the expected ranges would indicate an unrealistic structure. Similarly, the YASARA energy minimization would not be useful if it resulted in AARE models outside the expected triad CA-CA ranges.

Table 2. The α-carbon (CA) distances between Ser587, Asp675 and His707 at the active exopeptidase site of human (h) and rat (r) models of acylamino-acid-releasing enzyme (AARE)

Model Server	Active Site Triad - CA distances (Å)		
	Asp-His	Asp-Ser	His-Ser
Distances (Å) calculated from initial protein structure prediction models			
h-I-TASSER*	4.9	10.4	7.7
r-I-TASSER	5.0	10.6	8.2
h-Phyre2	9.8	14.8	13.2
h-M4T	4.8	11.2	8.4
Distances (Å) after YASARA energy minimization			
h-I-TASSER	5.1	10.0	7.7
r-I-TASSER	6.6	10.5	7.3
h-Phyre2	4.6	10.8	8.0
h-M4T	5.3	11.4	7.5
Distances (Å) for Porcine Dipeptidyl Peptidase IV (CD26)			
From PDB	4.7	10.8	8.1

* This column specifies (with the exception of porcine dipeptidyl peptidase IV) whether the predicted model is for human (h) or rat (r) AARE as well as the webserver (I-TASSER, Phyre2, etc.) used to obtain the predicted model. For porcine dipeptidyl peptidase IV, the distances were calculated from the known X-ray structure (1ORVA.PDB).

With the exception of the Phyre2 model, the CA-CA active site residue distances obtained for the various models before and after YASARA energy minimization were similar (see Table 2) and close to the values observed for serine proteinases in general. For the Phyre2 model, the CA-CA distances before YASARA energy minimization were unreasonably high. YASARA energy minimization resulted in a convergence of the CA-CA distances towards distances typical of serine proteases. The results provided by the I-TASSER server lists 1ORVA.PDB as a top enzyme homolog of hAARE and rAARE. 1ORVA.PDB is a dipeptidyl peptidase IV and the CA-CA active site distances for this protein are also provided in Table 2. Encouragingly, these distances are also close to the distances calculated for the AARE models after YASARA energy minimization, which provides an additional assurance that the models have the correct active site geometry.

Ramachandran Plot Quality, YASARA Energy Minimization and the Spatial Distribution of Conserved Amino Acid Residues in AARE Models

To further evaluate the structural quality of the homology models, the three-dimensional locations of the highly conserved AARE residues (those with POLYVIEW-3D conservation scores higher then 7 were viewed since they are key determinants of structure/function and likely to be most important in our subsequent *in silico* protein-ligand docking studies. As anticipated, the catalytic triad of Ser587, Asp675 and His707 in hAARE is highly conserved. Moreover, of the remaining twelve highly conserved residues, 66.6% are Gly, five of which (Gly508, Gly509, Gly585, Gly589 and Gly590) are clustered around the active site (see Figure 4A), which is consistent with the notion that these Gly residues are essential for providing conformation flexibility near the active site by preventing steric hindrance [58]. Moreover, the spatial arrangement of the highly conserved residues in hAARE is remarkably similar before (IT-hAARE see Figure 4A) and after YASARA energy minimization (ITY-hAARE see Figure 4B). Analogous results were found for rAARE, which showed a spatial distribution of conserved residues very similar to that of hAARE.

These findings suggest that the marked improvement in the Ramachandran plot quality provided by YASARA energy minimization is not achieved at the expense of major alterations in the spatial distribution of conserved amino acid residues, which are primarily located near the catalytic triad. Moreover, the model structures predicted by the I-TASSER server exhibit the expected spatial clustering of Gly residues near the active site, which is a characteristic of POP serine proteases such as AARE [58].

I-TASSER Results in More Detail and with MolProbity Scores Suggesting Reasonable Models

The data present above suggest that AARE I-TASSER models, after YASSARA energy minimization, had the best structural quality. The top threading templates used by I-TASSER for both rat and human AARE models include 4HXE.PDB (Pyrococcus horikoshii AARE), 4A5S.PDB (human dipeptidyl peptidase 4 soluble form), 4HXF.PDB (Pyrococcus horikoshii acylaminoacyl peptidase in complex with Z-Gly-Gly-Phe-chloromethyl ketone) and 3AZO.PDB (Streptomyces morookaensis puromycin hydrolase). These crystal structures are all fairly recent (2011-2013). 4HXE.PDB is a hexameric AARE and its crystal structure suggests that substrate specificity for AAREs is achieved through this multimerization [36].

Using the top templates, the I-TASSER provides five top models and each is assigned a confidence-score (or C-score) which is an estimate of model prediction accuracy [59]. Typical C-scores are in the range of -5 to 2. A higher C-score value suggests a model with better accuracy. In the case of hAARE the best model (model 1) had a C-score of -0.15 and the other four models (models 2-5) has C-scores between -2.08 and -1.67. A C-score > -1.5 indicates a model with the correct fold. This means that model 1 was considerably more accurate than the next four possible models (models 2-5) which did not have C-scores > -1.5. Model 1 was, therefore, the sole model used in subsequent refinement and ligand-binding calculations. Moreover, model 1 had a TM-score of 0.69 ± 0.12. The TM-score is a scale that measures the structural similarity between two structures. A TM-score >0.5 indicates a model of correct topology (as found for model 1) while a TM-score< 0.17 suggests a random similarity [59]. The I-TASSER results for rat AARE was very similar with best model (model 1) having a C-score of -0.23 and a TM-score of 0.68± 0.12.

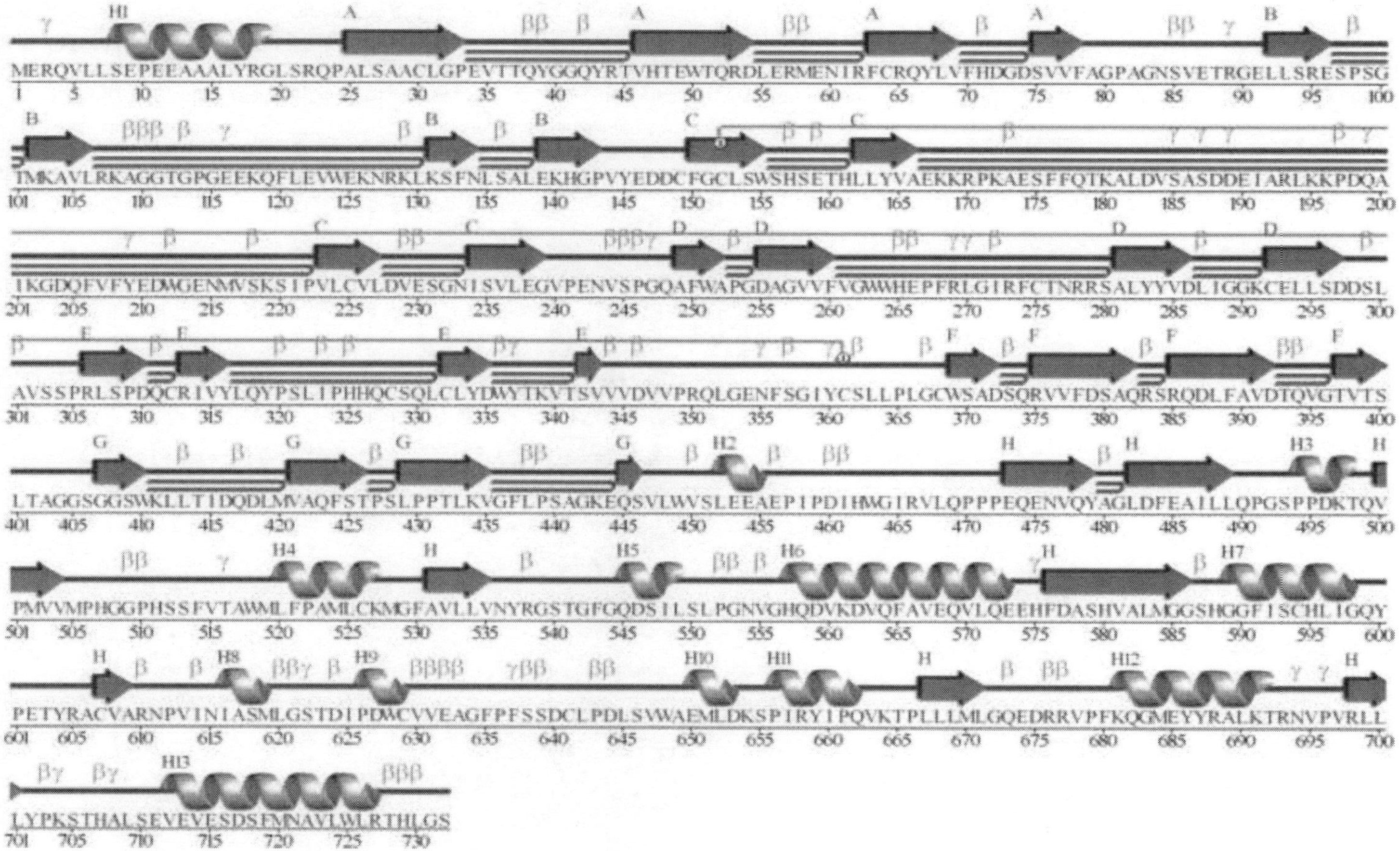

Figure 5. The wiring diagram forthe I-TASSER human acylamino-acid-releasing enzyme model after YASARA energy minimization (ITY-hAARE). This diagram shows the sequence locations of the ITY-hAARE's secondary structure (-helix and - strand), helices are labeled H1to H13 and strands by their sheets (A to H). Motifs are: β turn, γ turn, - beta hairpin. The labeled helices are also shown in the three-dimension model (3D) in Figure 7. There is a disulfide bond ( ) between Cys152 and Cys361.

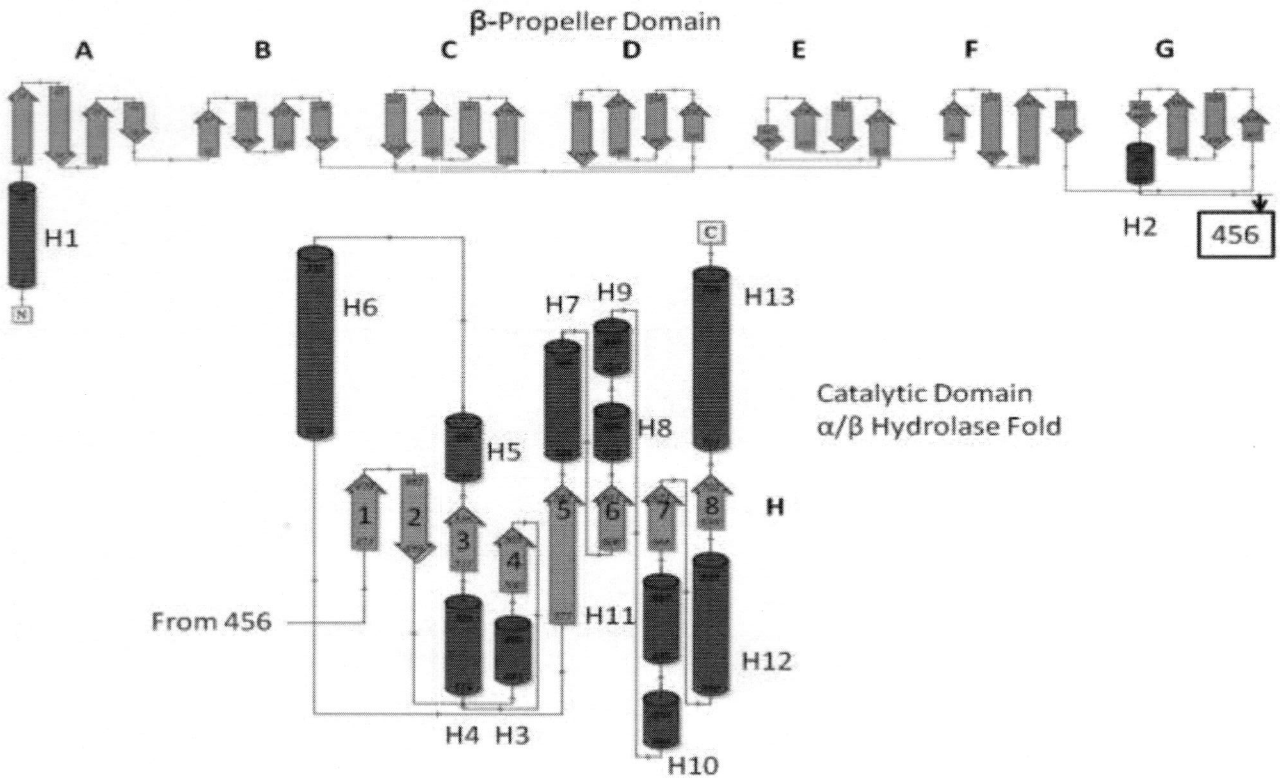

Figure 6. The topology diagram for the I-TASSER human acylamino-acid-releasing enzyme model after YASARA energy minimization (ITY-hAARE). This diagram illustrates how the β- strands (large arrows) align to form the β-sheets labeled A through H (also shown in Figure 5): small arrows indicate the direction of the protein chain. The locations of the α-helices (cylinders with labels H1 to H13), relative to the β-sheets, are also indicated and also shown in Figure 5 as well as the 3D model in Figure 7). The upper part of the figure (the β–propeller domain) shows the topology from residues 1-456 and, the lower part, the topology from residues 457 to 732 (the α/β-hydrolase domain). The N-terminal region shows a typical β-propeller domain and the C-terminal region shows a typical α/β-hydrolase fold with the catalytic domain. The eight β-strands of the α/β-hydrolase fold (sheet H) are also indicated.

As indicated above, the best I-TASSER model was further refined using the YASARA energy minimization with considerable improvement in the Ramachandran plot and the Z-score. As a final confirmation of the structural quality, we also submitted the ITY-hAARE and the ITY-rAARE models to the MolProbity structure-validation web service [47]. MolProbity scores of 1.82 and 2.14 were found for ITY-h-AARE and ITY-rAARE, respectively. Scores of 1.82 and 2.14 indicates that the structures were in the 84thand 68th and percentile, respectively (with the 100th percentile being the best quality X-ray structures). These data further support the conclusion that the proposed final models of human and rat are of reasonable quality to permit further protein-ligand docking calculations.

Structural Features of the Optimal AARE Models

The "wiring" diagram for ITY-hAARE, provided by the PDBsum server (http://www.ebi.ac.uk/pdbsum/), is shown in Figure 5 which shows the sequence locations of the protein's secondary structure, β-turns, γ-turns and β-hairpins [60-62]. A schematic summary of the secondary structure topology [60-62], also provided by the PDBsum server (http://www.ebi.ac.uk/pdbsum/), is shown in Figure 6 and is qualitatively similar to that reported by Bartmam *et al.* [35] for apAARE and Menyhard *et al.* [36] for phAARE. These bacterial AAREs have a β-propeller domain with seven blades, corresponding to β sheets A to G in Figure 6 for ITY-hAARE. All the β-propeller blades have four antiparallel strands. A second domain has the catalyticα/β-hydrolase fold with eight mostly parallel strands connected by helices, with only the second β-strand being antiparallel, corresponding to β sheet H in Figure 6.

As expected for an α/β hydrolase fold [63], the catalytic triad of ITY-hAARE shows a His residue (707) near the end of β-strand 8, an acidic residue (Asp675) near the end of β-strand 7, and a nucleophile (Ser587) near the end of β-strand 5. Moreover, Ser587 at the active site of ITY-hAARE is situated at a turn between β-strand 5 and helix H7 (see Figures 6 and 7) as found in other AAREs [36]. A disulfide bridge was identified by the PDBsum server, based on the criteria of two cysteine residues (Cys152 and Cys361) whose sulfur atoms are less than 3Å apart. This particular disulfide was classified as a right-handed hook (RHH) type based on the internal chi angles.

Figure 7 shows the 3D location of each helix (H1 to H13) in ITY-hAARE with Ser587 and Asp675, at the active site, shown as spheres. The β-strand 5 of sheet H is also shown in this Figure 7 where it can be seen ending in Ser587 at a very sharp turn, i.e., the nucleophile "elbow" typical of α/β hydrolase fold enzymes [63].

Although the optimal models of hAARE and rAARE models presented here have a structural quality comparable to many crystal structures they are, nevertheless, subject to the intrinsic limitations of protein structure prediction tools [53].

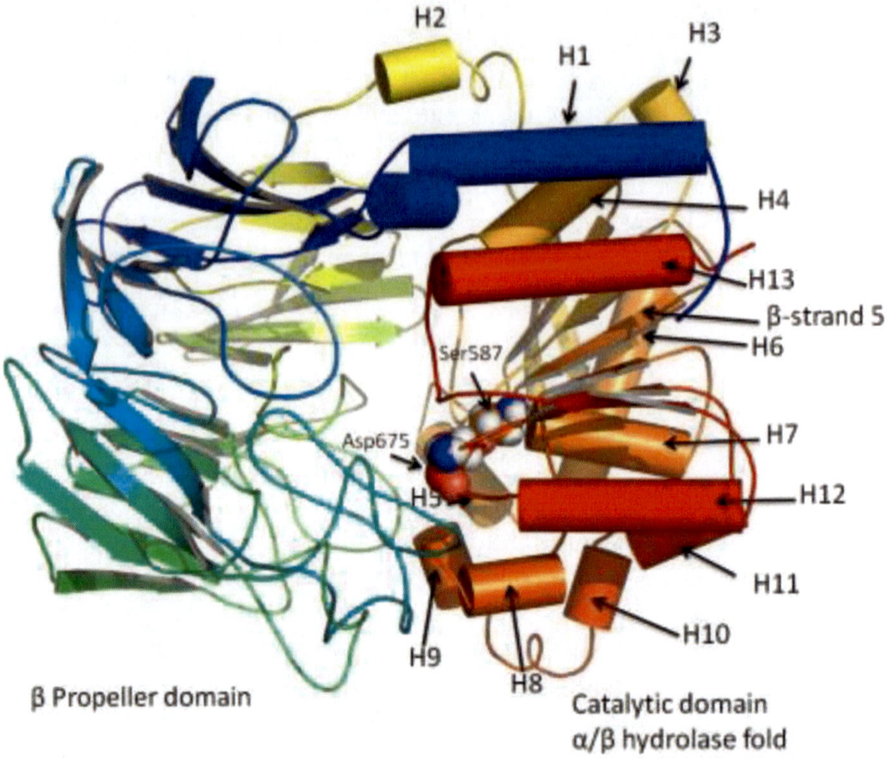

Figure 7. PyMOL rendering of the I-TASSER human acylamino-acid-releasing enzyme model after YASARA energy minimization (ITY-hAARE). This figure shows the 3D location of the (solid) helices labeled in Figure 6 (H1 to H13). The peptide chain and helices are rainbow colored from blue at N-terminus (N) to red at C-terminus (C). Ser587 and Asp675, at the active site, are shown as spheres. For β-sheet H of the α/β-hydrolase fold, the fifth β-strand is labeled (as also shown in Figure 6).

Blind Docking Calculations Show that Both N-acetyl-L-alanine-4-nitroanilide (AANA) and the Prototype QM Donating Analogue of AANA (NPAA) Bind at the Active Site of Human and Rat ITY-AARE Models with Reasonable Affinities

The next goal was to determine if the ligand-binding calculations showed that N-acetyl-L-alanine-4-nitroanilide (AANA), a specific substrate for AARE (see Figure 8A), bound at the expected AARE catalytic hydrolase domain with a reasonable affinity. We also evaluated the binding site location and affinity of AARE towards NPAA, a prototype QM donating analogue of AANA (see Figure 8B). We focused on the hAARE and rAARE I-TASSER models after YASARA energy minimization, i.e., the optimal models. The ligand-binding grid (or search space) for all the AutoDock Vina docking calculations was set to encompass the entire AARE protein. This "blind" docking approach does not, therefore, bias the subsequent docking calculations and enables the software (alone) to select the optimal binding site(s).

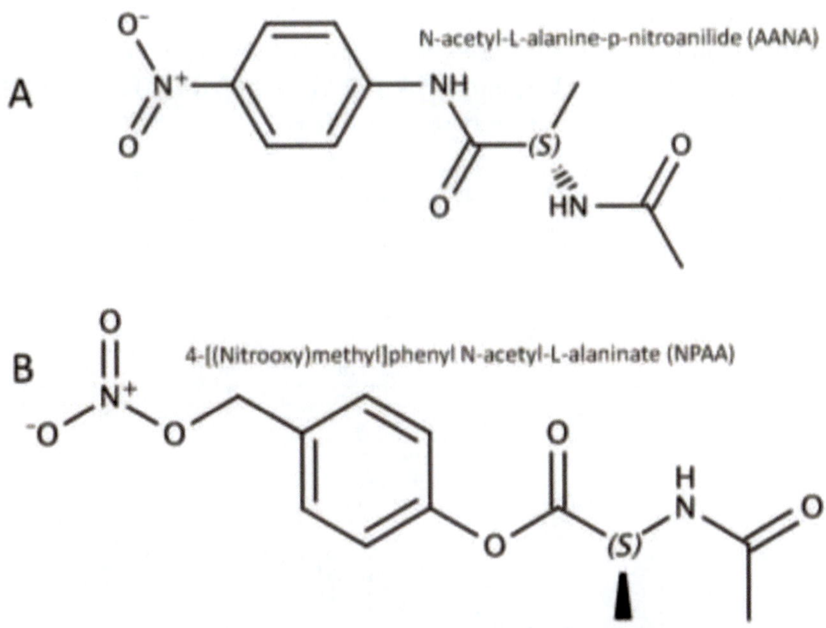

Figure 8. The ligand structures used in protein docking studies. Panel A shows the structure of the N-acetyl-L-alanine-p-nitroanilide (AANA), which is a specific substrate for AARE. Panel B show the structure of 4-[(Nitrooxy) methyl]phenyl N-acetyl-L-alaninate (NPAA) a potential anticancer prodrug similar in structure to both AANA and NO-ASA (see Figure 2). The (S)- label in the above structures refers to the configuration of the chiral center using the R-S-system. Our *in silico* protein-ligand docking suggests that both AANA and NPAA bind to the active site of human and rat AARE models derived from the I-TASSER protein structure prediction webserver.

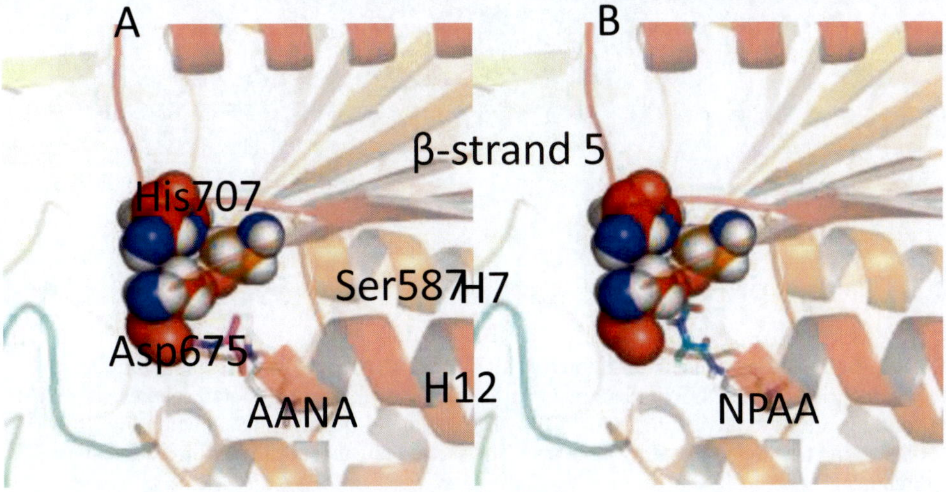

Figure 9. Ligand-docking studies with human AARE (ITY-hAARE). Panel A shows a PyMOL rendering of ITY-hAARE with the lowest energy pose of the AANA ligand (a specific AARE substrate) shown as sticks. The image is centered on Ser587and also shows Asp675 and His707 (the catalytic triad). The AARE orientation is the same as provided in Figure 7 and also shows the fifth β-strand of β-sheet H as well as helices H7 and H12. Panel B shows the lowest energy pose of the NPAA ligand, a prototype QM releasing anticancer prodrug. Both AANA and NPAA were found to bind at the AARE active site with very similar poses.

Table 3. The calculated binding affinities of N-acetyl-L-alanine-4-nitroanilide (AANA) and 4-[(nitrooxy)methyl]phenyl N-acetyl-L-alaninate (NPAA) to the I-TASSER (IT) models of human (ITY-hAARE) and rat AARE (ITY-rAARE) after YASARA(Y) energy minimization

Models	Prodrug used a ligand for *in silico* docking	
	ANNA	NPAA
	Binding affinity (kcal/mol)	
(kcal/mol)		
IT-hAARE	-7.5	-8.1
IT-rAARE	-8.4	-6.9

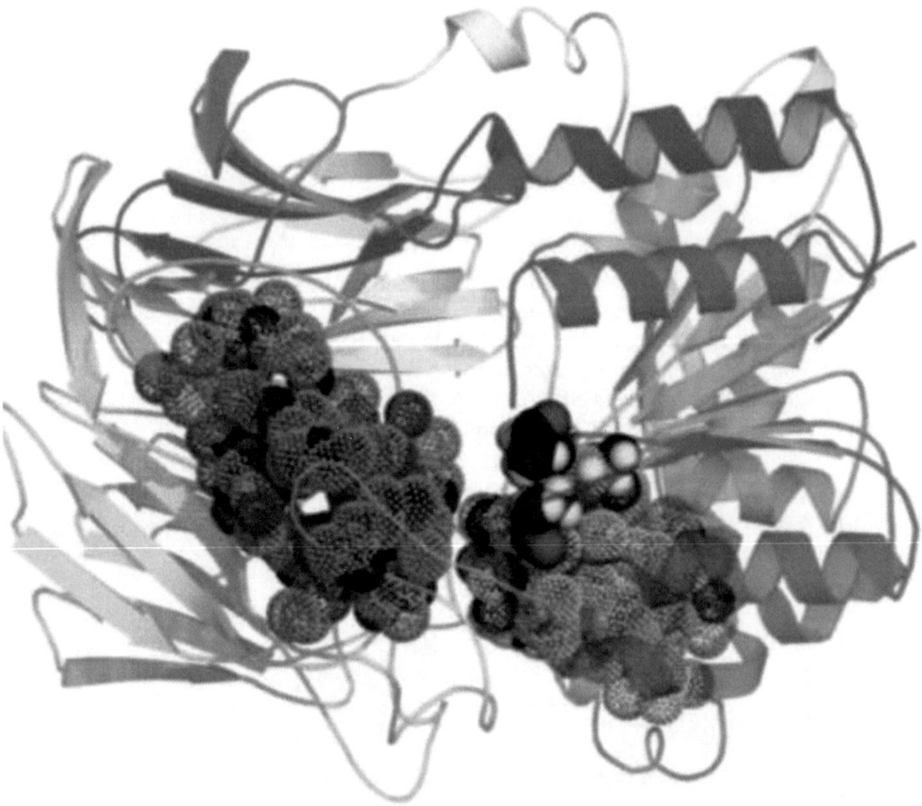

Figure 10. Druggable binding pockets for human AARE (ITY-hAARE). Two druggable binding pockets were identified by the DoGSiteScorer server and are shown as sets of doted spheres. The right-most drug-binding pocket totally encloses the α/β-hydrolase ligand-binding site shown in Figure 9. Both AANA and NPAA bind to this druggable site. The second left-most drug-binding site is in the β-propeller domain.

As shown in Figure 9A, the AutoDock Vina located AANA in a binding pocket in the immediate vicinity of the catalyticα/β-hydrolase domain. The binding pocket for NPAA (Figure 9B) was similarly located, thereby supporting the notion that this QM donating compound is a reasonable chemical analog of AANA. The AutoDock Vina software provides nine poses for each ligand. The poses in Figure 9A and 9B have the highest affinity (lowest energy) but are representative of the other high affinity poses which all cluster at the same location shown in Figure 9. We found that the binding pocket location and the poses of AANA and NPAA to ITY-rAARE, are similar to that discussed above for ITY-hAARE. The binding affinities for AANA and NPAA to ITY-hAARE and ITY-hAARE are provided in Table 3 and these data suggest that both ligands have reasonably strong affinities to hAARE. As indicated in Table 3, the results for rAARE are similar to those obtained for hAARE.

The Binding Site for AANA and NPAA in ITY-hAARE and ITY-rAARE Is in a Pocket with a High Druggability Score

We further investigated the binding site for AANA and NPAA in the ITY-hAARE and ITY-rAARE models using the DoGSiteScorer server, which predicts druggable pockets based on their calculated size, shape and chemical features. A score of "0" of indicates an undruggable pocket and a score of "1" indicates a highly druggable pocket. The two best pockets selected by the DoGSiteScorer server for ITY-hAARE are shown in Figure 10 as two sets of spherical dots. The pocket to the left has a score of 0.55 and overlaps with the catalyticα/β-hydrolase domain containing the AANA and NPAA binding sites provided by AutoDock Vina. The second druggable site is in the β-propeller domain and has a druggable score of 0.72. Similar results were found for ITY1-rAARE. These results could be useful for future studies aimed at optimizing cancer drugs targeted to human AARE.

Proof of Concept for the Glutathione (GSH) Depleting Ability of NPAA in the Presence of rAARE

Since our *in silico* studies suggest that NPAA binding to hAARE or rAARE is similar to that of the ANNA, our next objectives were to synthesize NPAA and then determine if rAARE could decrease *in vitro* GSH levels in the presence of NPAA. NPAA (Figure 8) is structurally similar to nitric oxide donating acetylsalicylic acid (NO-ASA as shown in Figure 2) and its hydrolysis yields the identical QM chemical species as the hydrolysis of NO-ASA. NPAA was synthesized (Figure 2) and its purity checked by TLC and HR-ESI-TOF. Both ^{1}H and ^{13}C NMR spectra were used to validate the chemical structure of NPAA and also served as an additional confirmation of purity.

AARE was purified as describe above and incubated with GSH and NPAA in the presence or absence of DFP, an irreversible inhibitor of serine proteases, including rAARE [15]. DFP covalently binds to Ser587. As indicated in Figure 11, rAARE catalyzed the *in vitro* consumption of GSH, an effect that was completely abolished in the presence of DFP. In the absence of rAARE there is also no consumption of GSH (data not shown). These data are consistent with the hypothesis that AARE can hydrolyze NPAA to form a QM, which can deplete GSH levels by a covalent reaction in a manner completely analogous to that proven for NO-ASA (Figure 2). RP nano-LC-MS/MS showed that none of the proteins in the semi-purified rAARE contained another enzyme with a known protease or hydrolase activity.

Conclusion

Exploiting the Esterase Activity of AARE for Pro-oxidant Anticancer Prodrug Activation

As outlined in Figure 1, the work presented here suggests a potentially new approach for exploiting a newly recognized weakness in the molecular armamentarium that cancer cells utilize to maintain an aggressive cancer phenotype, i.e., a high level of intrinsic oxidative stress due to the activation of the Akt kinase cascade. Akt kinase is a cardinal node for a diverse set of signaling cascades important for regulating cell survival, cell growth, glucose metabolism, cell motility and angiogenesis [7]. Akt activation is caused by mutations in components of its signaling cascade and results in cancer cells with an increased ability to escape apoptosis and proliferate. This, however, is a "double-edged sword" since Akt activation also causes an increased production of ROS as well as an increased sensitivity to pro-oxidant drugs causing ROS-induced apoptosis [3].

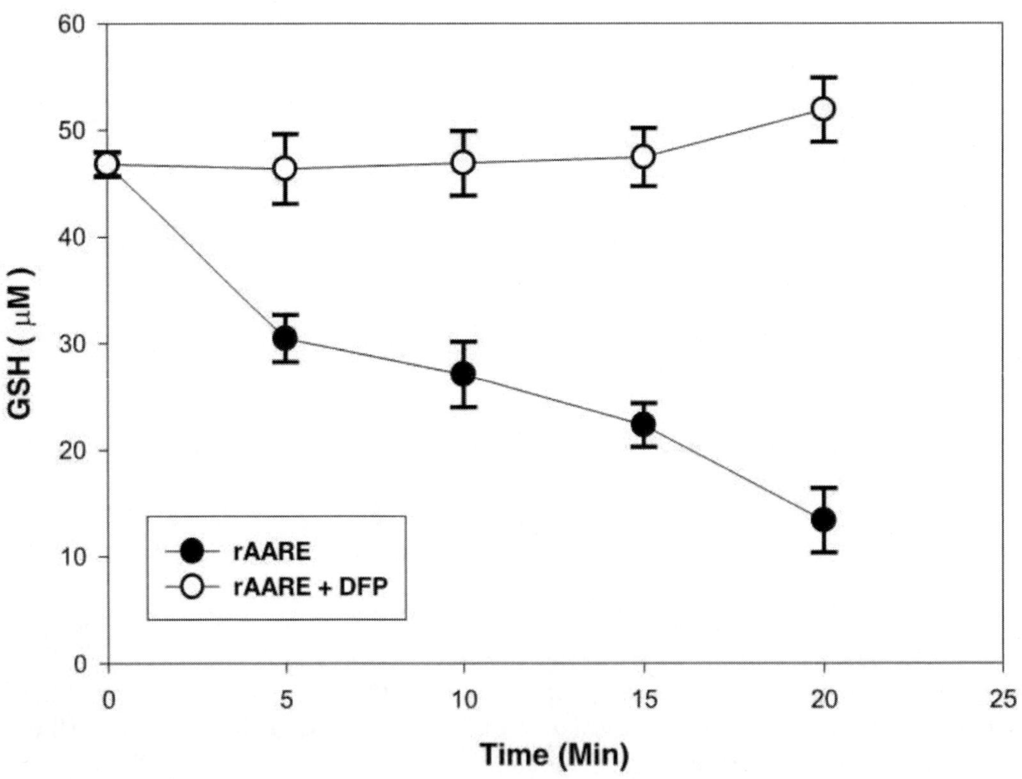

Figure 11. Rat acylamino-acid-releasing enzyme (rAARE) catalyzed *in vitro* consumption of glutathione (GSH). The *in vitro* consumption of GSH was measured in the presence of semi-purified rAARE as a function of incubation time (in triplicate ± SD). When rAARE is treated with DFP, a serine protease inhibitor, there is no consumption of GSH. All data points beyond 5 min are statistically different ($P < 0.05$).

The work presented here suggests that the esterase activity of AARE can be exploited as a potential target for the activation of a novel pro-oxidant nitrooxy N-acetyl-L-alaninate prodrug, NPAA, that depletes GSH in a manner completely analogous to that of NO-ASA, a well-characterized anti-cancer drug with minimal *in vivo* toxicity. NO-ASA is thought to exert its potent anticancer effect by depleting intracellular GSH and causing oxidative stress induced apoptosis by activation of the intrinsic death pathway [24]. As proof of concept, we have found (Figure 11) that rAARE can deplete GSH in the presence of NPAA.

We have recently reported that hAARE is overexpressed in the human LNCaP tumorigenic prostate cell line compared to control human nontumorigenic RWPE-1 prostate epithelial cells [64]. Moreover, cellular lysates of LNCaP cells were more effective than the cellular lysates of RWPE-1 cells at *in vitro* GSH depletion, which is consistent with the overexpression of hAARE found in LNCaP cells compared to RWPE-1 cells. LNCaP cells treated with NPAA were also found to have a greater loss of cell viability and greater depletion of intracellular GSH than similarly treated RWPE-1 cells. Collectively, our findings are significant since they potentially provide a molecular basis for selecting those cancer patients most likely to respond to NPAA –like prodrugs, i.e., those with activated Akt and AARE overexpression.

The Potential Utility of Having 3D AARE Models for the Design of Anticancer Drugs

The 3D models of hAARE and rAARE presented here have proven useful in the design of a potential prototype chemotherapeutic prodrug, NPAA, that is activated by the hydrolase activity of AARE. It should be noted, however, that drugs that inhibit the hydrolase activity of AARE could also be important as anticancer therapeutics.

The removal of N-acetyl groups from acetylated proteins by the hydrolase activity of AARE is thought to play a key role in the protein degradation by ubiquitin-proteasome system [12]. N-acetylated proteins are not substrates for N-ubiquitylation, which requires a free primary amino group [65]. Small molecule inhibitors of AARE have been found to induce proteasomal down-regulation, which is an important mechanism known to induce apoptosis in broad range of cancers and thereby block cancer progression [66]. The mammalian AARE models presented here could be useful in the design optimal AARE inhibitors. We are currently exploring this avenue of research.

Acknowledgment

This work was funded (in part) by a grant from the East Tennessee State University Research Development Committee Small Grants Program (to WLS and YLJ).

References

[1] Nogueira V, Park Y, Chen CC, Xu PZ, Chen ML, Tonic I, et al. Akt determines replicative senescence and oxidative or oncogenic premature senescence and sensitizes cells to oxidative apoptosis. *Cancer Cell* 2008 Dec 9;14(6):458-470.

[2] Watson J. Oxidants, antioxidants and the current incurability of metastatic cancers. *Open Biol* 2013 Jan 8;3(1):120144.

[3] Dolado I, Nebreda AR. AKT and oxidative stress team up to kill cancer cells. *Cancer Cell* 2008 Dec 9;14(6):427-429.

[4] Kumar B, Koul S, Khandrika L, Meacham RB, Koul HK. Oxidative stress is inherent in prostate cancer cells and is required for aggressive phenotype. *Cancer Res* 2008 Mar 15;68(6):1777-1785.

[5] Pelicano H, Carney D, Huang P. ROS stress in cancer cells and therapeutic implications. *Drug Resist Updat* 2004 Apr;7(2):97-110.

[6] Govindarajan B, Sligh JE, Vincent BJ, Li M, Canter JA, Nickoloff BJ, et al. Overexpression of Akt converts radial growth melanoma to vertical growth melanoma. *J Clin Invest* 2007 Mar;117(3):719-729.

[7] Testa JR, Tsichlis PN. AKT signaling in normal and malignant cells. *Oncogene* 2005 Nov 14;24(50):7391-7393.

[8] Benbrook DM, Masamha CP. The pro-survival function of Akt kinase can be overridden or altered to contribute to induction of apoptosis. *Curr Cancer Drug Targets* 2011 Jun;11(5):586-599.

[9] Singh S, Khan AR, Gupta AK. Role of glutathione in cancer pathophysiology and therapeutic interventions. *J Exp Ther Oncol* 2012;9(4):303-316.

[10] Schnelldorfer T, Gansauge S, Gansauge F, Schlosser S, Beger HG, Nussler AK. Glutathione depletion causes cell growth inhibition and enhanced apoptosis in pancreatic cancer cells. *Cancer* 2000 Oct 1;89(7):1440-1447.

[11] Mena S, Benlloch M, Ortega A, Carretero J, Obrador E, Asensi M, et al. Bcl-2 and glutathione depletion sensitizes B16 melanoma to combination therapy and eliminates metastatic disease. *Clin Cancer Res* 2007 May 1;13(9):2658-2666.

[12] Palmieri G, Bergamo P, Luini A, Ruvo M, Gogliettino M, Langella E, et al. Acylpeptide hydrolase inhibition as targeted strategy to induce proteasomal down-regulation. *PLoS One* 2011;6(10):e25888.

[13] Protein Atlas version 9.0 - 2011.11.11; Available at: http://www.proteinatlas.org/ENSG00000164062/cancer, 2012.

[14] Gade W, Brown JL. Purification and partial characterization of alpha-N-acylpeptide hydrolase from bovine liver. *J Biol Chem* 1978 Jul 25;253(14):5012-5018.

[15] Kobayashi K, Smith JA. Acyl-peptide hydrolase from rat liver. Characterization of enzyme reaction. *J Biol Chem 1987 Aug* 25;262(24):11435-11445.

[16] Harmat V, Domokos K, Menyhard DK, Pallo A, Szeltner Z, Szamosi I, et al. Structure and catalysis of acylaminoacyl peptidase: closed and open subunits of a dimer oligopeptidase. *J Biol Chem 2011 Jan* 21;286(3):1987-1998.

[17] Nakai A, Yamauchi Y, Sumi S, Tanaka K. *Role of acylamino acid-releasing enzyme/oxidized protein hydrolase in sustaining homeostasis of the cytoplasmic antioxidative system.* Planta 2012 Mar 8.

[18] Shimizu K, Ikegami-Kawai M, Takahashi T. Increased oxidized protein hydrolase activity in serum and urine of diabetic rat models. *Biol Pharm Bull* 2009 Sep;32(9):1632-1635.

[19] Shimizu K, Kiuchi Y, Ando K, Hayakawa M, Kikugawa K. Coordination of oxidized protein hydrolase and the proteasome in the clearance of cytotoxic denatured proteins. *Biochem Biophys Res Commun* 2004 Nov 5;324(1):140-146.

[20] Kikugawa K. Defense of living body against oxidative damage. *Yakugaku Zasshi* 2004 Oct;124(10):653-666.

[21] Xiao M, Yang HS, Klein SM, Muenyi CM, Stone WL, Jiang YL. *Novel Synthesis of NCX 4040 in Mild Conditions and Biological Evaluation Against Prostate Cancer.* Bioorganic & Medicinal Chemistry Letters 2007;submitted for publication.

[22] Razavi R, Gehrke I, Gandhirajan RK, Poll-Wolbeck SJ, Hallek M, Kreuzer KA. Nitric oxide-donating acetylsalicylic acid induces apoptosis in chronic lymphocytic leukemia cells and shows strong antitumor efficacy in vivo. *Clin Cancer Res* 2011 Jan 15;17(2):286-293.

[23] Dunlap T, Chandrasena RE, Wang Z, Sinha V, Wang Z, Thatcher GR. Quinone formation as a chemoprevention strategy for hybrid drugs: balancing cytotoxicity and cytoprotection. *Chem Res Toxicol* 2007 Dec;20(12):1903-1912.

[24] Gao J, Liu X, Rigas B. Nitric oxide-donating aspirin induces apoptosis in human colon cancer cells through induction of oxidative stress. *Proc Natl Acad Sci* U S A 2005 Nov 22;102(47):17207-17212.

[25] Gao L, Williams JL. Nitric oxide-donating aspirin induces G2/M phase cell cycle arrest in human cancer cells by regulating phase transition proteins. *Int J Oncol* 2012 Jul;41(1):325-330.

[26] Khan NI, Cisterne A, Baraz R, Bradstock KF, Bendall LJ. Para-NO-aspirin inhibits NF-kappaB and induces apoptosis in B-cell progenitor acute lymphoblastic leukemia. *Exp Hematol* 2012 Mar;40(3):207-215.e1.

[27] Rigas B. Novel agents for cancer prevention based on nitric oxide. *Biochem Soc Trans* 2007 Nov;35(Pt 5):1364-1368.

[28] Sun Y, Chen J, Rigas B. Chemopreventive agents induce oxidative stress in cancer cells leading to COX-2 overexpression and COX-2-independent cell death. *Carcinogenesis* 2009 Jan;30(1):93-100.

[29] Sun Y, Rigas B. The thioredoxin system mediates redox-induced cell death in human colon cancer cells: implications for the mechanism of action of anticancer agents. *Cancer Res* 2008 Oct 15;68(20):8269-8277.

[30] Hulsman N, Medema JP, Bos C, Jongejan A, Leurs R, Smit MJ, et al. Chemical insights in the concept of hybrid drugs: the antitumor effect of nitric oxide-donating aspirin involves a quinone methide but not nitric oxide nor aspirin. *J Med Chem* 2007 May 17;50(10):2424-2431.

[31] Rigas B, Williams JL. NO-donating NSAIDs and cancer: an overview with a note on whether NO is required for their action. *Nitric Oxide* 2008 Sep;19(2):199-204.

[32] Dunlap T, Abdul-Hay SO, Chandrasena RE, Hagos GK, Sinha V, Wang Z, et al. Nitrates and NO-NSAIDs in cancer chemoprevention and therapy: in vitro evidence querying the NO donor functionality. *Nitric Oxide* 2008 Sep;19(2):115-124.

[33] Feese M, Scaloni A, Jones WM, Manning JM, Remington SJ. Crystallization and preliminary X-ray studies of human erythrocyte acylpeptide hydrolase. *J Mol Biol* 1993 Oct 5;233(3):546-549.

[34] Wright H, Kiss AL, Szeltner Z, Polgar L, Fulop V. Crystallization and preliminary crystallographic analysis of porcine acylaminoacyl peptidase. *Acta Crystallogr Sect F Struct Biol Cryst Commun* 2005 Oct 1;61(Pt 10):942-944.

[35] Bartlam M, Wang G, Yang H, Gao R, Zhao X, Xie G, et al. Crystal structure of an acylpeptide hydrolase/esterase from Aeropyrum pernix K1. *Structure* 2004 Aug;12(8):1481-1488.

[36] Menyhard DK, Kiss-Szeman A, Tichy-Racs E, Hornung B, Radi K, Szeltner Z, et al. A Self-compartmentalizing Hexamer Serine Protease from Pyrococcus Horikoshii: Substrate Selection Achieved through Multimerization. *J Biol Chem* 2013 Jun 14;288(24):17884-17894.

[37] Roy A, Kucukural A, Zhang Y. I-TASSER: a unified platform for automated protein structure and function prediction. *Nat Protoc* 2010 Apr;5(4):725-738.

[38] Zhang Y. I-TASSER: fully automated protein structure prediction in CASP8. *Proteins* 2009;77 Suppl 9:100-113.

[39] Zhang Y. I-TASSER server for protein 3D structure prediction. *BMC Bioinformatics* 2008 Jan 23;9:40.

[40] Kelley LA, Sternberg MJ. Protein structure prediction on the Web: a case study using the Phyre server. *Nat Protoc* 2009;4(3):363-371.

[41] Fernandez-Fuentes N, Madrid-Aliste CJ, Rai BK, Fajardo JE, Fiser A. M4T: a comparative protein structure modeling server. *Nucleic Acids Res* 2007 Jul;35(Web Server issue):W363-8.

[42] Fernandez-Fuentes N, Rai BK, Madrid-Aliste CJ, Fajardo JE, Fiser A. Comparative protein structure modeling by combining multiple templates and optimizing sequence-to-structure alignments. *Bioinformatics* 2007 Oct 1;23(19):2558-2565.

[43] Rykunov D, Steinberger E, Madrid-Aliste CJ, Fiser A. Improved scoring function for comparative modeling using the M4T method. *J Struct Funct Genomics* 2009 Mar;10(1):95-99.

[44] Krieger E, Joo K, Lee J, Lee J, Raman S, Thompson J, et al. Improving physical realism, stereochemistry, and side-chain accuracy in homology modeling: Four approaches that performed well in CASP8. *Proteins* 2009;77 Suppl 9:114-122.

[45] Lovell SC, Davis IW, Arendall WB,3rd, de Bakker PI, Word JM, Prisant MG, et al. Structure validation by Calpha geometry: phi,psi and Cbeta deviation. *Proteins* 2003 Feb 15;50(3):437-450.

[46] Wiederstein M, Sippl MJ. ProSA-web: interactive web service for the recognition of errors in three-dimensional structures of proteins. *Nucleic Acids Res* 2007 Jul;35(Web Server issue):W407-10.

[47] Chen VB, Arendall WB,3rd, Headd JJ, Keedy DA, Immormino RM, Kapral GJ, et al. MolProbity: all-atom structure validation for macromolecular crystallography. *Acta Crystallogr D Biol Crystallogr* 2010 Jan;66(Pt 1):12-21.

[48] Trott O, Olson AJ. AutoDock Vina: improving the speed and accuracy of docking with a new scoring function, efficient optimization, and multithreading. *J Comput Chem* 2010 Jan 30;31(2):455-461.

[49] Volkamer A, Kuhn D, Rippmann F, Rarey M. DoGSiteScorer: A web-server for automatic binding site prediction, analysis, and druggability assessment. *Bioinformatics* 2012 May 23.

[50] Tsunasawa S, Narita K, Ogata K. Purification and properties of acylamino acid-releasing enzyme from rat liver. *J Biochem* 1975 Jan 1;77(1?):89-102.

[51] Roy A, Xu D, Poisson J, Zhang Y. A protocol for computer-based protein structure and function prediction. *J Vis Exp* 2011 Nov 3;(57):e3259. doi(57):e3259.

[52] Wu S, Szilagyi A, Zhang Y. Improving protein structure prediction using multiple sequence-based contact predictions. *Structure* 2011 Aug 10;19(8):1182-1191.

[53] Roy A, Zhang Y. *Protein Structure Prediction.* eLS 2012.

[54] Scaloni A, Jones WM, Barra D, Pospischil M, Sassa S, Popowicz A, et al. Acylpeptide hydrolase: inhibitors and some active site residues of the human enzyme. *J Biol Chem* 1992 Feb 25;267(6):3811-3818.

[55] Mitta M, Miyagi M, Kato I, Tsunasawa S. Identification of the catalytic triad residues of porcine liver acylamino acid-releasing enzyme. *J Biochem* 1998 May;123(5):924-931.

[56] Hedstrom L. Serine protease mechanism and specificity. *Chem Rev* 2002 Dec;102(12):4501-4524.

[57] Iengar P, Ramakrishnan C. Knowledge-based modeling of the serine protease triad into non-proteases. *Protein Eng* 1999 Aug;12(8):649-656.

[58] Venalainen JI, Juvonen RO, Mannisto PT. Evolutionary relationships of the prolyl oligopeptidase family enzymes. *Eur J Biochem* 2004 Jul;271(13):2705-2715.

[59] Roy A, Kucukural A, Zhang Y. I-TASSER: a unified platform for automated protein structure and function prediction. *Nat Protoc* 2010 Apr;5(4):725-738.

[60] Laskowski RA. PDBsum new things. *Nucleic Acids Res* 2009 Jan;37(Database issue):D355-9.

[61] Laskowski RA. PDBsum: summaries and analyses of PDB structures. *Nucleic Acids Res* 2001 Jan 1;29(1):221-222.

[62] Laskowski RA, Chistyakov VV, Thornton JM. PDBsum more: new summaries and analyses of the known 3D structures of proteins and nucleic acids. *Nucleic Acids Res* 2005 Jan 1;33(Database issue):D266-8.

[63] Nardini M, Dijkstra BW. Alpha/beta hydrolase fold enzymes: the family keeps growing. *Curr Opin Struct Biol* 1999 Dec;9(6):732-737.

[64] Novel prodrugs to target cancers cells overexpressing oxidized protein hydrolase. *Society for Free Radical Research International 16th Biennial Meeting;* September 6-9, 2012; ; 2012.

[65] Chen X, Chi Y, Bloecher A, Aebersold R, Clurman BE, Roberts JM. N-acetylation and ubiquitin-independent proteasomal degradation of p21(Cip1). *Mol Cell* 2004 Dec 3;16(5):839-847.

[66] Crawford LJ, Walker B, Irvine AE. Proteasome inhibitors in cancer therapy. *J Cell Commun Signal* 2011 Jun;5(2):101-110.

In: Free Radicals
Editor: Bill Stone

ISBN: 978-1-63117-177-2

Chapter VII

The Role of the Antioxidant Defense System in the Pathogenesis of Colorectal Cancer

Martina Perše, DVM, PhD *
Institute of Pathology, Medical Experimental Centre,
Faculty of Medicine, University of Ljubljana, Slovenia

Abstract

Numerous reports have shown that excessive and uncontrollable production of free radicals may be implicated in various diseases. It is known that high amounts of free radicals can modulate gene expression and cause cellular damage, such as injuries to DNA, lipids, proteins as well as cellular structures and organelles. When these injuries cannot be eliminated or properly repaired, they may be responsible for various diseases, including carcinogenesis. Because living organisms are constantly exposed to a variety of challenging conditions that affect free radical production, cells possess an enormous and powerful antioxidative protective mechanism to counteract the deleterious effects of free radicals. Antioxidative protective mechanisms are composed of different levels of antioxidant defense. The first level is directed towards the prevention of Fenton's reaction, the second level uses the detoxification and antioxidant system to reduce/ neutralize the production of free radicals and the third level uses various repair systems to eliminate damage caused by free radicals that escaped the first two levels of defense. The aim of this chapter is to summarize the literature demonstrating the enormous power of antioxidative protective mechanisms in colorectal cancer prevention and to review the literature on the role and failure of the antioxidant defense system in colorectal cancer development.

Keywords: antioxidant, antioxidant defense, protective mechanisms, gut, colorectal carcinogenesis

* Corresponding author: Martina Perše, DVM, PhD. Institute of Pathology, Medical Experimental Centre, Faculty of Medicine, University of Ljubljana, Zaloška 4, 1000 Ljubljana, Slovenia. E-mail: martina.perse@mf.uni-lj.si.

Abbreviations

AOM	azoxymethane
BER	base excision repair
CAT	catalase
CRC	colorectal cancer
DMH	dimethylhydrazine
DSS	dextran sodium sulfate
GGR	global genome repair
GPx	glutathione peroxidase
GR	glutathione reductase
GSH	glutathione
GSSG	glutathione disulfide
IBD	inflammatory bowel disease
MMR	mismatch repair
NER	nucleotide excision repair
PRXD	peroxiredoxin
ROS	reactive oxygen species
Sel	selenoprotein
SNP	single nucleotide polymorphism
SOD	superoxide dismutase
TCR	transcription-coupled repair
TXNRD	thioredoxin reductase

Introduction

Free radicals, more generally known as reactive oxygen species (ROS) and reactive nitrogen species, are known to be vitally important for the normal functioning of cells and the body. They are implicated in various physiological processes. Free radicals and their derivatives play important roles as intracellular signaling molecules. Under homeostatic conditions they are critical in multiple signal transduction pathways by acting as second messengers. Through cellular signaling, they regulate key cellular functions, such as proliferation, differentiation, growth and apoptosis. Under conditions of oxidative stress, free radicals and their derivatives can be detrimental for the cell itself, leading to uncontrolled proliferation, inflammation or apoptosis [1-10]. In addition to modulating gene expression, excessive production of free radicals may cause injuries to lipids and, consequently, affect the fluidity of cell membranes, reducing the capacity to maintain an equilibrated gradient of concentration and increasing membrane permeability and inflammation [11]. Injuries to proteins lead to structural alterations or alteration of enzyme functions, which can have a wide range of downstream functional consequences, such as inhibition of enzymatic and binding activities, increased or decreased uptake by cells, inactivation of DNA repair enzymes and loss of fidelity of damaged DNA polymerases in replicating DNA [12]. Free radicals and their derivatives may also cause injuries to DNA, such as G → T transversions and DNA hypomethylation, which may lead to carcinogenesis (reviewed in [13]).

It is becoming clear that the balance in ROS levels is essential for a cell's survival. An increased amount of ROS may affect physiological functions of cells in terms of cellular damage, aberrant cell signaling or cell death (necrosis or apoptosis).

On the other hand, decreased production of ROS may decrease cell signaling and cell function in terms of a decreased proliferative response or defective host defense capacity. Since the generation of free radicals is a constituent part of normal physiological processes in the body and their balance is of vital importance, cells have evolved a powerful antioxidant defense mechanism to control free radical production and to counteract and neutralize their detrimental effects when overproduced.

Antioxidative Protective Mechanisms

There are various protective mechanisms in cells to maintain the homeostatic balance of ROS and they can be divided into different levels of defense.

The first level of antioxidant defense is directed towards prevention of Fenton's reaction, the second level uses a detoxification and antioxidant system to reduce/neutralize the production of free radicals and the third level uses various repair systems to eliminate damage caused by free radicals that escaped the first two levels of defense (Figure 1) [14].

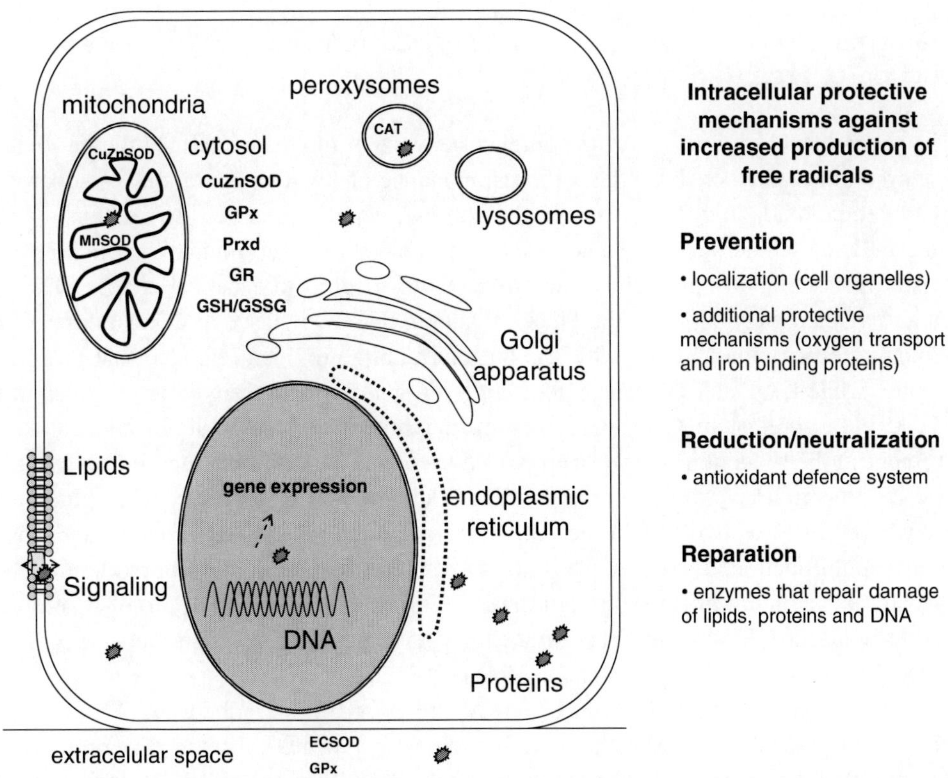

Figure 1. Shematic representation of intracellular protective mechanisms against oxidative stress.

Mechanisms Directed towards the Prevention of Production of Free Radicals

It is important to note that under normal conditions the production of free radicals is a carefully controlled process. Cells possess various cell organelles or subcellular compartments, in which specific oxidative processes take place. For example, mitochondria are specific cell organelles in which the production of superoxide can be elevated due to cellular respiration or the electron transport chain process. Peroxisomes are cell organelles in which the breakdown of very long chain fatty acids takes place, resulting in high production of hydrogen peroxide. Localization of these reactions in subcellular compartments is an important part of cell protection against damage. In addition to membrane-bound localization of cells' reactions, these organelles are also adequately protected by other mechanisms that minimize the ability to produce ROS and, consequently, minimize the risk of exposure to oxidative stress. For instance, mitochondria contain iron, copper and flavocoenzymes that are tightly bound to proteins to maintain very low concentrations of free iron and copper. This is of very great importance because in an environment with high concentrations of superoxide or peroxide (in mitochondria), these ions can catalyze a reaction known as Haber-Weiss or Fenton's reaction, which results in the production of hydroxyl radicals, which is a very powerful oxidant that can cause a variety of damage in the cell, as mentioned above [15, 16].

Mechanisms Directed towards Reduction/Neutralization of Increased Production of Free Radicals

The second level of defense is the complex network of molecules termed the antioxidant defense system and this level regulates the maintenance of low concentrations of superoxide and hydrogen peroxide in different subcellular compartments. The antioxidant defense system is composed of numerous enzymatic and non-enzymatic antioxidants, which exhibit synergistic interactions by protecting each other from specific free radical attacks. The best known and studied enzymatic antioxidants are superoxide dismutase (SOD), catalase (CAT) and glutathione peroxidase (GPx). SOD is an important antioxidant enzyme that eliminates superoxide, while CAT and GPx are important hydrogen peroxide-removing enzymes in the cell [17-19]. In contrast to CAT, GPx has a dual function in the cell. In addition to its involvement in the reduction of hydrogen peroxide to water, it is implicated in the reduction of lipid hydroperoxides to the corresponding alcohols. GPx, together with glutathione reductase (GR), is also involved in the regulation of glutathione (GSH) content. GSH is an important multifunctional intracellular non-enzymic water soluble antioxidant, which regulates redox signaling by altering both the level of total GSH and the ratio of its oxidized (GSSG) to reduced (GSH) forms. The intracellular level of GSH is responsive to ROS levels and reflects the balance between use and synthesis [17, 20].

Very important, although less well-known, are thioredoxin reductases (TXNRD) and thioredoxins. Humans have three thioredoxin reductases, which work in different cellular compartments. There are also other proteins involved in the antioxidant defense network, such as selenoproteins, a group of ~25 proteins with incorporated selenocysteine. They are implicated in various protective mechanisms against oxidative stress. For instance, selenoprotein P (SePP) is mostly present in blood and plasma.

Its key function is delivery of selenium from the liver to extra-hepatic tissues. Selenoprotein S (SelS), SelH Sel15 and SelM are endoplasmic reticulum selenoproteins that appear to be involved in redox balance and removal of the unfolded protein response [21]. In addition to all the above mentioned antioxidants, cells possess numerous other antioxidants (endogenous or nutritionally derived) that are involved in the antioxidant defense network and help maintain the redox state of the cell, such as vitamin E, vitamin C, β-carotene, uric acid, bilirubin and albumin.

Mechanisms Directed towards Repair or Elimination of Damage Caused by Free Radicals

The third level of defense includes enzymes that repair oxidative damage to lipids, proteins, carbohydrates and nucleic acids [14]. Some of these enzymes are various proteolytic enzymes, glycosylases, endo- and exonucleases, DNA ligases, DNA polymerases etc.

For example, repair and removal of DNA containing oxidized bases *in vivo* is regulated by DNA glycosylases [22], mainly through base excision repair (BER), although certain types of oxidative lesions also appear to be repaired by nucleotide excision repair (NER) and mismatch repair (MMR) [13]. Cells possess a complex DNA repair system composed of BER, NER, global genome repair (GGR) and transcription-coupled repair (TCR) [23].

The Role and Failure of Antioxidative Protective Mechanisms in the Pathogenesis of Cancer

As demonstrated above, antioxidative protective mechanisms are complex and work on different levels. Most of the current understanding of the role or failure of a particular enzyme employed in antioxidant defense results from transgenic mice models. Current knowledge about the role of some important enzymes implicated in antioxidative defense is briefly introduced below.

In humans, three forms of SOD have been identified. One that contains copper and zinc is termed CuZn-SOD or SOD1 or cytosolic SOD, because it is located mostly in the cytosol of cells, although it is also found in the mitochondrial intermembrane space. The second one, which contains manganese, is Mn-SOD or SOD2 or mitochondrial SOD due to its localization in the mitochondrial matrix. The third is located in the extracellular space and is termed ECSOD or SOD3 or extracellular SOD [16, 24].

The importance of the function of all three forms of SOD has been investigated in mice with the deletion of specific SODs. Mice with complete SOD1 deletion (*Sod1*$^{-/-}$) showed a high level of oxidative stress, increased DNA mutation levels in the liver and were prone to hepatocellular carcinoma [24]. Total dysfunction of the MnSOD (SOD2) enzyme has been shown to be of vital importance. Mice carrying total deletion of MnSOD (*Sod2*$^{-/-}$) died in the first three weeks of their lives. An even smaller dysfunction of the MnSOD enzyme has been shown to have harmful consequences for cells. It was found that *Sod2*$^{+/-}$ mice (which possess one wild type and one deleted allele) had decreased MnSOD activity by 50% and developed a higher tumor burden with age.

Interestingly, decreased activity of MnSOD in mice did not result in a compensatory increase in the activity of the GPx1 or CuZn-SOD enzyme. Based on current experimental results, it seems that total dysfunction of SOD3 is less harmful. *Sod3*$^{-/-}$ mice are viable and fertile; they are only more sensitive to hyperoxia than wild type mice [24].

CAT is mostly found in membrane-bound cell organelles such as peroxisomes. Mice deficient in CAT (*Cat*$^{-/-}$) grow normally and do not develop any pathology [25]. Another enzyme important in decomposing hydrogen peroxide is GPx. Eight different isoforms of glutathione peroxidase (GPx1-8) have been identified in humans. GPx isoforms vary in tissue distribution, cellular location and substrate specificity. The most abundant isoform is GPx1, which reduces hydrogen peroxide. In contrast, GPx4 has a high preference for lipid hydroperoxides. Both isoforms are expressed in the cytoplasm of all mammalian cells. GPx2 and GPx3 are extracellular enzymes expressed in the intestine and in plasma, respectively. *GPx1*$^{-/-}$ or *GPx2*$^{-/-}$ mice do not show a strong deleterious phenotype but *GPx1*$^{-/-}$*GPx2*$^{-/-}$ double knockout mice develop lethal intestinal inflammation [24]. The role of GPx3 failure in colon carcinogenesis has been recently demonstrated in an animal model [26]. When GPx3 deficient mice were treated with azoxymethane (AOM) and dextran sodium sulfate (DSS) (agents used to induce a model for inflammatory colon carcinogenesis), they developed an increased tumor number along with a higher degree of dysplasia, increased inflammation, increased proliferation, hyperactive Wnt signaling and increased DNA damage [26]. Less well-known enzymes that are implicated in the decomposition of hydrogen peroxide are peroxiredoxins, a thioredoxin peroxidase found in most tissues. Based on current results, they seem to be even more important antioxidant enzymes than CAT or GPx. Mice deficient in peroxiredoxin 1 (*Prxd1*$^{-/-}$) have an increased risk of cancer incidence and reduced lifespan, while *Prxd1*$^{+/-}$ heterozygous mice have increased tumor burden but no decrease in life span (similarly as *Sod2*$^{+/-}$ mice) [24]. Mice with peroxiredoxin 2 deletion (*Prxd2*$^{-/-}$) have a milder phenotype than *Prxd1*$^{-/-}$ mice [24]. There are also reports on the role of enzymes involved in the DNA repair process. One of the known major oxidative products of DNA is 8-oxo-dG, which leads to G to T transversions during replication unless the damage is repaired by base excision repair (reviewed in [13]). Two enzymes are importantly involved (Ogg1 and Myh) in this base excision repair (removal of dA mispared to 8-oxo-dG). When they work in conjunction, they prevent formation of G to T mutations. It is interesting that mice with complete deletion of one of these two enzymes (i.e., *Ogg1*$^{-/-}$ or *Myh*$^{-/-}$) do not develop a deleterious phenotype, while mice with double knockout for both enzymes, *Ogg1*$^{-/-}$ *Myh*$^{-/-}$, develop massive carcinogenesis and have a dramatic reduction in life span [24]. All the above mentioned data demonstrate that antioxidant enzymes are very important for living organisms and can contribute to various pathologies when their function is disturbed.

The Role and/or Failure of Antioxidative Protective Mechanisms in the Pathogenesis of Colorectal Cancer

Research has also recently been focused on the genetic level of antioxidant protective machinery in humans. The role of enzymes involved in antioxidant defense in humans is evaluated by looking for an association between genetic polymorphisms/variation in a particular enzyme and risk of colorectal cancer (CRC).

Literature on the association between certain polymorphisms in antioxidant genes and CRC risk is very recent and limited. Nevertheless, several single-nucleotide polymorphisms (SNPs) in genes involved in the antioxidative protective system that are associated with CRC risk have already been identified. For example, a study on 832 CRC patients and 705 healthy controls showed a significant association between SNPs in *SEPP1*, *GPX4* and *SELS* genes and risk of CRC [21]. Another study, on 827 patients with CRC and 733 healthy controls, found an association between SNPs in *SEP15* and *SELS* genes and altered risk of CRC [27]. It was found that genetic variation in various selenoprotein genes and other genes involved in the antioxidant defense system (mentioned above), such as *TXNRD1*, *TXNRD2*, *TXNRD3*, *SEPX1*, *SELN1*, *SEP15* [28], *SOD2* (MnSOD) [21, 27], *GPX3* [29], may influence susceptibility to CRC.

Genetic polymorphisms (SNPs) found in the above mentioned genes have been shown to have functional consequences that can lead to increased risk of CRC. It has been suggested that identified variants of these genes play a role in cancer development and may thus represent potential biomarkers for CRC risk [21]. Findings from two population-based case-control studies of colon (n=1555 cases, 1956 controls) and rectal (n=754 cases, 959 controls) cancer support an association between selenoprotein genes and CRC development and even survival after diagnosis [28]. The results also suggest that the impact of cancer susceptibility from genotype may be modified by lifestyle [28]. For instance, genetic variants in *TXNRD1* and *TXNRD2* interacted with aspirin or non-steroidal inflammatory drugs to influence CRC risk, genetic variants in *TXNRD2*, *SELS*, *SEP15* and *SELW1* interacted with estrogen to modify colon cancer risk, and *SEP15* and *SEPX1* influenced survival diagnosis with colon cancer [28].

All of the above mentioned studies demonstrate that the antioxidant capacity of a particular organism can be affected by the genetic variability of genes implicated in the antioxidative protective system. However, more studies need to be done before any conclusions can be reached.

In addition to enzymatic antioxidants, there are also micronutrient antioxidants, which compose an important part of the cell's antioxidative defense system by possessing free radical scavenging properties. As such, they are recognized to have an important role in the redox homeostasis of the cell. The beneficial role of micronutrient antioxidants has been investigated in various diseases and also in patients with different stages of colorectal carcinogenesis. One study found that patients with adenomatous polyps had significantly lower levels of all measured micronutrient antioxidants (α- and γ-tocopherol, lutein, β-cryptoxanthin, lycopene, and α- and β-carotene) in their colon mucosa than healthy control subjects, although the serum levels of these antioxidants were similar in both groups [30]. Another study investigating the levels of antioxidant enzymes, vitamins C and E, in the serum of colorectal cancer patients reported that colorectal cancer patients had significantly decreased levels of the measured parameters in serum than the corresponding healthy control group [31]. Based on these results (e.g., a higher level of antioxidants in normal colon mucosa vs. lower levels in adenomas and in the serum of cancer patients), it appears that micronutrient antioxidants may have a beneficial and/or protective role in the development of CRC. Nutritionally derived antioxidants, such as β-carotene [32], vitamins E and C, flavonoids and polyphenols, may provide a second line of defense against the production of

ROS. A number of vitamins and micronutrients are substrates and/or cofactors in the metabolic pathways regulating gene expression and DNA synthesis and repair mechanisms.

For example, it has been shown that deficiencies in vitamins C and E cause DNA oxidation and chromosomal damage. Vitamin D has been shown to stabilize chromosomal structure and prevent DNA double-strand breaks [33]. A growing number of experimental studies in animal and cell culture models have shown that selenium exerts anti-carcinogenic effects by multiple mechanisms. There are reviews that discuss the potential mechanisms through which selenium can suppress tumor initiation and growth and even suppress tumor migration, invasion, angiogenesis and overall metastasis in various cancers, including colon cancer [34]. Studies on animal models have likewise shown that antioxidants have beneficial effects in the battle against CRC. It has been shown that vitamin E (γ-tocotrienol) has antiproliferative properties in cancer cell lines [35], while various natural antioxidants, such as gallic acid [36], polyphenols [37], vitamin D [38] and vitamin A [39], have the potential to inhibit CRC development in the dimethylhydrazine (DMH) model, a well establish CRC animal model of human sporadic CRC [40].

Based on all of the above-mentioned results, one would expect that increased antioxidant intake or antioxidant therapy would result in a decreased risk of CRC. However, epidemiological studies evaluating the occurrence of polyps after supplementation with vitamin E and β-carotene have yielded mixed results [30]. Furthermore, a systematic review and meta-analysis investigating the effectiveness of antioxidants (vitamins A, C and E, selenium and β-carotene) in the prevention of colorectal carcinomas and/or adenomas in the general population demonstrated that these antioxidants did not reduce the formation of colorectal adenomas or carcinomas [41]. Interestingly, some studies have found that antioxidant supplementation might result in an increased risk of CRC and even overall mortality [41].

What could be the reason for such discrepancy between experimental and epidemiological studies?

The authors of this systematic review and meta-analysis discussed some of the potential limitations of their study that could have affected the results [41]. The length of follow-up of populations on the occurrence of CRC was stated as a key limitation. It ranged from 5 to 12 years, although it is known that the development of sporadic CRC is a long term process with a natural history of 10-15 years. The authors also reported a large variation in doses and combinations of antioxidants investigated, the duration of treatment and follow-up and differences in sample size and event numbers [41]. It is also possible that the results were affected by differences in the chemical form of the particular vitamin used in trials. For instance, there are eight forms of natural vitamin E (i.e., α-, β-, γ-, σ- tocopherols and α-, β-, γ-, σ-tocotrienols) and there are also supplements of vitamin E (such as all-rac-α-tocopheryl acetate or RRR-α-tocopherol) [42]. We found that the most frequently reported form of vitamin E used in trials was α-tocopherol, and RRR-α-tocopherol acetate was rarely reported. It has been reported that a high intake of RRR-α-tocopherol, synthetic α-tocopherol, which was found to be often commercially labeled natural vitamin E or α-tocopherol, may enhance the metabolism of other forms of natural vitamin E (γ- and σ- tocopherols) and, consequently, compromise the efficacy of α-tocopherol [42, 43]. It has also been demonstrated that supplementation of β-carotene may significantly interfere with the vitamin E (α-tocopherol) concentration in the colon [44]. The terminology, potential interactions between various antioxidants used in the same trial and different chemical forms of vitamins used among trials may thus be some of the additional factors responsible for confounding the results.

Homeostatic Mechanisms and the Antioxidant Paradox

The use of antioxidants to prevent cancer, including CRC, has attracted considerable interest. Despite their proposed role in the reduction of free radicals, results on the use of antioxidants in the prevention of any kind of cancer are contradictory. These contradictory results suggest that a closer and more careful approach to the theory of free radicals, antioxidants and oxidative stress is warranted. Many questions have been asked about the role and implication of free radicals in various disorders, such as "Is it that the importance of free radical formation has been overestimated or is it because these agents are not very effective in reducing free radicals?" [41]. Additional knowledge and research are needed to address these questions. However, there are some major points that are already known and need to be taken into account when investigating antioxidant defense mechanisms.

First of all, the antioxidant defense system is very important for living organisms and is thus very complex, with many mechanisms to balance and maintain the redox state of cells. It is therefore very unlikely that failure of antioxidant protection could be attributed to a single component (unless there is a genetic predisposition), because all are affected by an oxidative challenge.

Second, it is known that free radicals are not involved only in pathological processes but are necessary for many physiological functions of living organisms. Similarly, it should be noted that antioxidants are not involved only in protection against oxidative stress but can also promote oxidative reactions. Depending on the dose and type, antioxidants can protect against or contribute to oxidative stress.

Third, there are additional mechanisms that need to be taken into account when addressing this issue, e.g., knowledge of the homeostatic mechanisms of a particular tissue and the wider picture of CRC development. They are briefly introduced in the next section.

Protective Mechanisms of the Gut

All of the mechanisms mentioned and explained above are protective mechanisms that mostly take place in the cells and are mainly devoted to protecting cells. In addition to cell protective mechanisms, there are also strong homeostatic organ/tissue specific protective mechanisms. These protective mechanisms are a vitally important first line of defense against deleterious conditions of a particular organ. Their purpose is to counteract numerous challenges in the environment and to protect cells and their function.

In the case of a healthy gut, homeostasis is ensured by a complex system composed of the intracellular antioxidative protective system and extracellular protective mechanisms of the gut. In this section, we provide a brief description of these homeostatic mechanisms in the gut to help explain their complexity and interplay. Protective mechanisms of the gut are intrinsically linked in a complex physiology and therefore need to be considered together in both health and disease. The antioxidative defense system is too often considered in isolation, without considering tissue specific protective characteristics.

Mammals are in direct contact with the environment through their skin and the gastrointestinal tract. Since direct contact with environment is very challenging, specific protective mechanisms in these organs have been evolved.

The gut mucosa is composed of a layer of epithelial cells and the underlying non-epithelial tissue, composed of inflammatory cells, connective tissue etc. [45]. It is too often forgotten or not considered that epithelial cells in the gut mucosa of a healthy individual are not in direct contact with the luminal content or gut microbiota. The epithelial layer is covered with a secreted mucus layer, which is very thick (~800 μm in a rodent colon) and provides both a physical and chemical barrier to microbes and other factors. Its main function is to keep the mucosal surface well hydrated and to lubricate the luminal content [45]. There are also inflammatory cells that protect the gut from various kinds of injuries, help to eliminate various factors that could harm the morphology and normal function of the gut, and collaborate in tissue repair. Furthermore, it has been recently recognized that the gut microbiota (termed microflora) have an important role in protection of the gut. The gut microbiota contain a broad spectrum of microorganisms, which reside in the gastrointestinal tract and play important roles in human health and disease (reviewed in [46]. They are essential for the host's wellbeing in terms of nutrition and mucosal immunity. Certain members of the gut microbiota have been shown to promote the host's health, while some members of the gut microbiota may be implicated in the development of CRC, due to various mechanisms, including generation of reactive metabolites (*E.faecalis*) [47] and carcinogens, alterations in host carbohydrate expression and induction of chronic mucosal inflammation [48].

Finally, the intestinal mucosa is challenged with various harmful effects of some endogenous and exogenous factors, such as a diverse mixture of bile, mucus, desquamated epithelial cells, various microorganisms and their fermentation products, undigested or unabsorbed food and its metabolic products, such as metals, salts, toxins, mutagens, carcinogens, dissolved gases (like nitrogen, hydrogen, carbon dioxide, methane, oxygen), as well as various beneficial and modifying factors (for example healthy food, exercise), which can counteract the deleterious effects of harmful challenges (Figure 2) [49].

All these components of the gut are intrinsically linked in a complex physiology and provide important protection and defense against detrimental factors, including free radicals.

Colorectal Carcinogenesis

Colorectal cancer (CRC) is one of the most common cancers worldwide, with the highest incidence rates in western countries [50]. Most cases of CRC occur sporadically (70-80%) and are attributable to various environmental and lifestyle factors, such as dietary habits, obesity and physical inactivity [51].

Recent evidence has suggested that the generation of ROS may play an important role in all phases of carcinogenesis, i.e., initiation, promotion and progression stages [52]. However, there are currently no scientific results to indicate whether oxidative stress is a cause or a consequence in the pathogenesis of CRC [53].

Colorectal carcinogenesis is a multistage process. The first microscopically visible lesions in the multistep development of CRC are aberrant crypt foci (ACF). ACF is a term for morphologically and histologically altered colon crypts (composed of 1 or up to 100 crypts), which have the potential to progress to advanced adenomas and then transform further into adenocarcinomas [54].

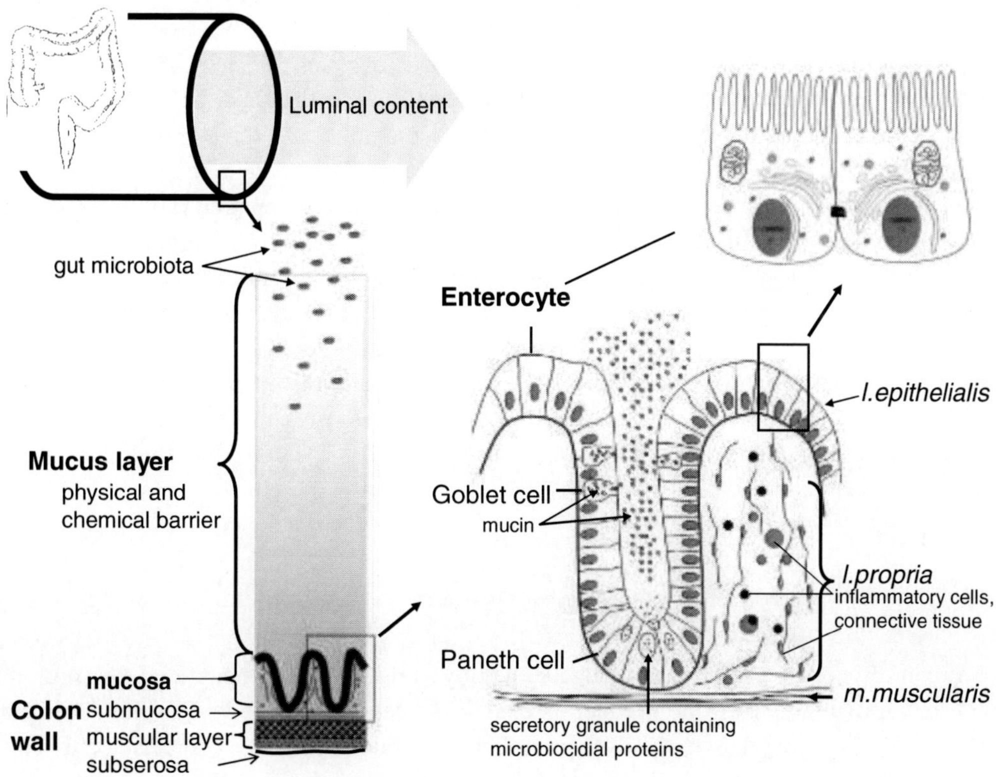

Figure 2. Shematic representation of the colon structure and its protective mechanisms.

Evidence from experimental and clinical studies demonstrates that ACF share similar histological and molecular features with colonic tumors (i.e., adenomas and adenocarcinomas) [40, 55, 56]. Today, high-magnification chromoscopic colonoscopy allows the detection and biopsy of ACF *in vivo* in humans. It also provides the opportunity to investigate and characterize the earliest genetic and molecular alterations in CRC development in humans. It has been found that ACF exhibit many of the molecular and genetic abnormalities that form the basis for the adenoma-carcinoma sequence in CRC. Genetic alterations found in human ACF include mutations in tumor suppressor genes, microsatellite instability, aberrant methylation, as well as aberrant expression of proteins. To date, three molecular pathways of CRC development have been identified and described, i.e., chromosomal instability, microsatellite instability and CpG island methylator phenotype [57]. All three types of molecular alteration have also been found in ACF [56, 57]. The presence of various markers of oxidative stress in adenomas and adenocarcinomas demonstrates that oxidative stress is present in these stages of carcinogenesis but does not explain whether it is a cause or consequence of cancer. To address this issue, further investigation of all these steps of CRC development, including the initiation event, should be performed.

Namely, colorectal carcinogenesis is a multistage process that originates from the epithelial cells that line the large bowel. Epithelial cells multiply in the lower third of the crypts and differentiate in the upper two-thirds. It has been suggested that proliferating cells are putative target cells of colon carcinogenesis, because they are very sensitive to the redox environment, divide rapidly and have a high metabolic rate, which has been found to be a potential factor that may be responsible for increased oxidation of DNA [58]. Proliferating cells are also exceptionally sensitive to DNA damage because the DNA is present as a single strand in the S-phase of the cell cycle and serves as a template for the complement strand in daughter cells. It has been suggested that DNA damage in a single strand could lead to varying mutations in the DNA of daughter cells, which cannot be repaired [59]. DNA damage can result in either cell cycle arrest or induction of transcription, induction of signal transduction pathways, replication errors and genomic instability, all of which are associated with colon carcinogenesis [16]. However, as explained above, at the same time it is important to be aware that living organisms possess various defense and repair mechanisms to counteract the deleterious effects of oxidative stress provoked from either the inner or outer environment. These protective homeostatic mechanisms are present on different levels, i.e., cellular, tissue, organ and body levels, and therefore need to be considered together in both health and disease.

Conclusion

Living organisms are constantly challenged by various factors (beneficial, harmful etc.) that can significantly affect the production of free radicals in their body. Despite detrimental situations that cause excessive and uncontrollable production of free radicals for extended time periods, our body is still capable of counteracting these unfavorable conditions without that necessarily resulting in cancer. For instance, patients with inflammatory bowel disease (IBD) have a 6-fold higher risk of CRC than the general population. However, most patients with IBD do not develop CRC, despite excessive and long-term production of free radicals and oxidative stress. This indicates that excessive production of free radicals alone, over a long time period, does not necessarily lead to carcinogenesis. It also demonstrates that organisms have a very powerful protective system that ensures redox homeostasis in the organism, in spite of numerous disturbances or harmful factors with which the organism is constantly faced. It also suggests that the role of free radicals or oxidative stress in the initiation of carcinogenesis may be more complex and multidimensional than initially thought.

Acknowledgments

Gratitude is due to all the animals that contribute their part in the science field. This work was in part supported by ARRS (Slovenian Research Agency, Program P3-0054).

References

[1] Ji, L. L. Exercise-induced modulation of antioxidant defense. *Ann. N. Y. Acad. Sci.* 2002 Apr.;959:82-92.

[2] Ji, L. L., Gomez-Cabrera, M. C., Vina, J. Exercise and hormesis: activation of cellular antioxidant signaling pathway. *Ann. N. Y. Acad. Sci.* 2006 May;1067:425-35.

[3] Ji, L. L., Gomez-Cabrera, M. C., Vina, J. Role of nuclear factor kappaB and mitogen-activated protein kinase signaling in exercise-induced antioxidant enzyme adaptation. *Appl. Physiol. Nutr. Metab*. 2007 Oct.;32(5):930-5.

[4] Ji, L. L. Modulation of skeletal muscle antioxidant defense by exercise: Role of redox signaling. *Free Radic. Biol. Med.* 2008 Jan. 15;44(2):142-52.

[5] Kramer, H. F., Goodyear, L. J. Exercise, MAPK, and NF-kappaB signaling in skeletal muscle. *J. Appl. Physiol*. 2007 Jul.;103(1):388-95.

[6] Valko, M., Leibfritz, D., Moncol, J., Cronin, M. T., Mazur, M., Telser, J. Free radicals and antioxidants in normal physiological functions and human disease. *Int. J. Biochem. Cell Biol*. 2007;39(1):44-84.

[7] Marnett, L. J. Oxy radicals, lipid peroxidation and DNA damage. *Toxicology* 2002 Dec. 27;181-182:219-22.

[8] Uchida, K. 4-Hydroxy-2-nonenal: a product and mediator of oxidative stress. *Prog. Lipid Res*. 2003 Jul.;42(4):318-43.

[9] Uchida, K., Kumagai, T. 4-hydroxy-2-nonenal as a COX-2 inducer. *Mol. Aspects Med.* 2003 Aug.;24(4-5):213-8.

[10] Cejas, P., Casado, E., Belda-Iniesta, C., De, C. J., Espinosa, E., Redondo, A., et al. Implications of oxidative stress and cell membrane lipid peroxidation in human cancer (Spain). *Cancer Causes Control* 2004 Sep.;15(7):707-19.

[11] Finaud, J., Lac, G., Filaire, E. Oxidative stress : relationship with exercise and training. *Sports Med*. 2006;36(4):327-58.

[12] Shringarpure, R., Davies, K. J. Protein turnover by the proteasome in aging and disease. *Free Radic. Biol. Med*. 2002 Jun. 1;32(11):1084-9.

[13] Bjelland, S., Seeberg, E. Mutagenicity, toxicity and repair of DNA base damage induced by oxidation. *Mutat. Res*. 2003 Oct. 29;531(1-2):37-80.

[14] Radić, N., Injac, R., Djordjević, A., Štrukelj, B. Analysis of parameters significant for oxidative stress and cell injury. In: Injac, R., editor. *The analysis of pharmacologically active compounds in biomolecules in real samples*. Kerala, India: Transworld Research Network; 2009. p. 165-94.

[15] Valko, M., Izakovic, M., Mazur, M., Rhodes, C. J., Telser, J. Role of oxygen radicals in DNA damage and cancer incidence. *Mol. Cell Biochem*. 2004 Nov.;266(1-2):37-56.

[16] Valko, M., Rhodes, C. J., Moncol, J., Izakovic, M., Mazur, M. Free radicals, metals and antioxidants in oxidative stress-induced cancer. *Chem. Biol. Interact*. 2006;160(1):1-40.

[17] Valko, M., Rhodes, C. J., Moncol, J., Izakovic, M., Mazur, M. Free radicals, metals and antioxidants in oxidative stress-induced cancer. *Chem. Biol. Interact*. 2006 Mar. 10;160 (1):1-40.

[18] Valko, M., Leibfritz, D., Moncol, J., Cronin, M. T., Mazur, M., Telser, J. Free radicals and antioxidants in normal physiological functions and human disease. *Int. J. Biochem. Cell Biol*. 2007;39(1):44-84.

[19] Carr, W. J., Oberley-Deegan, R. E., Zhang, Y., Oberley, C. C., Oberley, L. W., Dunnwald, M. Antioxidant proteins and reactive oxygen species are decreased in a murine epidermal side population with stem cell-like characteristics. *Histochem. Cell Biol.* 2011 Mar.;135(3):293-304.

[20] Valko, M., Izakovic, M., Mazur, M., Rhodes, C. J., Telser, J. Role of oxygen radicals in DNA damage and cancer incidence. *Mol. Cell Biochem.* 2004 Nov.;266(1-2):37-56.

[21] Meplan, C., Hughes, D. J., Pardini, B., Naccarati, A., Soucek, P., Vodickova, L., et al. Genetic variants in selenoprotein genes increase risk of colorectal cancer. *Carcinogenesis* 2010 Jun.;31(6):1074-9.

[22] Henderson, P. T., Evans, M. D., Cooke, M. S. Salvage of oxidized guanine derivatives in the (2'-deoxy)ribonucleotide pool as source of mutations in DNA. *Mutat. Res.* 2010 Nov. 28;703(1):11-7.

[23] Parlanti, E., D'Errico, M., Degan, P., Calcagnile, A., Zijno, A., van, dP., I., et al. The cross talk between pathways in the repair of 8-oxo-7,8-dihydroguanine in mouse and human cells. *Free Radic. Biol. Med.* 2012 Dec. 1;53(11):2171-7.

[24] Muller, F. L., Lustgarten, M. S., Jang, Y., Richardson, A., Van, R. H. Trends in oxidative aging theories. *Free Radic. Biol. Med.* 2007 Aug. 15;43(4):477-503.

[25] Ho, Y. S., Xiong, Y., Ma, W., Spector, A., Ho, D. S. Mice lacking catalase develop normally but show differential sensitivity to oxidant tissue injury. *J. Biol. Chem.* 2004 Jul. 30;279(31):32804-12.

[26] Barrett, C., Ning, W., Chen, X., Smith, J. J., Washington, M. K., Hill, K., et al. Tumor suppressor function of the plasma glutathione peroxidase Gpx3 in colitis-associated carcinoma. *Cancer Res.* 2012 Dec. 5.

[27] Sutherland, A., Kim, D. H., Relton, C., Ahn, Y. O., Hesketh, J. Polymorphisms in the selenoprotein S and 15-kDa selenoprotein genes are associated with altered susceptibility to colorectal cancer. *Genes Nutr.* 2010 Sep.;5(3):215-23.

[28] Slattery, M. L., Lundgreen, A., Welbourn, B., Corcoran, C., Wolff, R. K. Genetic variation in selenoprotein genes, lifestyle, and risk of colon and rectal cancer. *PLoS One* 2012;7(5):e37312.

[29] Haug, U., Poole, E. M., Xiao, L., Curtin, K., Duggan, D., Hsu, L., et al. Glutathione peroxidase tagSNPs: associations with rectal cancer but not with colon cancer. *Genes Chromosomes Cancer* 2012 Jun.;51(6):598-605.

[30] Nair, S., Norkus, E. P., Hertan, H., Pitchumoni, C. S. Serum and colon mucosa micronutrient antioxidants: differences between adenomatous polyp patients and controls. *Am. J. Gastroenterol.* 2001 Dec.;96(12):3400-5.

[31] Chang, D., Wang, F., Zhao, Y. S., Pan, H. Z. Evaluation of oxidative stress in colorectal cancer patients. *Biomed. Environ. Sci.* 2008 Aug.;21(4):286-9.

[32] Palozza, P., Calviello, G., Serini, S., Maggiano, N., Lanza, P., Ranelletti, F. O., et al. beta-carotene at high concentrations induces apoptosis by enhancing oxy-radical production in human adenocarcinoma cells. *Free Radic. Biol. Med.* 2001 May 1;30(9): 1000-7.

[33] Arigony, A. L., de Oliveira, I. M., Machado, M., Bordin, D. L., Bergter, L., Pra, D., et al. The influence of micronutrients in cell culture: a reflection on viability and genomic stability. *Biomed. Res. Int.* 2013;2013:597282.

[34] Chen, Y. C., Prabhu, K. S., Mastro, A. M. Is selenium a potential treatment for cancer metastasis? *Nutrients* 2013 Apr.;5(4):1149-68.

[35] Zhang, J. S., Li, D. M., Ma, Y., He, N., Gu, Q., Wang, F. S., et al. gamma-Tocotrienol induces paraptosis-like cell death in human colon carcinoma SW620 cells. *PLoS One* 2013;8(2):e57779.

[36] Giftson, J. S., Jayanthi, S., Nalini, N. Chemopreventive efficacy of gallic acid, an antioxidant and anticarcinogenic polyphenol, against 1,2-dimethyl hydrazine induced rat colon carcinogenesis. *Invest New Drugs* 2010 Jun.;28(3):251-9.

[37] Femia, A. P., Caderni, G., Vignali, F., Salvadori, M., Giannini, A., Biggeri, A., et al. Effect of polyphenolic extracts from red wine and 4-OH-coumaric acid on 1,2-dimethylhydrazine-induced colon carcinogenesis in rats. *Eur. J. Nutr.* 2005 Mar.;44(2): 79-84.

[38] Pence, B. C., Buddingh, F. Inhibition of dietary fat-promoted colon carcinogenesis in rats by supplemental calcium or vitamin D3. *Carcinogenesis* 1988 Jan.;9(1):187-90.

[39] Delage, B., Groubet, R., Pallet, V., Bairras, C., Higueret, P., Cassand, P. Vitamin A prevents high fat diet-induced ACF development and modifies the pattern of expression of peroxisome proliferator and retinoic acid receptor m-RNA. *Nutr. Cancer* 2004; 48 (1):28-36.

[40] Perse, M., Cerar, A. Morphological and molecular alterations in 1,2 dimethylhydrazine and azoxymethane induced colon carcinogenesis in rats. *J. Biomed. Biotechnol.* 2011; 2011:473964.

[41] Papaioannou, D., Cooper, K. L., Carroll, C., Hind, D., Squires, H., Tappenden, P., et al. Antioxidants in the chemoprevention of colorectal cancer and colorectal adenomas in the general population: a systematic review and meta-analysis. *Colorectal Dis.* 2011 Oct.;13(10):1085-99.

[42] Huang, H. Y., Caballero, B., Chang, S., Alberg, A., Semba, R., Schneyer, C., et al. Multivitamin/mineral supplements and prevention of chronic disease. *Evid. Rep. Technol. Assess.* (Full Rep.) 2006 May;(139):1-117.

[43] Huang, H. Y., Appel, L. J. Supplementation of diets with alpha-tocopherol reduces serum concentrations of gamma- and delta-tocopherol in humans. *J. Nutr.* 2003 Oct.; 133(10):3137-40.

[44] Simone, F., Pappalardo, G., Maiani, G., Guadalaxara, A., Bugianesi, R., Conte, A. M., et al. Accumulation and interactions of beta-carotene and alpha-tocopherol in patients with adenomatous polyps. *Eur. J. Clin. Nutr.* 2002 Jun.;56(6):546-50.

[45] McGuckin, M. A., Eri, R., Simms, L. A., Florin, T. H., Radford-Smith, G. Intestinal barrier dysfunction in inflammatory bowel diseases. *Inflamm. Bowel Dis.* 2009 Jan.;15 (1):100-13.

[46] Prakash, S., Tomaro-Duchesneau, C., Saha, S., Cantor, A. The gut microbiota and human health with an emphasis on the use of microencapsulated bacterial cells. *J. Biomed. Biotechnol.* 2011;2011:981214.

[47] Huycke, M. M., Moore, D. R. In vivo production of hydroxyl radical by Enterococcus faecalis colonizing the intestinal tract using aromatic hydroxylation. *Free Radic. Biol. Med.* 2002 Sep. 15;33(6):818-26.

[48] Hope, M. E., Hold, G. L., Kain, R., El-Omar, E. M. Sporadic colorectal cancer--role of the commensal microbiota. *FEMS Microbiol. Lett.* 2005 Mar. 1;244(1):1-7.

[49] Guz, J., Foksinski, M., Siomek, A., Gackowski, D., Rozalski, R., Dziaman, T., et al. The relationship between 8-oxo-7,8-dihydro-2'-deoxyguanosine level and extent of

cytosine methylation in leukocytes DNA of healthy subjects and in patients with colon adenomas and carcinomas. *Mutat. Res.* 2008 Apr. 2;640(1-2):170-3.

[50] Jemal, A., Bray, F., Center, M. M., Ferlay, J., Ward, E., Forman, D. Global cancer statistics. *CA Cancer J. Clin.* 2011 Mar.;61(2):69-90.

[51] Johnson, I. T., Lund, E. K. Review article: nutrition, obesity and colorectal cancer. *Aliment Pharmacol. Ther.* 2007 Jul. 15;26(2):161-81.

[52] Valko, M., Leibfritz, D., Moncol, J., Cronin, M. T., Mazur, M., Telser, J. Free radicals and antioxidants in normal physiological functions and human disease. *Int. J. Biochem. Cell Biol.* 2007;39(1):44-84.

[53] Perse, M. Oxidative stress in the pathogenesis of colorectal cancer: cause or consequence? *Biomed. Res. Int.* 2013;2013:725710.

[54] Tanaka, T. Colorectal carcinogenesis: Review of human and experimental animal studies. *J. Carcinog.* 2009;8:5.

[55] Pretlow, T. P., Pretlow, T. G. Mutant KRAS in aberrant crypt foci (ACF): initiation of colorectal cancer? *Biochim. Biophys. Acta* 2005 Nov. 25;1756(2):83-96.

[56] Cheng, L., Lai, M. D. Aberrant crypt foci as microscopic precursors of colorectal cancer. *World J. Gastroenterol.* 2003 Dec.;9(12):2642-9.

[57] Orlando, F. A., Tan, D., Baltodano, J. D., Khoury, T., Gibbs, J. F., Hassid, V. J., et al. Aberrant crypt foci as precursors in colorectal cancer progression. *J. Surg. Oncol.* 2008 Sep. 1;98(3):207-13.

[58] Foksinski, M., Rozalski, R., Guz, J., Ruszkowska, B., Sztukowska, P., Piwowarski, M., et al. Urinary excretion of DNA repair products correlates with metabolic rates as well as with maximum life spans of different mammalian species. *Free Radic. Biol. Med.* 2004 Nov. 1;37(9):1449-54.

[59] Oberreuther-Moschner, D. L., Rechkemmer, G., Pool-Zobel, B. L. Basal colon crypt cells are more sensitive than surface cells toward hydrogen peroxide, a factor of oxidative stress. *Toxicol. Lett.* 2005 Dec. 15;159(3):212-8.

In: Free Radicals
Editor: Bill Stone

ISBN: 978-1-63117-177-2

Chapter VIII

Oxidative Stress Imbalance in the Development of Prostate Cancer

Trevor Memmott, Evita Weagel, Chris Hamilton, Richard A. Robison, PhD and Kim L. O'Neill, PhD*
Department of Microbiology and Molecular Biology, Brigham Young University, Provo, UT, US

Abstract

Reactive oxygen species (ROS) and reactive nitrogen species (RNS) are key constituents of crucial physiological processes, but in excess they contribute to various prostatic disease states such as benign prostatic hyperplasia, prostate intraepithelial neoplasia, and prostate cancer. ROS and RNS play a vital role in establishing a microenvironment conducive to prostate cancer development. Prostate cancer is the second leading cause of cancer death in men. The balance between antioxidants and pro-oxidants has been intensely investigated by researchers due to the important effect these molecules have in regulating many cellular functions. Naturally, ROS and RNS are products of essential cellular processes such as the electron transport chain, other metabolic pathways, and inflammation, but they may also result from exposure to certain chemicals and cigarette smoke. Their production is also influenced by gene expression. When vital cellular systems become disrupted, as in mitochondrial leakage, infection, aging, etc., the balance between pro-oxidants and antioxidants is disturbed. The disturbance leads to increased damage by ROS and RNS through free radical chain reactions. These reactions take place due to the decreased amount or activity of antioxidants, and therefore, decreased deactivation of potentially harmful free radicals.

Damage from ROS and RNS, such as hydroxyl radicals, peroxide, superoxide, and nitric oxide, generated by endogenous factors as well as exogenous factors, accumulates over time. When an imbalance of sufficient intensity results, whether through overproduction of pro-oxidants, increased persistence of free pro-oxidants, a reduction in antioxidants, or a combination of these three, the microenvironment shifts to an oxidative stress state which in turn leads to damage of many key macromolecules such as DNA,

* Corresponding author e-mail: kim_oneill@byu.edu

proteins, and lipids. This oxidative stress appears to be a primary factor in the development of malignant prostate cancer and other diseases. It has been shown in prostate cancer specifically that ROS generation, rather than ROS accumulation, plays a key role in promoting an aggressive phenotype. For this reason, ROS and RNS play a key role in shifting the microenvironment to a state that permits prostate cancer development and progression.

Keywords: oxidative stress, prostate cancer, reactive oxygen species, cancer, pro-oxidant

Abbreviations

ROS:	Reactive oxygen species
RNS:	Reactive nitrogen species
PSA:	prostate specific antigen
DRE:	digital rectal exam
DHT:	dihydrotestosterone
AR:	androgen receptor
BPH:	benign prostatic hyperplasia
PIN:	prostate intraepithelial neoplasia
LGPIN:	low grade prostate intraepithelial neoplasia
HGPIN:	high grade prostate intraepithelial neoplasia
SOD:	superoxide dismutase
$NO^{\bullet}$:	nitric oxide radical
NF-κB:	nuclear factor κB
HIF-1:	hypoxia induced factor 1
SOD1:	superoxide dismutase 1
SOD2:	superoxide dismutase 2
GST:	glutathione transferases
GSTP1:	glutathione S transferase P1
GSH:	glutathione
VEGF:	vascular epidermal growth factor
miRNA:	microRNA
Rb:	retinoblastoma
IGF:	insulin growth factor
EGF:	epidermal growth factor
NGF:	nerve growth factor
PTEN:	phosphatase and tensin homologue
eNOS:	endothelial nitric oxide synthase
mtDNA:	mitochondrial DNA
GRS:	glutathione redox system
ARE:	antioxidant response elements
USPSTF:	U.S. Preventive Services Task Force
NO:	nitric oxide
H_2O_2:	hydrogen peroxide
Fe(II):	iron (II)

$ROO^{\bullet}$:	peroxyl radical
Nox (1,2,4,5):	NAD(P)H oxidase (1,2,4,5)
O_2^{-}:	superoxide anion

Introduction

Prostate cancer is the most common cancer in men in the United States and the second leading cause of cancer death among men, after lung cancer [1]. Globally, prostate cancer is the sixth leading cancer-related killer [2]. A family history of prostate cancer, as well as lifestyle, can influence its development. A family history of prostate cancer increases the risk of developing prostate cancer by 15%. In its early stages, prostate cancer does not cause observable symptoms and is often hard to diagnose through prostate-specific antigen (PSA) screening and digital rectal exam (DRE) because these tests are not conclusive [3]. In most cases, prostate cancer is diagnosed at stage 3 through a biopsy, and after PSA screening and DRE show irregularities. Aging brings about many of the changes necessary for oxidative stress: serum androgen levels drop, androgen-estrogen ratios decrease, and antioxidant levels drop. While these changes have been the focus of much research, the role of each in prostate carcinogenesis requires additional investigation. Despite the work to be done, it has been shown that oxidative stress is a significant agonist in the progression of prostate cancer [4].

In this chapter, oxidative stress is defined as the imbalance of pro-oxidants and antioxidants due to an increase in either production or persistence of pro-oxidants resulting in cellular damage due to excess oxidative load. This shift overwhelms the normal antioxidant defenses of the microenvironment, resulting in damage to important macromolecules such as proteins, lipids, and DNA. DNA damage may lead to driver mutations in vital regulatory genes, which can lead to initiation and progression of cancer. Reactive oxygen species (ROS) and reactive nitrogen species (RNS) such as hydroxide radicals, peroxide radicals, superoxide radicals, hydroperoxy radicals, organic peroxide radicals, hydrogen peroxide, singlet oxygen, nitric oxide, and NO byproducts–nitrate, nitrite, and peroxynitrite–are the primary effectors of cellular damage [5,6]. Studies have shown that genetic mutations are not sufficient to generate deadly, metastatic disease, but require a properly conditioned microenvironment [7]. The tumor microenvironment must be appropriately conditioned to support and possibly promote the development of prostate cancer. This chapter attempts to more clearly identify the processes by which pro-oxidants contribute to the initiation and progression of prostate cancer.

Prostate Structure and Function

The prostate gland is an endodermal derived structure that completely develops by birth in humans. In the initial stages of development, the prostate is entirely dependent on androgens secreted by the testes, but this dependency diminishes with time [8]. The primary androgen responsible for hormonal regulation of the prostate is dihydrotestosterone (DHT), due to its increased affinity for androgen receptors (AR) over testosterone [9,10].

The healthy prostate is comprised of smaller glands, which have been categorized into three zones: the peripheral zone, the central zone, and the transitional zone. In addition to zones, there exists the stroma which is devoid of glandular tissue [11]. The peripheral zone is the posterior and inferior region of the gland where 60-70% of prostate cancers form. The central zone is the next largest portion of the prostate gland. This segment encloses the ejaculatory ducts and is generally the site of prostatitis. The transitional zone is the smallest portion of the prostate, but is significant due to it being the primary site of benign prostatic hypertrophy and nearly a quarter of all prostatic adenocarcinomas [11,12]. According to the McNeal anatomy of the prostate, the gland consists of stromal and epithelial cells–specifically neuroendocrine, basal, and secretory cells–in each zone, and fibroblasts, endothelial cells, and smooth muscle cells in the stroma.

The prostate is an accessory gland that plays a key role in the male reproductive system. The prostate's key function is to produce an alkaline secretion containing PSA, citric acid, and seminalplasmin. PSA has enzymatic activity in semen, citric acid is a nutrient for sperm, and seminalplasmin serves as an antibiotic against urinary tract infections [13]. This fluid contributes to the motility and viability of sperm during fertilization.

As the body ages, the prostate undergoes changes resulting in a sequence of disease states, possibly culminating in prostate cancer. Initial inflammation and damage in the prostate tissue produces benign prostatic hyperplasia (BPH). Although it has been argued that BPH is not indicative of guaranteed cancer development, it is a disease characterized by oxidative stress and ROS activity [4]. A more accepted precursor to prostate cancer is prostate intraepithelial neoplasia (PIN), which ranges from low grade prostate intraepithelial neoplasia (LGPIN) to high grade prostate intraepithelial neoplasia (HGPIN or more commonly PIN). This is characterized by a loss of proliferative capacity in the basal cells and an increased proliferative capacity in the secretory luminal cells. As PIN progresses from low grade to high grade, biomarkers specific to the basal cell population are overexpressed by the secretory epithelial cells [14]. The next step in prostate disease progression is the development of apoptotic disorders typical in cancer. Preliminary development of tumor cells in the transition zone accompanies this change, although there is little evidence of full-scale cancerous growth. After secretory luminal cell gene expression parallels that of neighboring cancer cells, the prostate cancer invades into the prostate stroma [15]. This invasion is facilitated by signals produced by the basement membrane which has been conditioned [7]. Neuroendocrine cells also play an important role in the process of tumor invasion in prostate cancer, due to the regulatory effect they exert.

Pro-Oxidants Lead to Oxidative Damage

ROS and RNS are products of many natural processes in the body. They can also result as byproducts from radiation, metal-catalyzed reactions, pollutants, the electron transport chain in mitochondria, and activated inflammatory cells such as macrophages, neutrophils and eosinophils. When activated, macrophages uptake increased levels of oxygen and produce superoxide anion, NO, and H_2O_2 [16]. In a macrophage oxidative burst, superoxide anion and NO may react producing peroxynitrite anion, which may cause DNA damage and lipid oxidation [17].

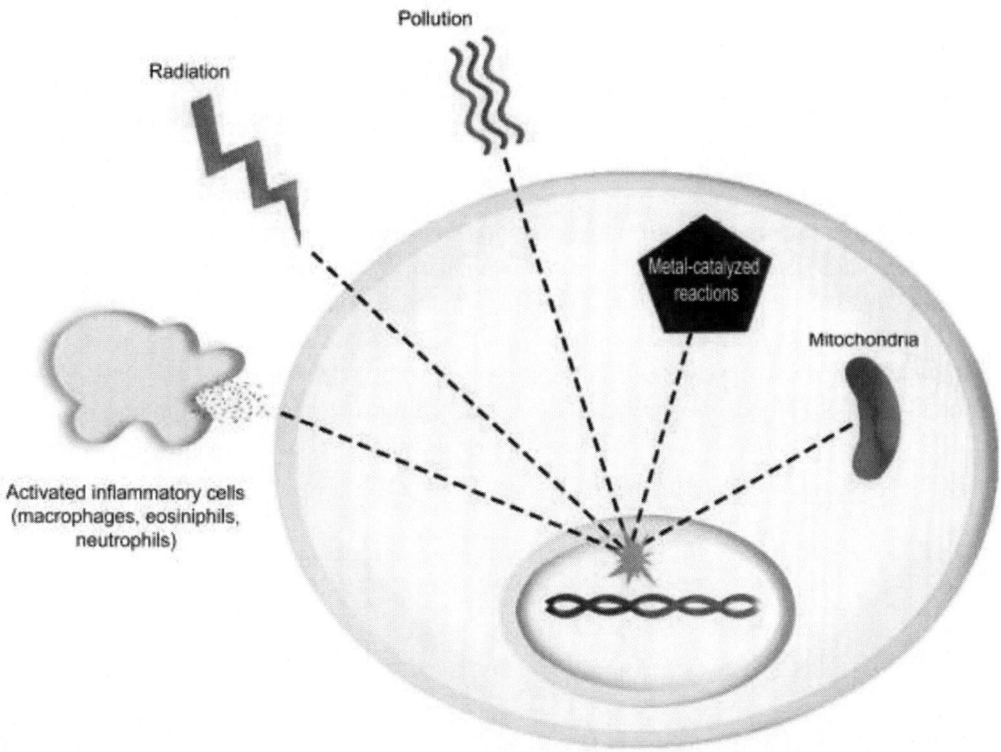

Figure 1. ROS Sources.
ROS are generated as a result of both exogenous and endogenous factors. This can result in significant DNA damage.

The free radicals generated by the mitochondria are manifest by the presence of H_2O_2. While H_2O_2 is not a radical species, it is the product of the enzyme superoxide dismutase (SOD). This enzyme converts its substrate, superoxide radicals, to H_2O_2 thereby making H_2O_2 indicative of superoxide production. Superoxide occurs in mitochondria at a rate of approximately 2-3 nmol/min per mg of protein, making the mitochondria the primary source of this radical [18]. H_2O_2 can alternatively produce hydroxyl radicals via Fenton chemistry.

The superoxide anion is considered to be a primary ROS or pro-oxidant which generates secondary ROS through radical chain reactions and enzyme-catalyzed or metal-catalyzed reactions [18]. This anion does not directly react with polypeptides or nucleic acids, rather the secondary ROS generated by it react with these molecules to induce damage. The superoxide anion alternatively produces oxidative damage when produced in excess. As superoxide anion levels rise, iron-containing molecules may release Fe(II), which subsequently reacts with H_2O_2 via the Fenton reaction, producing hydroxyl radicals. The superoxide anion also reacts with H_2O_2 in the Haber-Weiss reaction to produce hydroxyl radicals [19]. The hydroxyl radicals produced in these reactions have a half-life of less than 1 ns in an aqueous environment, and subsequently they damage the molecules nearest to them at the time of production [20]. Hydroxyl radicals and other reactive species have been estimated to assault one cell and its components approximately 1.5×10^5 times per day [21]. Common targets of hydroxyl radical reactions are DNA components, e.g., purine bases, pyrimidine bases, and the deoxyribose backbone [22]. Frequent forms of ROS-induced DNA damage are purine, pyrimidine, and deoxyribose alterations, single-strand and double-strand breaks, and DNA cross-linkage. This damage is a primary step in the processes of ageing, mutagenesis, and carcinogenesis.

Another oxygen-derived radical is the peroxyl radical ($ROO^{\bullet}$). Peroxyl radicals are high-energy ROS whose function depends on the R group, the microenvironment, the concentration of oxygen, and of other reactants [23]. While peroxyl radicals participate in a variety of reactions, the most frequent is lipid peroxidation. Additional peroxyl radical reactions include DNA cleavage and modification of protein structure. Peroxyl radicals also increase DNA damage by superoxide anion in a synergistic manner [18].

Nitric oxide ($NO^{\bullet}$) is a common RNS. This RNS is an important signaling molecule with a variety of functions across multiple biological systems. Specifically, NO plays a role in neurotransmission, blood pressure regulation, smooth muscle relaxation, immune regulation, and defense mechanisms [18,24]. $NO^{\bullet}$ may react with transition metals, but does not typically react with non-radicals. $NO^{\bullet}$ and peroxynitrites can also cause DNA mutations.

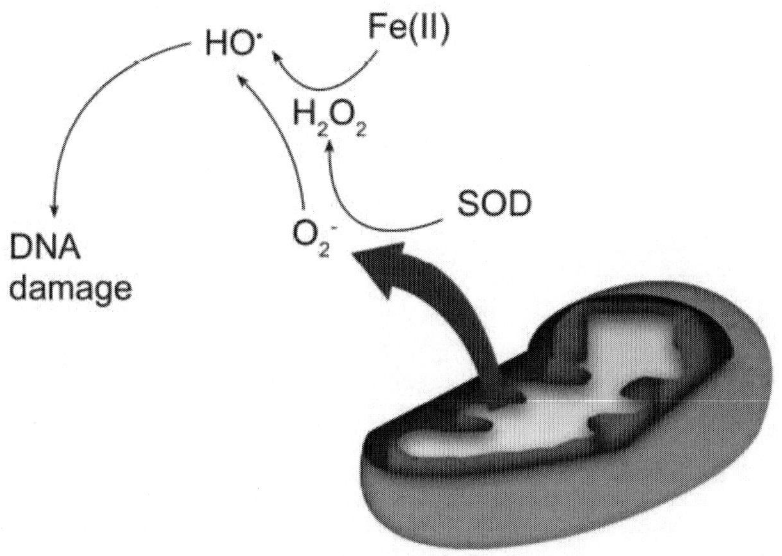

Figure 2. Role of Superoxide Anion in Oxidative Stress.
Superoxide anion is reduced to hydrogen peroxide by SOD. Hydrogen peroxide can subsequently react with either Fe(II) or superoxide anions to produce hydroxyl radicals which damage DNA.

Proteins are targets for damage from ROS generated by either ionizing radiation exposure or hydroxyl radicals produced by superoxide reactions with transition metals. In studies where ROS were generated by ionizing radiation, hydroxyl radicals removed hydrogen atoms from the polypeptide backbone [25]. This formed a carbon-centered radical which reacted with dioxygen under aerobic conditions to form peroxyl radicals. These peroxyl radicals reacted with protonated superoxide to form alkyl peroxides. Protein damage catalyzed by transition metals may be extensive and includes loss of histidine (His) residues, oxidative scission, bityrosine crosslinks, addition of carbonyls, and creation of protein-centered alkyl, alkoxyl, and alkylperoxyl radicals. Additional protein damage may be induced by hydroxyl radical attack of glutamic acid and proline residues. While protein damage is a generally repairable event, studies suggest that damage to the mitochondrial proteins aconitase and adenine nucleotide translocase may result in long-term oxidative damage [25].

Specific protein targets for oxidative damage are protein phosphatases, such as phosphotyrosine-, phospholipid-, and phosphoserine/threonine-phosphatases. Studies by Poli *et al.* and Thannickal *et al.* showed that the interactions likely occurred with the sulfhydryl groups of cysteine residues, causing formation of disulfide bonds [26,27]. These conformational changes resulted in increased activity in the signaling cascades that led to activation of the transcription factors nuclear factor κB (NF-κB) and hypoxia-inducible factor-1 (HIF-1), which have both been implicated in prostate cancer development.

Prostate Cancer Development

Benign Prostatic Hyperplasia

Benign prostatic hyperplasia is a condition common in many men and may be a precursor to prostate cancer. The exact etiology of the disease has yet to be elucidated, but ageing and oxidative stress have been implicated in the development of BPH [28]. BPH is so prevalent that estimates suggest 90% of males will have the condition by the time they are eighty years old [12]. Oxidative stress in BPH may result in insufficient DNA repair and increased DNA damage in response to increased generation of ROS [4]. Studies by Ahmad *et al.* established that oxidative stress is present in BPH, but their work did not identify whether the oxidative stress resulted from overproduction of ROS, reduction in ROS scavenging enzymes or their activity, or a combination of both [4].

Androgens have also been linked to BPH development and prostate cancer as well. Studies have shown that castration before puberty and genetic deficiencies in testosterone production and activity prevented BPH development in patients.

Prostatic Intraepithelial Neoplasia

Prostatic intraepithelial neoplasia (PIN) has a strong correlation to prostate cancer. This isn't to say that PIN always precedes prostate cancer; rather that it is a significant indicator in a pathway leading to carcinogenesis. Davidsson *et al.* found that death from prostate cancer was 89% more likely to occur in men diagnosed with PIN [29].

PIN is characterized by inflammation and the presence of infiltrating immune cells such as macrophages and neutrophils. Whether the presence of immune cells is due to foreign invaders or endogenous expression of inflammatory cytokines is not fully clear and may vary on a case-by-case basis. The presence of inflammatory cells in PIN does, however, provide a possible explanation for ROS generation and subsequent carcinogenesis.

An additional source of oxidative stress in PIN has been attributed to reduced production of SOD and catalase enzymes. Bostwick *et al.* observed decreased production of copper-zinc superoxide dismutase (SOD1), manganese superoxide dismutase (SOD2), and catalase in both PIN and prostate cancer. Additional immunohistochemical results also showed a similar number of immunoreactive cells in both PIN and prostate cancer [30]. Other enzymes that have been found to be downregulated in both PIN and prostate cancer are the glutathione transferases (GST). All enzyme subclasses showed lost or reduced expression in PIN and prostate cancer. These findings strengthen the evidence suggesting that ROS and oxidative stress in PIN are precursors for carcinogenesis.

Prostate Cancer

Several studies have shown that increased ROS production is inherent to prostate cancer. A study by Kumar and colleagues looked at the relationship between ROS production and prostate cancer aggressiveness [31]. They used PC3, DU145, and LNCaP cell lines and compared their ROS production with normal prostate cells. All prostate cancer cell lines showed higher ROS production than normal prostate cells and ROS levels correlated with prostate cancer aggressiveness. They also found that NAD(P)H oxidase (Nox) systems (extramitochondrial enzymes that convert molecular oxygen into O_2^- which is subsequently dismutated by SOD to form H_2O_2) have a crucial role in prostate cancer malignant phenotypes, and that inhibiting Nox ROS production decreases cell invasion and increases cell death [32]. Nox1 production propels angiogenesis, converting the prostate cancer from dormant to aggressive [33]. Studies by Khandrika *et al.* also discovered the isoforms Nox2, Nox4, and Nox5 in prostate cancer [34]. Inhibition of Nox 5 leads to growth inhibition and apoptosis. Additionally, castration results in increased expression of Nox1, Nox2, and Nox4 [35]. These findings are important because ROS production by the mitochondria is vital for cell metabolism, but targeting extramitochrondrial ROS sources such as Nox, could have therapeutic potential in prostate cancer.

Freitas and colleagues performed a study on ROS and antioxidant production in prostate cancer cells. They used RWPE1, HPV10, and PC3 cell lines, which are human normal prostate tissue, localized prostate carcinoma, and metastatic prostate carcinoma respectively. They analyzed the effect of ROS on cell growth and viability in each cell line. They found that higher H_2O_2 concentrations inhibited growth in RWPE1 cells, but PC3 growth persisted. This was due to higher glutathione (GSH) levels in PC3 cells. This suggests that PC3 cells use their antioxidant protection mechanisms to allow them to continue proliferating despite inhibitive ROS levels and increased oxidative stress [36].

Hypoxia in Prostate Cancer

Normal prostate tissue maintains sufficient oxygen levels to supply all the processes of aerobic metabolism. Non-cancerous tissue proliferates at a consistent pace that allows oxygen control to be maintained. When prostate tissue becomes cancerous, proliferation increases and oxygen is consumed faster than it is supplied. This imbalance triggers signaling pathways that perpetuate alternating oxygenated and hypoxic environments. This cycle results in an overall increase in HIF-1 in the cell over time through repeated intermittent hypoxic conditions. This differs from normal tissue, which degrades HIF-1 quickly to maintain control over cell processes.

HIF-1 is a transcription factor that is key in regulating oxygen availability in the cell and activating physiological responses. Galanis *et al.* report that HIF-1 has been found to control over 70 different physiological responses including metabolism, motility, and vascularization. Zhong *et al.* reported metastasis induced by this mechanism in several common cancers, including prostate cancer. Further evidence supports increased angiogenesis in tumor cells as a mechanism to further cancer aggressiveness in the prostate.

Vascular epidermal growth factor (VEGF) is mainly responsible for the induction of angiogenesis in tissue. Tumor development was demonstrated in PC-3 cells, an aggressive metastatic prostate cancer line, which was treated with insulin and stimulated to produce H_2O_2. H_2O_2 production (Zhou et al). H_2O_2 increased the levels of phosphorylated p70S6K1, which in turn increased levels of VEGF as a result of HIF-1 overexpression. When catalase was added, VEGF production was reduced. Catalase is an enzyme that quickly destroys H_2O_2. This demonstrates a role of ROS in HIF-1 induced angiogenesis [37].

Recent studies have also shown that microRNA (miRNA) expression is altered in multiple cell lines. The 23 miRNAs that were reported to be changed in hypoxic conditions exhibit high binding affinity to HIF-1, thus indicating that HIF-1 could play a significant role in altering miRNA expression in cancer tissue under hypoxic conditions [38].

Hormones in Prostate Cancer

Normal prostate function and regulation rely heavily on androgens and other hormones. Davis and Day have shown that luminal epithelial cells require testosterone to survive [39]. If testosterone levels decrease, apoptosis occurs. This relationship between androgen and androgen receptor (AR) is vital in the beginning stages of prostate cancer. Normal apoptosis in prostate epithelial cells occurs when stromal cells send a paracrine signal to initiate androgen withdrawal, but as is common in many cancers, prostate cancer cells have the capacity to avoid the apoptotic pathways and continue proliferating. Prostate cancer cells avoid apoptosis by losing their dependence on androgens for survival, while only maintaining their androgen dependence for growth [14]. Further mutations occur which promote androgen independence entirely. Current hypotheses for this evolution involve mutations in vital elements of the AR signaling pathway such as the receptor itself, ligands, kinases, or regulatory proteins. Studies have shown that prostate cancer becomes androgen-independent due to the heterogeneous mix of androgen-dependent and androgen-independent cells in the tumor. It has been proposed that androgen-independent cells are positively selected as a result of antiandrogen therapy, resulting in entire androgen-independent prostate tumors [14]. In prostate carcinoma, stromal AR dependence is altered to both androgen and estrogen dependence. This trend is due to AR mutations leading to an inactivated, down-regulated, absent, or alternatively activated receptor in advanced prostate cancers. Additional differences in androgen-independent prostate cancers are manifest in AR activation by growth factors and other regulatory signals, rather than androgens.

Studies by Ripple *et al.* have shown that androgen concentration has a powerful impact on androgen-dependent LNCaP prostate cancer cells. After exposure to increasing concentrations of DHT and synthetic androgen R1881, LNCaP growth exhibited a bell-shaped response. Subsequent analysis of ROS generation revealed an inverse response, with growth-promoting levels of androgen leading to reduced ROS levels and growth-inhibiting levels of androgen leading to increased ROS levels. A matter of interest in this regard is that other growth-inhibiting compounds did not induce ROS production.

Key enzymes were also affected in this study. A key enzyme in regulating GSH, γ-glutamyl transpeptidase, showed increased activity after exposure to androgen. This enzyme has been implicated in ROS generation via breakdown of extracellular glutathione [40]. According to Stark *et al.*, catabolism of GSH produces cysteinyl-glycine which reduces ferric iron (Fe(III)). The ROS produced in the process are superoxide and hydrogen peroxide. GSH breakdown, rather than decreased production, was observed as the limiting enzyme in GSH production, γ-glutamylcysteine synthetase, remained unaffected by androgen exposure. The activity of catalase, the enzyme responsible for converting hydrogen peroxide to water and oxygen, also increased when exposed to 1 n*M* R1881. This increase in activity suggests an increase in H_2O_2 production by superoxide dismutase as a result of increased superoxide (O_2^-) generation from androgen exposure [41].

Another key observation by Ripple and her team was the increase in mitochondrial activity of LNCaP cells after androgen exposure based on the MTT (3-(4,5-dimethylthiazol-2-yl)-2,5-diphenyltetrazolium bromide) reduction assay [41]. This assay detects both hydroxyl (OH^-) radicals and H_2O_2. Evidence to support the increase in mitochondrial activity is manifest by an increase in oxygen consumption. MTT can also be reduced by superoxide, which is also indicative of ROS generation and potential oxidative stress.

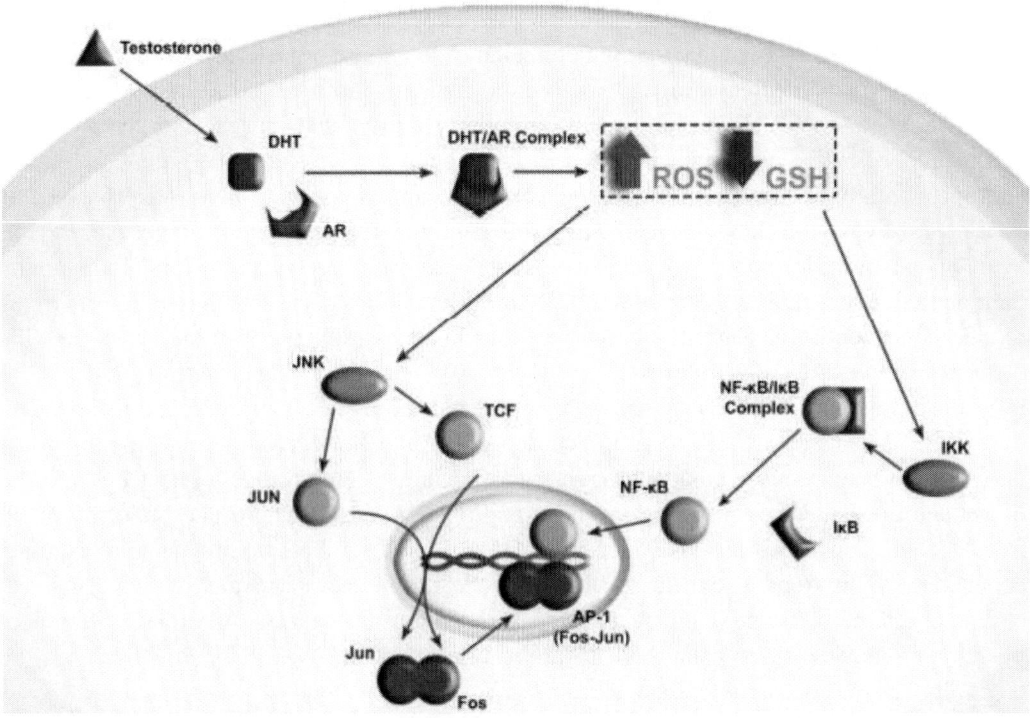

Figure 3. Androgen-mediated Gene Expression through GSH Regulation.
Androgen exposure leads to an imbalance in the GSH redox systems thereby promoting oxidative stress. This leads to gene activation by AP-1 and NF-κB.

On a molecular level, the effect of androgens on intracellular GSH levels may affect expression of certain genes and proteins without the androgen directly interacting with a promoter sequence. GSH is a necessary component in pathways involving the transcription factors NF-κB, Fos, and Jun [42,43]. As ROS increase in the cell, they tip the balance of the glutathione redox system, which preserves the balance between antioxidants and oxidants in the body; this imbalance in the GSH redox system promotes oxidative stress. This triggers the Jun *N*-terminal kinases/stress-activated protein kinase signaling pathway, which leads to gene activation and posttranslational protein modifications required for apoptosis [6].

Mitochondrial membrane permeability is also affected by androgens. Androgens lead to increased O_2^- levels in androgen-dependent prostate cancer, thereby increasing superoxide dismutase activity and H_2O_2 production. H_2O_2 activates caspase, via cytochrome c release from the mitochondria, which triggers apoptosis.

Androgens also play a role in cell cycle regulation in prostate cancer. Androgens' role is manifest as an upregulation of the cell cycle. Androgen-stimulated proliferation leads to apoptosis in the presence of a functioning retinoblastoma (Rb) tumor suppressor gene. When accompanied by mutations in the Rb tumor suppressor gene, androgen-stimulated proliferation bypasses apoptosis and leads to carcinogenesis.

As prostate cancer progresses, tumors may switch from androgen dependence to androgen independence. In many cases this androgen independence correlates with more aggressive tumors and metastasis. Androgen independent prostate tumors still rely on AR signaling for growth and development [44]. For this reason, androgen-refractory prostate cancer is a better identifier to denote the true nature of the disease. Androgen-refractory prostate cancer may depend on AR for continued development, or it may bypass AR entirely. These two alternatives are not independent from one another, and both may be seen in androgen-refractory prostate cancer.

The AR-dependent survival pathways function through amplified or mutated receptors, deregulated growth factors and cytokines, and altered coactivators [45]. An amplified AR gene was seen in a significant number of androgen-refractory prostate cancer patients, where none existed when the carcinomas were androgen dependent [45]. Mutated AR genes may lead to AR activation by anomalous ligands, but this is an uncommon occurrence. AR may also be activated by growth factors and cytokines such as insulin growth factor (IGF), epidermal growth factor (EGF), nerve growth factor (NGF), and interleukin 6 [34,45]. Activation of AR through these ligands happens as a result of altered function or expression of coactivators.

AR-independent survival pathways in androgen-refractory prostate cancer vary. Neuroendocrine cells in the prostate have the capacity to survive chemotherapeutic, endocrine, and radiation treatments. As a result, when these cells secrete neuropeptides that increase proliferation of adjacent tumor cells, the entire tumor grows independent of androgen exposure. Alternative AR-independent proliferation occurs when apoptotic genes are deregulated. Phosphatase and tensin homologue (PTEN) is a tumor suppressor gene that inhibits the phosphatidylinositol 3-kinase pathway, which is responsible for inactivation of Akt signaling. Akt is a protein responsible for inhibition of apoptosis via suppression of proteins that initiate cell death. In androgen-refractory prostate cancer, PTEN is inhibited, permitting Akt activity and inhibition of apoptosis [45]. ROS have been shown to inhibit the PTEN protein by forming a disulfide linkage in the active site [46].

Molecular Aspects of Prostate Cancer

Hereditary gene alterations that increase prostate cancer risk are found in germline genes such as *ELAC2* (*HPC2*), *MSR1*, and *RNASEL* (*HPC1*). The *ELAC2* (*HPC2*) gene encodes a 3' endonuclease and certain nonsense mutations that inhibit 3'-endonuclease activity, have been found in pedigrees of prostate cancer [47]. Inhibiting enzyme activity may not be the only factor that increases risk in prostate cancer, as unique silent mutations are also found in hereditary prostate cancer [48]. The *MSR1* gene (macrophage scavenger receptor 1) is a member of macrophage scavenger receptor genes found in the p22 band of chromosome 8, a common loci that is deleted in prostate cancer. Missense and nonsense mutations found in the *MSR1* gene have been shown to increase susceptibility in both hereditary and sporadic prostate cancer (Xu *et al.*, 2003). *RNASEL* (*HPC1*) gene encodes the 2'-5'- oligoadenylate (2–5 A)-dependent RNase L, which is an enzyme that regulates apoptosis and cell proliferation through the interferon-regulated 2–5 A pathway. Nonsense and frameshift mutations, as well as independent segregation of the *RNASEL* gene are significantly associated with early onset risk of prostate cancer in men of many races [47]. A recent study reported a recurrent but rare germline mutation (G84E) in the *HOXB13* gene (involved in prostate development) located on chromosome 17q21-22 that is also found to increase hereditary prostate cancer [49].

The majority of prostate cancer cases, however, occur because of a lifetime of acquired mutations. Some of these mutations lead to phenotypic changes in prostate cells. The prostate is an organ that has high cellular organization which includes epithelial stem cells, transiently proliferating cells, fully differentiated epithelial prostate cells, and neuroendocrine cells. In a cancerous prostate, a similar cellular organization is found, and a cancer cell can be traced to its origin through keratin expression patterns. These keratin expression patterns change with the stages of cell differentiation; therefore, it has been suggested that prostate cancer cells arise from a malignant mutation in intermediate stem cells [50].

Oncogenes and tumor suppressor genes are also involved in the development of prostate cancer. Oncogenes are usually dominant, meaning that only one copy of the gene is sufficient for its expression. Oncogenes are usually activated by translocations, point mutations, mutagenesis, and amplifications. No oncogene specific to prostate cancer has been identified, but other oncogenes present in several neoplasias such as *RAS*, *C-MYC*, *C-ERB-B2*, *RAF*, and *EZH2* also play a role in prostate cancer [51].

The *RAS* gene encodes GTPase signal transduction proteins of 21 kDa in size. Mutations in the *RAS* gene that result in overexpression of Ras inhibit the activity of p21–a protein responsible for cell-cycle inhibition. This *RAS* mutation can stimulate cell proliferation even when external signaling is absent, because its GTPase activity is continuously activated [52]. Mutations in the *RAS* gene are common in various cancers and may not have a prognosis potential for prostate cancer, and yet studying *RAS* variations and mutation rates may be important to understand cancer initiation and development [51].

C-myc is a DNA-binding protein that functions as a transcription factor that controls cell proliferation, cell cycle progression, apoptosis, differentiation, and cellular motility. Normal cells exhibit low levels of c-myc until they enter the cell cycle when c-myc levels increase and then decrease to basal level after cell cycle is completed. In cancer cells, c-myc levels are always high due to gene amplification [53]. Prostatic intraepithelial neoplasia as well as primary prostate cancer show elevated levels of c-myc. The level of amplification of c-myc correlates with malignancy, higher Gleason scores, early disease progression, and early cancer-related death [54]. Overexpression of c-myc can also predict recurrence of prostate cancer [55].

The *C-ERB-B2* oncogene (also known as *HER-2 NEU*) codes for a protein similar to the epidermal growth factor receptor [51]. *C-ERB-B2* is found overexpressed in several breast cancers but not in localized prostate cancer. However, it is found amplified on 60% of androgen-independent prostate cancer [56]. Amplification of *C-ERB-B2* correlates with shorter survival times and higher Gleason scores in prostate cancer, and may help to develop androgen independence [56–58].

The *RAF* oncogene family (*A-RAF*, *B-RAF*, and *C-RAF*) encodes serine/threonine kinases which are regulated by binding of Ras. Raf kinases activate MAPK or ERK kinases, which control cell division. All the malignant mutations in the *RAS* genes are found in their kinase domains, and cause Ras to continually phosphorylate MAPK/ERK causing uncontrollable cell division [59]. Ras inhibitors are used to treat prostate cancer, and have been shown to be effective in sensitizing cells to chemotherapy and radiotherapy. Ras inhibitors also suppress metastasis in prostate cancer [60]. A recent study by Palanisamy *et al.* looked at gene fusions that may affect the RAF kinase pathway in prostate cancer. These fusions may prevent Ras inhibitors from working. They suggested that tumor transcriptomes and genomes should be sequenced to identify prostate cancer patients who will actually benefit from Raf inhibitor therapy [61].

EZH2 is the enhancer of zeste homolog 2 and functions as a transcription repressor. It is activated in advanced prostate cancer and causes generalized reduction of transcription by increasing histone deacetylation. High concentrations of *EZH2* transcripts and protein predict poor prognosis in prostate cancer [62]. *EZH2* has been proposed as a molecular target for advanced prostate cancer treatments. *EZH2* inhibitors have been shown to induce apoptosis with high efficacy and low toxicity [63].

Tumor suppressor genes also play a role in the development of prostate cancer. Unlike oncogenes, tumor suppressor genes are recessive, meaning both copies of the gene must be defective to cause disease. The tumor suppressor genes involved in the development of prostate cancer are retinoblastoma (*Rb*), p53, *PTEN*, *E-CADHERIN*, *BRC1*, *BRC2*, Glutathione S transferase (*GST*), and Kruppel like factor 6 [51].

The *Rb* gene's function is to repress E2F transcription factors. E2F transcription factors regulate many genes but are mostly involved in the transcriptional regulation of genes involved in nucleotide synthesis, DNA replication, and cell cycle checkpoints. *Rb* is usually activated in between phases G1 and S in the cell cycle, and can halt the cell cycle at that point. Oxidative stress can activate *Rb* during S phase, where it regulates the E2F transcription factors involved in the mitotic checkpoint [64]. In prostate cancer, the loss of function of *Rb* contributes to tumor initiation, correlates with poor prognosis, and induces hormone therapy resistance [65].

The P53 gene codes for a 53 kDa phosphoprotein involved in cell cycle checkpoints in between G1 and S phases. Loss of P53 function can lead to genetic instability and tumorigenesis. Prostate cancer cell lines do not proliferate when there is a wild-type allele of P53 [66]. Recent studies have proposed that functional inactivation of the Rb and P53 pathways may be a mechanism by which the androgen receptor is overexpressed, and the gene transcription mediated by androgen receptors dysregulated, which leads to therapy-resistant prostate cancer [67].

GSTs are a family of isoenzymes involved in the detoxification of free radicals. When the cell experiences oxidative stress, glutathione S transferase P1 (GSTP1) is often invoked to prevent cellular damage from cytotoxic and carcinogenic agents [6]. In prostate cancer, GSTP1 expression is low due to promoter hypermethylation, which is found in 70% of prostatic intraepithelial neoplasias [68]. In a recent study, Re and colleagues suggested that the hypermethylation process that leads to GSTP1 silencing may be due to a complex formed between the estrogen receptor β and the endothelial nitric oxide synthase (eNOS) [69].

Mitochondrial DNA (mtDNA) mutations also contribute to prostate cancer. The mitochondria are responsible for energy production through oxidative phosphorylation, a process that produces ROS [70]. Cellular signaling relies on ROS products, and maintaining a balance between ROS and antioxidants is important to avoid cellular damage [6,26,71]. Severe mutations in mtDNA, especially those that inhibit oxidative phosphorylation, lead to increased ROS, which along with p53 inactivation, can lead to tumor development and proliferation [72]. Normal prostate cells have high concentrations of zinc in their mitochondria, which halts the Krebs cycle. These cells have terminal oxidation, and hence low production of ROS. In an early event of prostate cancer development, prostate cells decrease their zinc uptake, which prevents m-aconitase from completing citrate metabolism. This allows prostate cells to have higher respiration rates, and to generate high concentrations of ROS that may lead to mutations in the mtDNA [34]. Several studies have also shown that alterations in the mitochondrion IV subunit are significantly different between malignant prostate cells and normal prostate cells [73]. Recently, Petros and colleagues introduced pathogenic mutations in the mtDNA of PC3 cells through hybrid transfer, and injected the mutated PC3 cells into nude mice. They showed that tumors with mtDNA mutations were 7 times larger in size than the control tumors [70]. These data suggest that mtDNA mutations contribute to tumorigenicity in prostate cancer and that elevated ROS production plays a key role in early prostate cancer development.

Prevention of Prostate Cancer

Numerous epidemiological studies have identified an inverse correlation between intake of foods high in antioxidants and lower incidence of prostate cancer [74]. Natural defense systems, such as the glutathione redox system (GRS) and antioxidant response elements (ARE), help to minimize oxidative damage. *In vitro* evidence suggests that antioxidant compounds can enhance and supplement these defense systems to further prevent oxidative damage during high oxidative stress [74].

Several large scale clinical trials have been conducted with antioxidant supplements in order to investigate the possibility of preventative treatment for prostate cancer. During clinical trials investigating antioxidant supplements and prostate cancer incidence, many known antioxidant compounds found in fruits and vegetables showed little or no effect. These trials used artificial supplementation, which could suggest that protective effects of antioxidants are derived from food sources only. Resveratrol is commonly found in grapes, peanuts, and soy products. *In vivo* studies in mice have been done with resveratrol and have shown tumor growth delay without any signs of toxicity [75]. Flavonoids, another group of antioxidant compounds, have shown promise in clinical trials as well. A Phase II clinical trial was conducted on a cohort of men that had rising PSA levels and had recently received either surgery or radiotherapy. After treatment with pomegranate juice, a significant source of flavonoids, over the period of a few months, PSA doubling time was significantly delayed [76]. Genistein, another flavonoid found in soy, has been shown to increase transcription of certain genes which code for proteins involved in the body's antioxidant defense systems. Evidence suggests that genistein can reverse oxidative damage through this increased transcription [74]. This suggests that genistein and other soy flavonoids could delay the decreased functionality of antioxidant systems that comes with age, which would be significant for age-related cancers such as prostate cancer [74].

Detection of Prostate Cancer

Active screening programs can result in early detection of prostate cancer. The PSA test and the DRE are the most common tests used to detect prostate cancer. The prostate gland produces prostate-specific antigen, an enzyme that is part of the seminal fluid. PSA is mostly found in semen, but a small quantity can leak into the bloodstream and be detected in serum [77]. The PSA test consists of determining the amount of PSA present in the serum. Normal blood PSA levels are 4 ng/mL or lower. However, when cancer develops, PSA levels are elevated. Patients with elevated PSA levels are advised to repeat the testing or get an ultrasound-guided needle biopsy to accurately determine the presence of cancer [3,77].

PSA as a serum marker was first described in 1987 when Stamey and colleagues developed a radioimmunoassay for PSA to compare it to the one for prostatic acid phosphatase (PAP). They found that PSA levels were increased in prostate cancer patients who were recently diagnosed and in patients with suspected disease. They concluded that PSA testing was more sensitive than PAP testing but that neither marker was specific [78].

Serum PSA levels can vary depending on age, medical conditions such as benign prostatic hyperplasia, prostatitis, ejaculation, etc. [3]. Recent studies also showed that some single nucleotide polymorphisms are associated with increased levels of PSA in the serum, which is why the PSA test is not 100% accurate, and further testing is always needed to properly diagnose prostate cancer [79]. Furthermore, the U.S. Preventive Services Task Force (USPSTF) made a recommendation against PSA testing for prostate cancer because it may be misleading, but advised doctors to make decisions on a case-to-case basis [80].

The digital rectal exam (DRE) test is another option for detecting prostate cancer, but it has limitations including variability between results from different examiners and failure to diagnose if nothing is palpable [81]. The exam is usually performed by a doctor and is performed by introducing a finger into the patient's rectum to palpate the prostate for enlargement and abnormalities. The American Cancer Society considers the DRE test less effective than the PSA test, but after the USPSTF recommendation against PSA testing, the DRE test may become more important in the coming years [3,81].

A third alternative is an ultrasound-guided needle biopsy to test for prostate cancer. This is the most effective way to diagnose prostate malignancies, but it is intrusive and expensive. Further research needs to be done in the field of early detection and prognosis of prostate cancer.

Conclusion

Prostate cancer is inextricably linked to oxidative stress in the prostate microenvironment. Prostate cancer progression parallels other events such as aging and BPH, and as such, ROS are a necessary factor to be considered in targeting and treating prostate disease. Further work must be done to determine the extent to which ROS and oxidative stress affect prevention, detection, and treatment of prostate tumors. This may include determining detectable differences in the reactive species in different prostate diseases; e.g., ROS levels or species promoting oxidative stress in BPH versus PIN. As we come to more fully understand the role of ROS and oxidative stress in prostate cancer, we will be better equipped to prevent, detect, and treat this prevalent disease.

References

[1] CDC. *CDC - Cancer - Statistics by Demographic - Cancer Among Men.* 2013 [cited 2013 Jun 26]; Available from: http://www.cdc.gov/cancer/dcpc/data/men.htm

[2] Baade PD, Youlden DR, Krnjacki LJ. Review International epidemiology of prostate cancer: Geographical distribution and secular trends. Molecular Nutrition & Food Research. 2009;171–84.

[3] *American Cancer Society. Can prostate cancer be found early?* [Internet]. 2013 [cited 2013 Jun 26]. Available from: http://www.cancer.org/cancer/prostatecancer /detailedguide/prostate-cancer-detection

[4] Ahmad M, Suhail N, Mansoor T, Banu N, Ahmad S. Evaluation of Oxidative Stress and DNA Damage in Benign Prostatic Hyperplasia Patients and Comparison with Controls. *Indian Journal of Clinical Biochemistry* [Internet]. 2012 Jun 12 [cited 2013 Aug 14];27(4):385–8. Available from: http://link.springer.com/10.1007/s12291-012-0229-4

[5] Lam YW, Yuan Y, Isaac J, Babu CVS, Meller J, Ho S-M. Comprehensive identification and modified-site mapping of S-nitrosylated targets in prostate epithelial cells. *PloS one* [Internet]. 2010 Jan [cited 2013 Aug 14];5(2):e9075. Available from: http://www.pubmedcentral.nih.gov/articlerender.fcgi?artid=2816712&tool=pmcentrez &rendertype=abstract

[6] Gupta-Elera G, Garrett AR, Robison R a, O'Neill KL. The role of oxidative stress in prostate cancer. *European journal of cancer prevention: the official journal of the European Cancer Prevention Organisation* (ECP) [Internet]. 2012 Mar [cited 2013 Jul 1];21(2):155–62. Available from: http://www.ncbi.nlm.nih.gov/pubmed/21857523

[7] Rennebeck G, Martelli M, Kyprianou N. Anoikis and survival connections in the tumor microenvironment: is there a role in prostate cancer metastasis? *Cancer research* [Internet]. 2005 Dec 15 [cited 2013 Aug 14];65(24):11230–5. Available from: http://www.pubmedcentral.nih.gov/articlerender.fcgi?artid=2367317&tool=pmcentrez &rendertype=abstract

[8] Prins GS, Putz O. Molecular signaling pathways that regulate prostate gland development. Differentiation; research in biological diversity [Internet]. *International Society of Differentiation;* 2008 Jul [cited 2013 Aug 14];76(6):641–59. Available from:

http://www.pubmedcentral.nih.gov/articlerender.fcgi?artid=2824174&tool=pmcentrez &rendertype=abstract

[9] Wilson JD, Gloyna RE. The intranuclear metabolism of testosterone in the accessory organs of reproduction. *Recent progress in hormone research* [Internet]. 1970 Jan [cited 2013 Aug 14];26:309–36. Available from: http://www.ncbi.nlm.nih.gov/ pubmed /4990424

[10] Fang S, Anderson KM, Liao S. Receptor proteins for androgens. On the role of specific proteins in selective retention of 17-beta-hydroxy-5-alpha-androstan-3-one by rat ventral prostate in vivo and in vitro. *The Journal of biological chemistry* [Internet]. 1969 Dec 25 [cited 2013 Aug 14];244(24):6584–95. Available from: http://www.ncbi.nlm.nih.gov/pubmed/5361546

[11] Selman SH. The McNeal prostate: a review. *Urology* [Internet]. 2011 Dec [cited 2013 Aug 14];78(6):1224–8. Available from: http://www.ncbi.nlm.nih.gov/ pubmed /21908026

[12] Swindle P, Ramadan S, Stanwell P, McCredie S, Russell P, Mountford C. Proton magnetic resonance spectroscopy of the central, transition and peripheral zones of the prostate: assignments and correlation with histopathology. *Magnetic Resonance Materials in Physics, Biology and Medicine* [Internet]. 2008 Nov [cited 2013 Aug 14];21(6):423–34. Available from: http://www.ncbi.nlm.nih.gov/pubmed/18797949

[13] McKinley M, O'Loughlin VD. *Human Anatomy.* Third. McGraw Hill; 2011. p. 868.

[14] Farnsworth WE. Prostate Carcinogenesis is an Endogenous, Hypoxic Process. *UroOncology* [Internet]. 2004 Jun 1 [cited 2013 Aug 14];4(2):77–83. Available from: http://www.informaworld.com/openurl?genre=article&doi=10.1080/15610950410001720251&magic=crossref||D404A21C5BB053405B1A640AFFD44AE3

[15] Josson S, Matsuoka Y, Chung LWK, Zhau HE, Wang R. Tumor-stroma co-evolution in prostate cancer progression and metastasis. *Seminars in cell & developmental biology* [Internet]. 2010 Feb [cited 2013 Aug 14];21(1):26–32. Available from: http://www.pubmedcentral.nih.gov/articlerender.fcgi?artid=3388105&tool=pmcentrez &rendertype=abstract

[16] Conner EM, Grisham MB. Inflammation, free radicals, and antioxidants. *Nutrition* [Internet]. 1996 Apr [cited 2013 Aug 15];12(4):274–7. Available from: http://dx.doi.org/10.1016/S0899-9007(96)00000-8

[17] Carr AC, McCall MR, Frei B. *Oxidation of LDL by myeloperoxidase and reactive nitrogen species: reaction pathways and antioxidant protection. Arteriosclerosis, thrombosis, and vascular biology* [Internet]. 2000 Jul [cited 2013 Aug 15];20(7):1716–23. Available from: http://www.ncbi.nlm.nih.gov/pubmed/10894808

[18] Valko M, Rhodes CJ, Moncol J, Izakovic M, Mazur M. *Free radicals, metals and antioxidants in oxidative stress-induced cancer. Chemico-biological interactions* [Internet]. 2006 Mar 10 [cited 2013 Aug 7];160(1):1–40. Available from: http://www.ncbi.nlm.nih.gov/pubmed/16430879

[19] Liochev SI, Fridovich I. *The Haber-Weiss cycle -- 70 years later: an alternative view. Redox report: communications in free radical research* [Internet]. Maney Publishing; 2002 Jan [cited 2013 Aug 15];7(1):55–7; author reply 59–60. Available from: http://www.ingentaconnect.com/content/maney/rer/2002/00000007/00000001/art00010?token=00691ff6af1419a2da43a4968263c4a6f644a467c79675d7c4e4a47543c7e386f7e2a46762c6b635d7e666725702a765f246b573c

[20] Pastor N, Weinstein H, Jamison E, Brenowitz M. A detailed interpretation of OH radical footprints in a TBP-DNA complex reveals the role of dynamics in the mechanism of sequence-specific binding. *Journal of molecular biology* [Internet]. 2000 Nov 17 [cited 2013 Aug 15];304(1):55–68. Available from: http://dx.doi.org/ 10.1006/jmbi.2000.4173

[21] Beckman KB. Oxidative Decay of DNA. *Journal of Biological Chemistry* [Internet]. 1997 Aug 8 [cited 2013 Aug 15];272(32):19633–6. Available from: http://www. jbc.org/content/272/32/19633

[22] Dizdaroglu M, Jaruga P, Birincioglu M, Rodriguez H. *Free radical-induced damage to DNA: mechanisms and measurement* 1,2. 1This article is part of a series of reviews on "Oxidative DNA Damage and Repair." The full list of papers may be found on the homepage of the journal. 2Guest Editor: Miral Dizdaroglu. Free Radical Biology and Medicine [Internet]. 2002 Jun [cited 2013 Aug 15];32(11):1102–15. Available from: http://dx.doi.org/10.1016/S0891-5849(02)00826-2

[23] Barceloux DG, Barceloux DD. *Nickel. Informa* UK Ltd UK; 1999 Aug 6 [cited 2013 Aug 15]; Available from: http://informahealthcare.com/doi/abs/10.1081/CLT-100102423

[24] Alderton WK, Cooper CE, Knowles RG. *Nitric oxide synthases: structure, function and inhibition*. Portland Press Ltd.; 2001 Aug 1 [cited 2013 Aug 15]; Available from: http://www.biochemj.org/bj/357/bj3570593.htm

[25] Stadtman ER. Role of Oxidant Species in Aging. *Current Medicinal Chemistry* [Internet]. Bentham Science Publishers; 2004 May 1 [cited 2013 Aug 15];11(9):1105–12. Available from: http://www.ingentaconnect.com/content/ben/cmc/2004/00000011/ 00000009/art00004?token=005312bd95383a4b3b25702a7b607a6c6a42352046662a726 e2d58464340592f3f3b57b2227e4a42f6b

[26] Thannickal VJ, Fanburg BL. Reactive oxygen species in cell signaling. American journal of physiology. *Lung cellular and molecular physiology* [Internet]. 2000 Dec;279(6):L1005–28. Available from: http://www.ncbi.nlm.nih.gov /pubmed/ 11076791

[27] Poli G, Leonarduzzi G, Biasi F, Chiarpotto E. Oxidative Stress and Cell Signalling. *Current Medicinal Chemistry* [Internet]. Bentham Science Publishers; 2004 May 1 [cited 2013 Aug 15];11(9):1163–82. Available from: http://www.ingentaconnect.com/ content/ben/cmc/2004/00000011/00000009/art00008?token=005619f9ddfa9f9b941333 c4a2f7a3f6a43573a675d3e5534734f6d62222c227e3725303329764bb4c568c

[28] Timms BG, Hofkamp LE. Prostate development and growth in benign prostatic hyperplasia. *Differentation* [Internet]. 2011 [cited 2013 Aug 14];82(4-5):173–83. Available from: http://www.ncbi.nlm.nih.gov/pubmed/21939815

[29] Davidsson S, Fiorentino M, Andrén O, Fang F, Mucci L a, Varenhorst E, et al. Inflammation, focal atrophic lesions, and prostatic intraepithelial neoplasia with respect to risk of lethal prostate cancer. *Cancer epidemiology, biomarkers & prevention: a publication of the American Association for Cancer Research, cosponsored by the American Society of Preventive Oncology* [Internet]. 2011 Oct [cited 2013 Aug 14];20(10):2280–7. Available from: http://www.pubmedcentral.nih.gov/ articlerender .fcgi?artid=3671592&tool=pmcentrez&rendertype=abstract

[30] Bostwick DG, Alexander EE, Singh R, Shan A, Qian J, Santella RM, et al. Antioxidant enzyme expression and reactive oxygen species damage in prostatic intraepithelial

neoplasia and cancer. *Cancer* [Internet]. 2000 Jul 1;89(1):123–34. Available from: http://www.ncbi.nlm.nih.gov/pubmed/10897009

[31] Kumar B, Koul S, Khandrika L, Meacham RB, Koul HK. Oxidative stress is inherent in prostate cancer cells and is required for aggressive phenotype. *Cancer research* [Internet]. 2008 Mar 15 [cited 2013 May 23];68(6):1777–85. Available from: http://www.ncbi.nlm.nih.gov/pubmed/18339858

[32] Clark RA. Activation of the neutrophil respiratory burst oxidase. *The Journal of infectious diseases* [Internet]. 1999 Mar [cited 2013 Aug 15];179 Suppl S309–17. Available from: http://www.ncbi.nlm.nih.gov/pubmed/10081501

[33] Block K, Ricono JM, Lee D-Y, Bhandari B, Choudhury GG, Abboud HE, et al. Arachidonic acid-dependent activation of a p22(phox)-based NAD(P)H oxidase mediates angiotensin II-induced mesangial cell protein synthesis and fibronectin expression via Akt/PKB. *Antioxidants & redox signaling* [Internet]. Mary Ann Liebert, Inc. 2 Madison Avenue Larchmont, NY 10538 USA; 2006 Jan 20 [cited 2013 Aug 15];8(9-10):1497–508. Available from: http://online.liebertpub.com/doi/abs/ 10.1089 /ars.2006.8.1497

[34] Khandrika L, Kumar B, Koul S, Maroni P, Koul HK. Oxidative stress in prostate cancer. *Cancer letters* [Internet]. 2009 Sep 18 [cited 2013 Jun 28];282(2):125–36. Available from: http://www.pubmedcentral.nih.gov/articlerender.fcgi?artid= 2789743 &tool=pmcentrez&rendertype=abstract

[35] Tam NNC, Gao Y, Leung Y-K, Ho S-M. Androgenic regulation of oxidative stress in the rat prostate: involvement of NAD(P)H oxidases and antioxidant defense machinery during prostatic involution and regrowth. *The American journal of pathology* [Internet]. 2003 Dec [cited 2013 Aug 15];163(6):2513–22. Available from: http://www. pubmedcentral.nih.gov/articlerender.fcgi?artid=1892368&tool=pmcentrez&rendertype =abstract

[36] Freitas M, Baldeiras I, Proença T, Alves V, Mota-Pinto A, Sarmento-Ribeiro A. Oxidative stress adaptation in aggressive prostate cancer may be counteracted by the reduction of glutathione reductase. *FEBS open bio* [Internet]. 2012 Jan [cited 2013 Jul 22];2:119–28. Available from: http://dx.doi.org/10.1016/j.fob.2012.05.001

[37] Zhou Q, Liu L-Z, Fu B, Hu X, Shi X, Fang J, et al. Reactive oxygen species regulate insulin-induced VEGF and HIF-1alpha expression through the activation of p70S6K1 in human prostate cancer cells. *Carcinogenesis* [Internet]. 2007 Jan [cited 2013 Aug 14];28(1):28–37. Available from: http://www.ncbi.nlm.nih.gov/pubmed/16774940

[38] Galanis A, Pappa A, Giannakakis A, Lanitis E, Dangaj D, Sandaltzopoulos R. Reactive oxygen species and HIF-1 signalling in cancer. *Cancer letters* [Internet]. 2008 Jul 18 [cited 2013 Aug 13];266(1):12–20. Available from: http://www.ncbi.nlm.nih.gov/ pubmed/18378391

[39] Davis JN, Day ML. The convergence of hormone regulation and cell cycle in prostate physiology and prostate tumorigenesis. *Molecular biotechnology* [Internet]. 2002 Oct [cited 2013 Aug 15];22(2):129–38. Available from: http://www.ncbi.nlm.nih.gov/ pubmed/12405261

[40] Pompella A, Corti A, Paolicchi A, Giommarelli C, Zunino F. Gamma-glutamyltransferase, redox regulation and cancer drug resistance. *Current opinion in pharmacology* [Internet]. 2007 Aug [cited 2013 Aug 14];7(4):360–6. Available from: http://www.ncbi.nlm.nih.gov/pubmed/17613273

[41] Ripple M, Wilding G. Pro-oxidant-antioxidant shift induced by androgen treatment of human prostate carcinoma cells. *Journal of the National Cancer Institute* [Internet]. 1997 [cited 2013 Aug 14];89(1). Available from: http://jnci.oxfordjournals.org/ content/89/1/40.short

[42] Staal F. Intracellular Thiols Regulate Activation of Nuclear Factor B and Transcription of Human Immunodeficiency Virus. *Proceedings of the National Academy of Sciences* [Internet]. 1990 Dec 15 [cited 2013 Aug 15];87(24):9943–7. Available from: http://www.pnas.org/content/87/24/9943.abstract?ijkey=c4f17009e211c1e0076d1baa4e c217465ed20888&keytype2=tf_ipsecsha

[43] Bergelson S, Pinkus R, Daniel V. Intracellular Glutathione Levels Regulate Fos/Jun Induction and Activation of Glutathione S-Transferase Gene Expression. *Cancer Res.* [Internet]. 1994 Jan 1 [cited 2013 Aug 15];54(1):36–40. Available from: http:// cancerres.aacrjournals.org/content/54/1/36.abstract?ijkey=5ea9f8ce8a450c5c30b257d2 d465ea1ce4f81ebc&keytype2=tf_ipsecsha

[44] Saraon P, Jarvi K, Diamandis EP. Molecular alterations during progression of prostate cancer to androgen independence. *Clinical chemistry* [Internet]. 2011 Oct [cited 2013 Aug 14];57(10):1366–75. Available from: http://www.ncbi.nlm.nih.gov/ pubmed /21956922

[45] Debes JD, Tindall DJ. Mechanisms of androgen-refractory prostate cancer. *The New England journal of medicine* [Internet]. 2004 Oct 7;351(15):1488–90. Available from: http://www.ncbi.nlm.nih.gov/pubmed/15470210

[46] Chetram M a, Don-Salu-Hewage AS, Hinton C V. ROS enhances CXCR4-mediated functions through inactivation of PTEN in prostate cancer cells. *Biochemical and biophysical research communications* [Internet]. 2011 Jul 1 [cited 2013 Aug 14];410(2):195–200. Available from: http://www.pubmedcentral.nih.gov/ articlerender .fcgi?artid=3163383&tool=pmcentrez&rendertype=abstract

[47] Dong J-T. *Prevalent mutations in prostate cancer. Journal of cellular biochemistry* [Internet]. 2006 Feb 15 [cited 2013 Jun 6];97(3):433–47. Available from: http://www.ncbi.nlm.nih.gov/pubmed/16267836

[48] Camp NJ, Tavtigian S V. Meta-analysis of associations of the Ser217Leu and Ala541Thr variants in ELAC2 (HPC2) and prostate cancer. *American journal of human genetics* [Internet]. 2002 Dec [cited 2013 Jun 30];71(6):1475–8. Available from: http://www.pubmedcentral.nih.gov/articlerender.fcgi?artid=378598&tool=pmcentrez&r endertype=abstract

[49] Ewing CM, Ray AM, Lange EM, Zuhlke KA, Robbins CM, Tembe WD, et al. Germline Mutations in HOXB13 and Prostate-Cancer Risk. *The New England Journal of Medicine.* 2012;141–9.

[50] Schalken J a, van Leenders G. Cellular and molecular biology of the prostate: stem cell biology. *Urology* [Internet]. 2003 Nov [cited 2013 Jun 26];62(5):11–20. Available from: http://linkinghub.elsevier.com/retrieve/pii/S0090429503007581

[51] Karayi MK, Markham a F. Molecular biology of prostate cancer. *Prostate cancer and prostatic diseases* [Internet]. 2004 Jan [cited 2013 May 30];7(1):6–20. Available from: http://www.ncbi.nlm.nih.gov/pubmed/14999233

[52] Bos JL. *ras Oncogenes in Human Cancer: A Review. Cancer Res.* [Internet]. 1989 Sep 1 [cited 2013 Jun 30];49(17):4682–9. Available from: http://cancerres. Aacrjournals .org/content/49/17/4682.abstract

[53] Vita M, Henriksson M. The Myc oncoprotein as a therapeutic target for human cancer. *Seminars in cancer biology* [Internet]. 2006 Aug [cited 2013 Jun 12];16(4):318–30. Available from: http://dx.doi.org/10.1016/j.semcancer.2006.07.015

[54] Sato H, Minei S, Hachiya T, Yoshida T, Takimoto Y. Fluorescence in situ hybridization analysis of c-myc amplification in stage TNM prostate cancer in Japanese patients. *International journal of urology: official journal of the Japanese Urological Association* [Internet]. 2006 Jun [cited 2013 Jun 30];13(6):761–6. Available from: http://www.ncbi.nlm.nih.gov/pubmed/16834657

[55] Hawksworth D, Ravindranath L, Chen Y, Furusato B, Sesterhenn I a, McLeod DG, et al. Overexpression of C-MYC oncogene in prostate cancer predicts biochemical recurrence. *Prostate cancer and prostatic diseases* [Internet]. 2010 Dec [cited 2013 Jun 30];13(4):311–5. Available from: http://www.ncbi.nlm.nih.gov/pubmed/20820186

[56] Jorda M, Morales A, Ghorab Z, Fernandez G, Nadji M, Block N. Her2 expression in prostatic cancer: a comparison with mammary carcinoma. *The Journal of urology* [Internet]. 2002 Oct [cited 2013 Jul 1];168(4 Pt 1):1412–4. Available from: http://www.ncbi.nlm.nih.gov/pubmed/12352406

[57] Di Lorenzo G, Autorino R, De Laurentiis M, Cindolo L, D'Armiento M, Bianco AR, et al. HER-2/neu receptor in prostate cancer development and progression to androgen independence. *Tumori* [Internet]. 2004 [cited 2013 Jul 1];90(2):163–70. Available from: http://www.ncbi.nlm.nih.gov/pubmed/15237576

[58] Shi Y, Brands FH, Chatterjee S, Feng AC, Groshen S, Schewe J, et al. Her-2/neu expression in prostate cancer: high level of expression associated with exposure to hormone therapy and androgen independent disease. *The Journal of urology* [Internet]. 2001 Oct [cited 2013 Jul 1];166(4):1514–9. Available from: http://www.ncbi.nlm.nih.gov/pubmed/11547123

[59] Roovers K, Assoian RK. Integrating the MAP kinase signal into the G1 phase cell cycle machinery. *BioEssays: news and reviews in molecular, cellular and developmental biology* [Internet]. 2000 Sep [cited 2013 Jun 10];22(9):818–26. Available from: http://www.ncbi.nlm.nih.gov/pubmed/10944584

[60] Keller ET, Fu Z, Yeung K, Brennan M. Raf kinase inhibitor protein: a prostate cancer metastasis suppressor gene. *Cancer letters* [Internet]. 2004 Apr 30 [cited 2013 Jul 1];207(2):131–7. Available from: http://www.ncbi.nlm.nih.gov/pubmed/15151133

[61] Palanisamy N, Ateeq B, Kalyana-Sundaram S, Pflueger D, Ramnarayanan K, Shankar S, et al. Rearrangements of the RAF kinase pathway in prostate cancer, gastric cancer and melanoma. *Nature medicine* [Internet]. Nature Publishing Group; 2010 Jul [cited 2013 Jun 9];16(7):793–8. Available from: http://dx.doi.org/10.1038/nm.2166

[62] Varambally S, Dhanasekaran SM, Zhou M, Barrette TR, Kumar-Sinha C, Sanda MG, et al. The polycomb group protein EZH2 is involved in progression of prostate cancer. *Nature* [Internet]. 2002 Oct 10 [cited 2013 May 29];419(6907):624–9. Available from: http://www.ncbi.nlm.nih.gov/pubmed/12374981

[63] Yang YA, Yu J. EZH2, an epigenetic driver of prostate cancer. *Protein & cell* [Internet]. 2013 May [cited 2013 May 21];4(5):331–41. Available from: http://www.ncbi.nlm.nih.gov/pubmed/23636686

[64] Macleod KF. The RB tumor suppressor: a gatekeeper to hormone independence in prostate cancer? *The Journal of clinical investigation* [Internet]. 2010 Dec [cited 2013

Jul 1]; 120(12):4179–82. Available from: http://www.pubmedcentral.nih.gov/articlerender.fcgi?artid=2993607&tool=pmcentrez&rendertype=abstract

[65] Sharma A, Yeow W-S, Ertel A, Coleman I, Clegg N, Thangavel C, et al. The retinoblastoma tumor suppressor controls androgen signaling and human prostate cancer progression. *The Journal of clinical investigation* [Internet]. American Society for Clinical Investigation; 2010 Dec 1 [cited 2013 Jul 1];120(12):4478–92. Available from: http://www.jci.org/articles/view/44239

[66] Isaacs WB, Carter BS, Ewing CM. Wild-Type p53 Suppresses Growth of Human Prostate Cancer Cells Containing Mutant p53 Alleles. *Cancer Res.* [Internet]. 1991 Sep 1 [cited 2013 Jul 1];51(17):4716–20. Available from: http://cancerres.aacrjournals.org/content/51/17/4716.short

[67] Dean JL, Knudsen KE. The role of tumor suppressor dysregulation in prostate cancer progression. *Current drug targets* [Internet]. 2013 Apr [cited 2013 Jul 1];14(4):460–71. Available from: http://www.ncbi.nlm.nih.gov/pubmed/23410128

[68] Nakayama M, Gonzalgo ML, Yegnasubramanian S, Lin X, De Marzo AM, Nelson WG. GSTP1 CpG island hypermethylation as a molecular biomarker for prostate cancer. *Journal of cellular biochemistry* [Internet]. 2004 Feb 15 [cited 2013 May 22];91(3):540–52. Available from: http://www.ncbi.nlm.nih.gov/pubmed/14755684

[69] Re A, Aiello A, Nanni S, Grasselli A, Benvenuti V, Pantisano V, et al. Silencing of GSTP1, a prostate cancer prognostic gene, by the estrogen receptor-β and endothelial nitric oxide synthase complex. *Molecular endocrinology* (Baltimore, Md.) [Internet]. 2011 Dec [cited 2013 Jul 1];25(12):2003–16. Available from: http://www.pubmedcentral.nih.gov/articlerender.fcgi?artid=3231834&tool=pmcentrez&rendertype=abstract

[70] Petros JA, Baumann AK, Ruiz-pesini E, Amin MB, Sun CQ, Hall J, et al. mtDNA mutations increase tumorigenicity in prostate cancer. *Proceedings of the National Academy of Sciences of the United States of America.* 2014;102(3).

[71] Murphy MP. How mitochondria produce reactive oxygen species. *The Biochemical journal* [Internet]. 2009 Jan 1 [cited 2013 May 22];417(1):1–13. Available from: http://www.pubmedcentral.nih.gov/articlerender.fcgi?artid=2605959&tool=pmcentrez&rendertype=abstract

[72] Brandon M, Baldi P, Wallace DC. Mitochondrial mutations in cancer. *Oncogene* [Internet]. 2006 Aug 7 [cited 2013 May 24];25(34):4647–62. Available from: http://dx.doi.org/10.1038/sj.onc.1209607

[73] Chen JZ, Gokden N, Greene GF, Green B, Kadlubar FF. Simultaneous generation of multiple mitochondrial DNA mutations in human prostate tumors suggests mitochondrial hyper-mutagenesis. *Carcinogenesis* [Internet]. 2003 Sep 1 [cited 2013 Jun 28];24(9):1481–7. Available from: http://carcin.oxfordjournals.org/ content/24/9/1481

[74] Hamilton C, Aidukaitis L, Liu PG, Robison RA, O'Neill KL. *Dietary Antioxidants in Prostate Cancer.* 2012.

[75] Seeni A, Takahashi S, Takeshita K, Tang M, Sugiura S, Sato S, et al. Suppression of prostate cancer growth by resveratrol in the transgenic rat for adenocarcinoma of prostate (TRAP) model. *Asian Pacific journal of cancer prevention: APJCP* [Internet]. 2008;9(1):7–14. Available from: http://www.ncbi.nlm.nih.gov/pubmed/18439064

[76] Pantuck AJ, Leppert JT, Zomorodian N, Aronson W, Hong J, Barnard RJ, et al. Phase II study of pomegranate juice for men with rising prostate-specific antigen following surgery or radiation for prostate cancer. *Clinical cancer research: an official journal of the American Association for Cancer Research* [Internet]. 2006 Jul 1 [cited 2013 Aug 14];12(13):4018–26. Available from: http://www.ncbi.nlm.nih.gov/pubmed/16818701

[77] Giles GG. Prostate Cancer [Internet]. *International Encyclopedia of Public Health. Elsevier;* 2008 [cited 2013 Aug 8]. p. 323–31. Available from: http://dx.doi.org/10.1016/B978-012373960-5.00260-4

[78] Stamey TA, Yang N, Hay AR, McNeal JE, Freiha FS, Redwine E. Prostate-specific antigen as a serum marker for adenocarcinoma of the prostate. *The New England journal of medicine* [Internet]. 1987 Oct 8 [cited 2013 Aug 8];317(15):909–16. Available from: http://www.ncbi.nlm.nih.gov/pubmed/2442609

[79] Helfand BT, Loeb S, Hu Q, Cooper PR, Roehl KA, McGuire BB, et al. Personalized prostate specific antigen testing using genetic variants may reduce unnecessary prostate biopsies. *The Journal of urology* [Internet]. 2013 May [cited 2013 Aug 1];189(5):1697–701. Available from: http://dx.doi.org/10.1016/j.juro.2012.12.023

[80] Moyer VA. Screening for prostate cancer: U.S. Preventive Services Task Force recommendation statement. Annals of internal medicine [Internet]. *American College of Physicians;* 2012 Jul 17 [cited 2013 Aug 9];157(2):120–34. Available from: http://annals.org/article.aspx?articleid=1216568

[81] Tourville EA, Nguyen MM. Prostate Cancer Detection by Using Digital Rectal Examination: Contemporary Practice Patterns in the United States. *Clinical genitourinary cancer* [Internet]. 2013 May 3 [cited 2013 Aug 9];11(3). Available from: http://dx.doi.org/10.1016/j.clgc.2013.04.013

In: Free Radicals
Editor: Bill Stone
ISBN: 978-1-63117-177-2

Chapter IX

Registering Superoxide Production in Live Neuronal Cultures by EPR

***Matthew E. Pamenter*[1,2] *and Sameh S. Ali*[*3,4]**
[1]Department of Zoology, University of British Columbia, Vancouver, BC, Canada
[2]School of Medicine (Division of Physiology), University of California San Diego, La Jolla, CA, US
[3]Center for Aging and Associated Diseases, Helmy Institute of of Medical Sciences, Zewail City of Science and Technology, Giza, Egypt
[4]School of Medicine (Division of Geriatrics), University of California San Diego, La Jolla, CA, US

Abstract

Reactive oxygen species (ROS) are common cellular and intracellular messengers that can also act deleteriously to exacerbate a wide variety of pathophysiologies. In particular, deleterious ROS generation can directly damage proteins and DNA, among other cellular targets, and improper ROS generation has been implicated as a key signal in ischemia-related pathologies, aging, and cancer. Therefore, the accurate determination of ROS generation is necessary to elucidate the etiology of a wide variety of cellular interactions and stress responses. Until recently, such examinations have relied upon fluorescent probes to measure ROS generation. Unfortunately, such fluorescent probes typically provide poor spatial and temporal resolution of ROS production due to the extremely rapid decay of unstable reactive species. Moreover, optical methods are non-specific and the identification of the radical species is usually not possible. Recent advances have paired spin-trap reagents with electron paramagnetic resonance (EPR) to yield a technique that effectively prolongs the dwell-time of ROS and permits extremely rapid and fine-scale measurements of ROS generation; however, these techniques have primarily been utilized to measure ROS from cells or mitochondria in suspension. In this chapter, we describe a method that permits the measurement of ROS production from

[*] Corresponding author Email: ssali@ucsd.edu

cultured cells, including synaptically connected nerve cells, and compare this approach to other industry standard ROS measurement techniques. This approach permits highly accurate measurements of ROS production from cells in a more physiologically relevant preparation as well as exploration of the intracellular signaling capabilities of ROS. As a proof of principle of this approach, we present data examining the effects of ischemia on neuronal ROS production and demonstrate how this method can be employed to determine the cellular source of ROS generation and the specific species of ROS produced. EPR has become the "gold standard" of ROS measurements and our methodology extends the applicability of this technique to a wider range of experimental preparations and research questions.

Keywords: reactive oxygen species; spin-trap; mitochondria, cell culture

Abbreviations

ACSF	–	artificial cerebral spinal fluid
CrOx	–	chromium oxalate
DIPPMPO	-	5-(diisopropoxyphosphoryl)-5-methyl-1-pyrroline-N-oxide
EPR	–	electron paramagnetic resonance
H_2O_2	–	hydrogen peroxide
IS	–	ischemic solution
MAPK	-	mitogen activated protein kinase
Nox	–	NAPDH oxidase
$O_2^{\bullet-}$	-	superoxide
ROS	–	reactive oxygen species
SOD	–	superoxide dismutase

Introduction

Reactive oxygen species (ROS), such as hydrogen peroxide (H_2O_2) and superoxide ($O_2^{\bullet-}$), are chemically reactive molecules that are formed as a byproduct of the cellular catabolism of oxygen. Physiologically, ROS are primarily produced during mitochondrial respiration. Due to the high sensitivity of this process to O_2 levels, ROS are excellent candidates to regulate cellular responses to changes in systemic or tissue-level oxygen availability. Indeed, ROS are important second messengers that regulate a myriad of intra- and extracellular signaling pathways [1]. For example, ROS are able to function as signaling molecules by modifying target proteins via the oxidation of reactive -thiol groups. This process results in the formation of disulfide bonds, which reversibly alter protein structure and thus function [2]. Examples of such target proteins include phosphatases that modify signal transduction pathways (e.g., mitogen-activated protein kinases (MAPKs), proteins that regulate embryogenesis, nuclear transcription factors, RNA-binding proteins that effect DNA methylation, and also proteins involved in processes related to histone acetylation, deacetylation, or methylation (i.e., epigenetic modifications), among many others [3-7]. ROS are also central to immune system host-defense responses and also play a key role in wound repair (e.g., platelet attraction to wound sites, scar formation, etc.) [8, 9].

In addition to such roles as potent biomessengers, ROS also frequently act deleteriously on cells or organelles during periods of environmental or metabolic stress, communicating cellular distress or inducing damage directly. For example, in mammalian stroke pathology, ROS production from neurons peaks during the reperfusion phase. This spike in ROS production leads to local DNA damage and also deleteriously activates cell death pathways in surrounding tissue (the penumbra) [1, 10, 11]. Furthermore, ROS generated following ischemic stroke contribute to the breakdown of the blood brain barrier, inducing edema and facilitating penumbral spread following stroke [12]. Therefore, ROS generation during ischemia plays an important role in the initiation of cell death pathways and the spread of cell death via myriad cellular and intercellular interactions. Furthermore, ROS are also involved in intercellular signaling and the spread of cancerous tumor cells [13, 14]; and are thought to contribute to the biology of aging by damaging DNA, RNA, and proteins [15], which contributes to senescence at the cellular level and loss of memory at the functional level [16], among other deleterious side effects. Historically it has been suggested that the primary form of ROS generated in cells is mitochondria-derived $O_2^{\bullet -}$ [17], which is converted to H_2O_2 by superoxide dismutase (SOD) in the cytosol [18]. In addition, plasma membrane-bound proteins, such as the NADPH oxidase (Nox), are another important source of free radical generation. Nox are a principle enzyme for cellular $O_2^{\bullet -}$ generation and are critical to intracellular signals that induce cell death during ischemic stress [12, 19, 20]. Given the myriad of positive and deleterious signaling and direct effects of ROS generation and transmission throughout biology, accurate measurement of the quantity, cellular source, and free radical form of ROS generated in response to a wide variety of stressors and signals, and in numerous cell types, is of pressing scientific and clinical interest. Unfortunately, the accurate measurement of ROS production in living cells has historically proven to be a difficult undertaking due to the extremely rapid degradation, transformation, and transmission of ROS within and between cells. Indeed, by definition ROS are inherently unstable molecules that are rapidly produced, easily transmitted between cellular compartments and cells themselves, and rapidly converted to more stable forms due to interactions with scavengers (e.g., SOD), other free radicals, or cellular components such as proteins. Previously, researchers have relied upon fluorescent probes to evaluate ROS production; however, such indicators are notoriously blunt tools that are incapable of detecting fine-scale and rapid changes of ROS production, and that cannot differentiate between ROS produced in various cellular compartments. Electron paramagnetic resonance (EPR) spectroscopy is a technique that overcomes these limitations and represents the present "gold standard" of ROS detection technology. The EPR technique utilizes spin-trapping reagents (i.e., spin-probes), which are organic molecules that form more stable secondary free radical adducts when reacting with a specific radical species. The resulting changes to the EPR spectra provide information about the quantity and identity of the reactive oxygen species bound to the specific probe. In this fashion, the rapid decay of unpaired electrons on ROS is coupled to the reagent, which preserves the signal long enough for its detection and examination, allowing extremely rapid, real-time measurement of species-specific ROS production in living cells. Previously, EPR has been employed to examine ROS production from suspensions of disconnected cells and organelles; however, we have developed a technique that enables us to examine ROS production from adherent cells that have maintained there normal cellular connections in culture, which is a considerably more physiologically relevant preparation. In this chapter, we describe a method for the detection, quantification, and identification of real-time ROS production from live cell cultures. To demonstrate the utility of this approach we also examine the effect of ischemic stress on the generation of ROS from cultured murine hippocampal neurons and determine the source and species of ROS generated. This technique is suitable for the investigation of a wide variety of biological questions and pathophysiological processes in numerous cell types.

Experimental Protocol

1. Preparation of Culture Media and Cell Cultures

1.1) Make 500 ml of complete cell culture media (normal growth media) and filter sterilize. The composition of this media will vary depending on the cell type chosen for investigation by the individual researcher. For HT22 hippocampal neuronal cell line, utilize media supplemented with 10% bovine calf serum and 100 U/ml penicillin/streptomycin. Sterile-filtered media may be stored at 4 °C for several weeks.

1.2) Equilibrate approximately 50 ml of media in a cell culture incubator in vented-top sealed cell culture flasks overnight. This will allow the media to reach the temperature and pH of the incubator settings (typically 37 °C and 5% CO_2) without compromising the sterility of the solution.

1.3) Thaw an aliquot of frozen cell suspension by rapidly rubbing the cryovial between hands. Suspend the contents of the cryovial in an appropriate volume of pre-warmed culture media equilibrated in the incubator overnight (approximately 5, 10, or 20 ml of media for 25, 75, or 150 cm^2 flasks, respectively) and add this suspension to the appropriate cell culture flask. Place the flask in the incubator and allow cells to adhere and divide.

1.4) Feed cells 2-3 times per week and split cells when they reach approximately 70-80% confluence (feeding rate, cell growth, desired confluence, etc. will vary depending on the cell line used. Please refer to the suppliers' instructions for this information).

2. Preparation of Coverslips

2.1) Prepare 50 μg/ml solution of poly-D-lysine by adding 5 mg poly-D-lysine powder (Sigma-Aldrich, St. Louis, MO) to 100 ml of sterile tissue culture grade H_2O and mixing until dissolved by pipetting. Allow mixture to sit for 30 min and then mix again by pipetting. Poly-D-lysine solution can be stored for several days at 2-8 °C or divided into aliquots in sterile tubes and stored long-term at -20 °C (only thaw once).

2.2) Precisely cut plastic coverslips (Thermanox Plastic Coverslips (22x60mm), Fischer Sci., Toronto, CAN) to 4 mm width x 22-25 mm length using straight blade surgical scissors. It is not necessary to utilize sterile techniques at this stage. Coverslips may be handled by their edges using fine forceps. Note: Care should be taken at all times to avoid scratching or scoring the surface of the coverslips.

2.3) Transfer coverslips to Petri dishes or multiwall plates with sufficient bottom surface area to allow coverslips to be arrayed flat on the bottom of the dish without overlapping. Multiple coverslips should be placed in each container to cover the bottom of the dish/well and minimize the quantity of poly-D-lysine used (see next step).

2.4) Add sufficient poly-D-lysine solution to each dish/well to cover the surface of coverslips at a depth of approximately 0.5-1 mm. Coverslips may float up in this solution and can be gently pushed back to the bottom of the dish/well with forceps.

2.5) Incubate dishes containing coverslips at room temperature under UV light (ideally in a laminar flow fume hood) for 1-1.5 hrs.

2.6) Aspirate poly-D-lysine solution from each dish/well and rinse the plate 3x with sterile tissue culture grade H_2O.

2.7) Allow the coverslips to air dry in a laminar flow fume hood with the Petri dish lid off (~ 2 hrs). When dried, transfer coverslips to a clean Petri dish and seed cells (see below). Alternatively, coverslips in a Petri dish may be sealed by wrapping with Parafilm, and stored at 4-8 °C until use (some loss of function of Poly-D-lysine may occur with long-term storage).

3. Seeding Cells onto Coverslips

3.1) On the day before the experiment, carefully place 2-4 sterile poly-D-lysine coated coverslips into each well of standard 6-well plates.

3.2) Detach cells from the growth matrix (use 0.05% trypsin with EDTA for HT22 neurons but the appropriate lysis agent and concentration will vary between cell type).

3.3) Re-suspend cells in ~ 5 volumes of normal growth media in a 15 ml falcon tube (the serum in the media inactivates the trypsin and prevents unwanted cell lysis), and centrifuge this suspension at 125 x g for 5-7 min at room temperature. Aspirate the supernatant.

3.4) Re-suspend the cell pellet in normal growth media diluted to the desired seeding density. The desired seeding density will vary depending on the growth rate and desired confluency of the cells at the time of experimentation. Typically, it is ideal to seed cells at a density such that following 24 hrs (overnight growth) they will be at the desired density for experimentation. It will be necessary to determine this density for each cell type used.

3.5) Add sufficient cell suspension to each well of the 6-well plates to coat the coverslips to a depth of ~ 1 mm (about 2 ml suspension/well). Note: it is important to have an even distribution of cells across the coverslips, and for this reason it is preferable to seed cells in this manner as opposed to pipetting smaller volumes directly onto the coverslips.

3.6) As before, coverslips may tend to float to the surface of the cell suspension. Coverslips may be gently pushed back to the bottom of the well using forceps and will stay at the bottom once the electrostatic charge of the fluid meniscus has been broken by the coverslip.

3.7) Replace the lid of the 6-well plates and incubate the cells and coverslips overnight in the normal tissue culture incubator.

3.8) (Optional). 2-16 hrs prior to experimentation, replace normal growth media with serum-free media to halt cell division and phase-lock cells.

4. Treating Cells for Experimentation

4.1) On the day of experimentation, view coverslips in the 6-well plates under a microscope to ensure that cells are evenly distributed across the coverslip, that coverslips are not scratched or scored, and that cells appear healthy.

4.2) To test the effects of various solutions or pharmacological agents on the production of free radicals from their cells, aspirate the media in individual wells of 6-well plates and replace it with an equal volume of the treatment media. Save a small volume (approximately 1-2 ml) of each treatment media for use in EPR recordings (see below).

4.3) Incubate samples on coverslips for the desired experimental period in the various treatment media. Each EPR sample takes approximately 20-30 min to prepare and read following treatment, so stagger experimental treatments appropriately to maintain consistent treatment durations between samples.

4.4) Picking up and moving coverslips is a tricky process and occasionally the forceps may slip and score the cultured cells or the surface of the coverslip. For this reason prepare 2-3 coverslips per well to provide multiple backups for each treatment replicate (a single well of the plate). Plan to use a single coverslip from each well of their dish, as loss or damage of samples during transfer is common!

5. EPR Measurement of Superoxide Production from Living Cells

5.1) Immediately before measurement by EPR, mix 20 μl of the same treatment media used to treat the individual sample to be examined with 20 μl of the spin trap reagent: (diisopropoxyphosphoryl)-5-methyl-1-pyrroline-N-oxide (DIPPMPO, Axxora Life Sci. Inc., Flemingdale, NY) dissolved in phosphate buffered saline (PBS). Pipette this mixture into the ~ 30 mm x 5 mm x 0.5 mm groove in the EPR tissue chamber.

5.2) Carefully grasp the slide from the edges while avoiding any contact with cells using a pair of sharp-edged forceps. Place the coverslip in the EPR cell (GZ 170 tissue cell, Magnettech GmbH, Berlin, GER) so that the neurons are facing the media/spin trap mixture.

5.3) Tightly cover the EPR cell to avoid media leakage and insert the cell into the spectrometer (MiniScope MS300 Benchtop Spectrometer, Magnettech), which maintains temperature at 37°C.

5.4) Record EPR spectra using the following settings: microwave power, 5 mW; modulation amplitude, 2 G; modulation frequency, 100 kHz; sweep width, 150 G centered at 3349.0 G; scan rate, 7.5 G s^{-1}. Each measurement takes approximately 20-25 min to complete, including the time required to insert and remove the coverslips.

6. Data Analysis

6.1) Perform spectral simulations using WinSim software (http://www.niehs.nih.gov /research/resources/software/tox-pharm/tools/index.cfm) and published parameters for the DIPPMPO adducts with various biologically relevant radicals to identify the free radical species from each sample [21].

6.2) Quantify the free radical concentration by calculating the mean of the amplitudes of the four spectral peaks p1-p4 as defined in Figure 5.

Representative Results

The ability of this assay to accurately quantify ROS production to allow for comparison between samples and treatments relies upon the initial use of healthy cells in equal quantities that are evenly distributed across the coverslip and not damaged by transfer to the EPR.

Once multiple samples of healthy cells have been produced and treated, samples are ready for loading into the custom EPR chamber. Figure 1 shows the EPR chamber designed to hold the custom-cut coverslips and attached cells with sufficient volume to include enough treatment media to cover the cells and prevent dehydration. The EPR chamber is sealed with the glass cover (also shown) to prevent media leakage or disturbance of the cells and the chamber is then inserted into the bench top EPR spectrophotometer for experimentation.

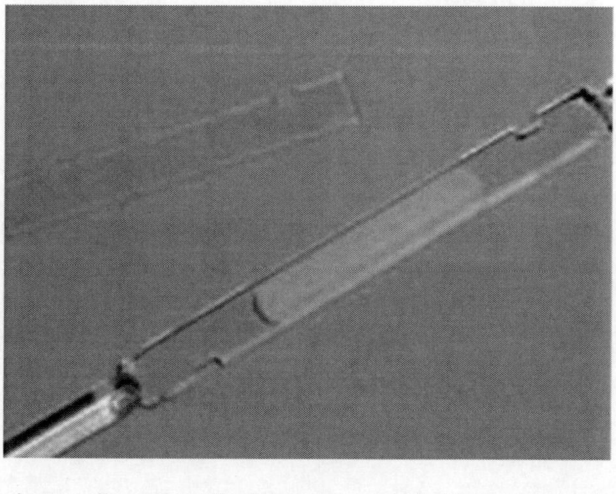

Figure 1. The GZ 170 tissue cell consists of a flat part (sample holder) with the dimensions 65 x 7 x 2 mm having two holders in axial direction (bottom length of holder 20 mm, upper length 85 mm). The flat part has a milled deepening (length 30 mm, width 5 mm, depth 0.5 mm) which serves to hold the sample. The cell includes one cover slide and two clamps for fixing the cover slide.

The research questions explored with this technique will vary between laboratories. For our representative experiments, we are interested in the effect of an *in vitro* mimic of the ischemic penumbra on ROS generation from hippocampal neurons [22-25]. Prior to EPR analysis, neurons were treated with either artificial cerebral spinal fluid (ACSF), or our novel ischemic solution (IS) for 2 hrs. Samples were loaded into the EPR chamber along with the spin-trap reagent mixed in the respective treatment medias (ACSF or IS), and EPR spectra were examined. Figure 2 shows representative traces of EPR spectra from our cells treated in ACSF (control) or IS. In general, we found that ROS generation in IS-challenged neurons increased approximately 75% relative to controls.

To demonstrate the utility of this method, we also asked whether the source of the IS-induced ROS generation was cellular or extracellular. To determine this, we treated samples with chromium oxalate (CrOx, 1.25 μg/μl, which is a cell-impermeable paramagnetic broadening agent that dissipates the resonance signal of any extracellular ROS (by broadening the EPR spectrum) or superoxide dismutase (CuZn-SOD), 100 U/ml, which scavenges extracellular superoxide (CuZn-SOD generates H_2O_2 as a bi-product of superoxide scavenging but the H_2O_2 can be scavenged with the addition of catalase) [26]. Figure 3 demonstrates that in controls, perfusion of either CrOx or SOD each decreased ROS generation ~ 35%.

These results indicate that at rest, ROS accumulation due to generation from intracellular versus extracellular sources occurs at a ratio of 2:1. Interestingly, in neurons treated with either CrOx or SOD we observed that the ischemic increase in ROS generation and total ROS generation was entirely abolished relative to controls. These data indicate that the ischemic change in ROS generation is due to extracellular accumulation of ROS. Figure 4 demonstrates the site of action of a variety of pharmacological tools whose usage enables dissection of the source and mode of action of detected ROS.

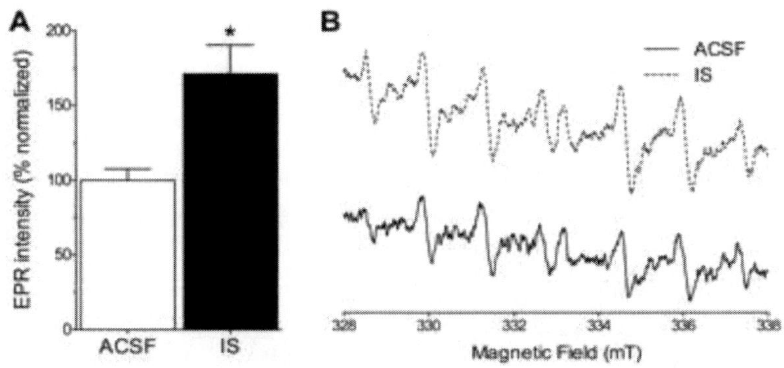

Figure 2. IS increases free superoxide production from neurons. (A) Summary of EPR-revealed changes in superoxide production from neurons treated with ACSF or ischemic solution (IS) for 2-hrs. (B) Raw EPR traces from (A). Data are mean ± SEM normalized to control experiments in ACSF. Asterisks (*) indicate significant difference from control ($p < 0.05$).

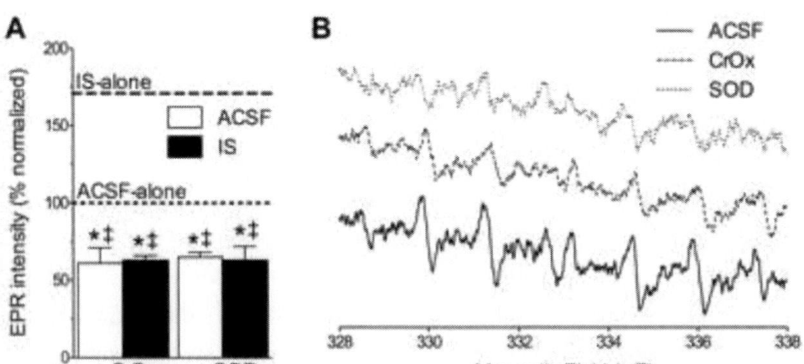

Figure 3. IS-mediated ROS production is extracellular in origin. (A) Summary of EPR-revealed changes in superoxide production from neurons treated with ACSF ± chromium oxalate (CrOx) or superoxide dismutase (SOD) for 2-hrs. (B) Raw EPR traces from (A). Data are mean ± SEM normalized to control experiments in ACSF (see Figure 2). Dashed lines indicate ACSF and IS controls from Figure 2A, respectively. Asterisks (*) indicate significant difference from ACSF control (Figure 2A); double daggers indicate significant difference from IS-alone (Figure 2A; $p < 0.05$).

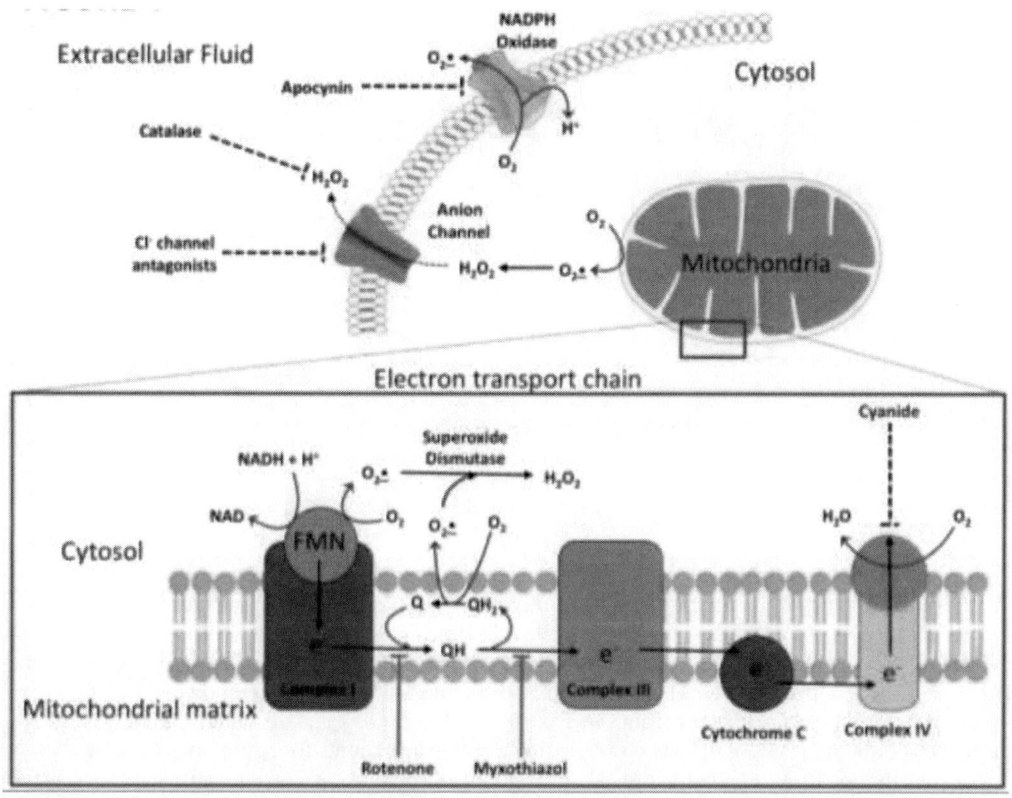

Figure 4. Schematic of cellular sites of ROS production and pharmacological means of manipulation. *ROS production and cycling*: ROS are primarily generated in the mitochondria via the electron transport chain (ETC) in the course of oxidative metabolism. Within the mitochondrial ETC, ROS are generated when electrons (e^-) are transferred between complexes. Specifically, superoxide ($O_2^{\bullet-}$) can be generated at the complex I flavin mononucleotide (FMN) center and from the ubisemiquinone radical (·QH) produced in the Q-cycle. Mitochondria-derived $O_2^{\bullet-}$ are rapidly converted to hydrogen peroxide (H_2O_2) in the cytosol and $O_2^{\bullet-}$ or H_2O_2 can exit the cell via active anion channels. Superoxide can also be generated directly to the extracellular space by plasma membrane-bound NADPH oxidases. *Pharmacological ROS manipulation*: To determine the specific mitochondrial complexes involved in ROS production electron transfer from complex I to ubiquinone (Q) can be inhibited by rotenone. Myxothiazol inhibits electron transfer from ubiquinol (QH_2) to complex III, and cyanide inhibits complex IV (cytochrome oxidase). Intracellular and extracellular ROS can be scavenged with superoxide dismutase or catalase, respectively (among other scavenging agents). Cytosolic ROS efflux can be inhibited by antagonists of anion channels, and NADPH-derived ROS can be analyzed by antagonizing the NADPH oxidase with apocynin. Pharmacological agents and their sites of action are indicated by red text and lines. Modified from Pamenter et al., 2007 (43).

To determine the species of free radicals produced in our experiments and also to quantify the magnitude of ROS production, we performed computer simulations that indicated that the observed signal was due primarily to spin trapping of $O_2^{\bullet-}$ along with the formation of a negligible concentration of hydroxyl radical.

An example is given in Figure 5, in which we simulated the experimental spectrum by calculating DIPPMPO-OH + DIPPMPO-OOH radical adducts using parameters published previously [21, 27].

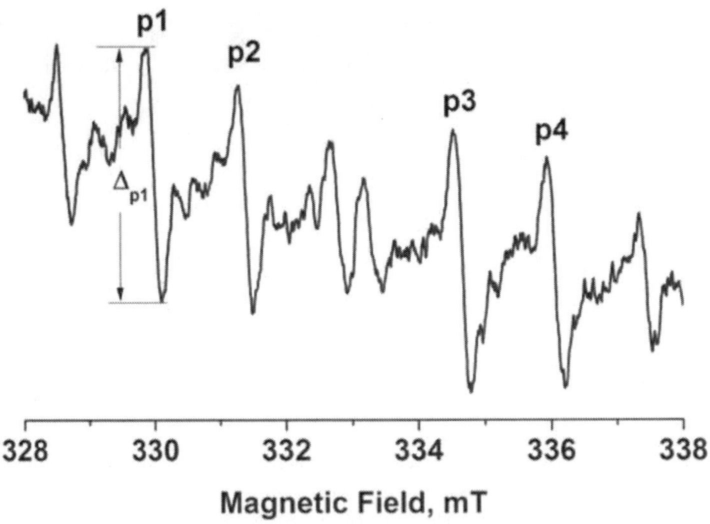

Figure 5. Sample image of EPR spectra analysis. To identify the free radical species we carry out spectral simulations using WinSim software: (http://www.niehs.nih.gov/research/resources/software/tox-pharm/tools/index.cfm) and published parameters for the DIPPMPO adducts with various biologically relevant radicals (21). Here we have simulated the experimental spectrum by calculating DIPPMPO-OH + DIPPMPO-OOH radical adducts using parameters published previously. Here, the hydroxyl radical adduct originates from superoxide adduct as SOD quenched both signals effectively. From the simulation result of this spectrum, hydroxyl radical accounts for approximately 94% with minor contribution from superoxide radicals (6%) to the observed signal. To quantify the free radical concentration, we calculate the mean of the amplitudes of the four spectral peaks p1-p4.

Conclusion

In this chapter, we describe a method to precisely measure reactive oxygen species production from cultured cells using the "gold standard" of ROS measurement: electron paramagnetic resonance. Relative to other methods for measuring cellular ROS production, the EPR technique allows for more accurate and fine-scale measurement of ROS generation, as well as spatial, and temporal determination of the free radicals produced. Furthermore, this technique permits the simultaneous measurement and differentiation of multiple species of ROS (e.g., $O_2^{\bullet-}$, H_2O_2, $^{\bullet}OH$). Finally, although previous researchers have utilized EPR to measure ROS production from suspensions of cells or organelles (e.g., mitochondria), our approach is the first to describe a method to measure ROS from cell cultures adhered to a level matrix. This approach is a significant improvement over previous EPR techniques in that it allows for ROS measurement from a wider variety of cell types and preparations, and because it permits measurement of ROS production from synaptically connected cells and cellular networks [24, 28].

There are numerous significant advantages provided by the use of EPR spectroscopy relative to the use of fluorescence-based measurement of ROS [29-31]. First, in the preparation of samples, the loading of fluorescent probes requires that samples be incubated in the fluorescent dye for significant periods of time, and also for the dye to be rinsed out with several washes to remove background fluorescence. For cell suspensions, this requires numerous cycles of centrifugation and re-suspension in various media, which can damage cells or induce cellular stress signals such as ROS and may thus confound experimental results. For samples of adherent cells, the use of fluorescent probes is further complicated by the inherent difficulties of adequately washing adherent cells without disrupting their connections to the matrix, and also by the general autofluorescence properties of many types of commonly used coverslips, which can increase the signal to noise ratio of the desired fluorescent signal. Furthermore, fluorescent probes are prone to bleaching when they are exposed to light, and thus the fluorescent baseline is frequently shifted by the very act of measuring the fluorescent signal. Second, in addition to these general complications, which are common to the use of fluorescent probes, indicators designed to detect changes in ROS are notoriously poor in quality and often require the occurrence of large changes in ROS to induce a measureable change in fluorescence [29-31]. Third, due to the rapid generation, transmission, and transmutation of ROS within and between cells, fluorescent probes generally do not respond rapidly enough to detect temporally distinct changes in ROS generation, and are better suited for measuring bulk changes in free radicals between treatments [30]. Fourth, ROS are rapidly interconverted to different free radical forms in the cell and therefore the slow temporal response and non-specific measurement of ROS with fluorescent dyes is not suitable for the determination of the spatial resolution of ROS production between mitochondrial or other cellular sources, nor for the determination of the exact species of free radical generated (e.g., $O_2^{\cdot-}$, H_2O_2,$^{\cdot}OH$, etc) [2, 29-31]. Indeed, the EPR technique permits the simultaneous detection of all forms of free radicals produced from a population of cells, whereas fluorescent dyes detect only one from of free radical (e.g., ROS or reactive nitrogen species). Thus EPR provides a more complete picture of the redox state of a population of cells; and therefore overall, the EPR technique is a significant improvement over fluorescent indicators of ROS generation due to reduced sample preparation requirements, improved signal to noise ratios, and far more precise spatial and temporal resolution of ROS measurements.

Previously, the use of EPR approaches has largely been confined to the measurement of ROS production from cell or organelle suspensions contained in a capillary tube [32-35]. One of the primary advantages of the technique described in this chapter is the use of a custom-designed EPR "cell" in which cells grown on coverslips can be recorded from without detaching adherent cells or disrupting cellular connections and networks. This permits the measurement of ROS from cells in a far more physiologically relevant situation [24]. Furthermore, many cell lines and types of cells are naturally adherent and begin to attach to available surfaces or to clump together shortly after being suspended in solution. Measurements from such cells in capillary tubes is therefore difficult as they tend to clump up within the 15-20 min required for measurement with the EPR, and a uniform suspension of cells is critical to accurate EPR measurements in such a configuration. Therefore, our approach is suitable for the measurement of ROS from a wider variety of cell types and cell lines than previous EPR techniques, and when combined with the use of Poly-D-lysine or other matrix substrates, permits similar measurements from poorly adherent cells as well.

Beyond the practical and technical advantages offered by our methodology, a key advantage of our overall technique is that it can be combined with pharmacological approaches to determine the site of production of ROS and also of the transmission of ROS within and between cells [24, 36-38]. In this chapter we demonstrate this utility by scavenging extracellular $O_2^{\cdot-}$ with SOD or by blocking the EPR detection of extracellular ROS with CrOx. Using these approaches, we can then subtract the resulting ROS production from control experiments to determine what percentage of ROS production occurs from extracellular sources relative to intracellular sources, and what species of free radical is produced from each source. Similar approaches can be used to determine the source of ROS generation by blocking commonly studied cellular sites of ROS production such as various components of the mitochondrial electron transport chain or Nox proteins [24, 36]. Indeed, there are many additional pharmacological approaches that could be combined with this technique to further study the source of ROS generation. Different scavengers may be used to target individual species of extracellular ROS. For example, catalase targets H_2O_2, whereas CuZn-SOD targets $O_2^{\bullet-}$. Using such modulators alone or in combination during EPR experiments allows researchers to better determine the species of extracellular ROS generated and also the interactions between forms of extracellular ROS as they are scavenged and transmuted extracellularly. Similarly, since this system is optimized for use in cell lines and primary cell cultures, genetic approaches aimed at over-expressing or knocking out cytosolic or mitochondrial SOD isoforms may be combined with our method to explore the roles of specific intracellular ROS scavenging mechanisms in a given biological response. Genetic approaches are also suitable for exploring the role of specific ROS and NOS generating proteins, such as components of the electron transport chain or membrane-bound Nox. In addition, the extracellular extrusion of cellularly derived ROS can be blocked by anion channel antagonists to determine whether ROS are acting intracellularly or are being extruded to act on neighboring cells [24]. Therefore this technique, in combination with well thought out pharmacological or genetic manipulations, permits researchers to explore almost any facet of ROS production and handling in a variety of cells and across a range of biological questions.

The main limitation of this technique is that it is designed for cell culture systems and is not suitable for use in whole-tissues or whole-animals. Therefore the preparations involved are somewhat less physiologically relevant. In addition, the system as currently designed is not amenable to flow-through experiments, so bulk changes in the perfusate or addition of drugs to the system once measurements have begun are not feasible. As a result, experiments must be done on separate populations of cells and changes must be compared between groups as opposed to within single samples. Lastly, the system utilizes a sealed chamber, which is not amenable to changes in oxygen availability beyond the initial gas saturation of the media at the start of the experiment. Modifications are currently being designed that will permit researchers to manipulate oxygen delivery to the system during an experiment, which will be an important advantage for many research systems, particularly as ROS production is inherently linked to oxygen availability.

In the present chapter, we have demonstrated the utility of this system by examining ischemia-related questions in cultured neurons; however, this system is also well suited to the study of many important questions related to the role of free radicals in tumor formation, cancer biology, and therapeutics targeting various cancers. The interplay of reactive oxygen species in cancer is an area of intensive research and beyond the scope of the present chapter; however, this topic has been expertly reviewed recently and interested researchers may read further in other chapters of this book [see also 39, 40]. Briefly, irregular ROS generation due to environmental factors (such as cigarette smoke, radiation, or hypoxia), aging, hormonal changes, etc., induces oxidative damage to DNA that leads to mutations and tumor formation during normal cell division [40], and antioxidant treatment has been shown to prevent tumor formation [41]. Moreover, antioxidant treatment can increase the dose of chemotherapeutics that patients can withstand by reducing deleterious ROS-related side effects [39]. Conversely, pro-oxidant therapy has also been proposed as a treatment option to increase the susceptibility of tumors to chemical therapeutic treatment [39], and indeed the cytotoxic effects of many chemotherapeutic approaches to cancer treatment currently in use are due to ROS generation [42]. The method of EPR detection described in this chapter offers considerable potential benefit to cancer researchers. For example, our methodology may allow for the determination of specific species of ROS that contribute to increased oxidative stress in cancer cells, or in the screening of potential pro-oxidant chemotherapy agents.

In summary, the EPR method of determining free radical production is currently considered the gold standard measure of ROS generation due to its low signal to noise resolution, high degree of spatial and temporal resolution, and the ability to simultaneously detect multiple forms of free radicals in the same preparation. Secondary pharmacological approaches allow researchers to determine the specific sites of ROS production and action. Our methodology extends the functionality of this technique by permitting the measurement of ROS from a wider variety of cells and from preparations wherein synaptic and network connections are maintained, which is a more representative of the *in vivo* situation. This approach may be extremely useful to a wide variety of redox-related research fields, and in particular to research related to ischemia, hypoxia, or cancer biology and treatment.

Acknowledgments

This work was supported in part by NIA 1K25AG026379 and Zewail City start-up funds to SSA, and a National Sciences and Engineering Research Council of Canada fellowship to MEP.

Disclosures

We have nothing to disclose.

References

[1] Kakkar P, Singh BK. Mitochondria: a hub of redox activities and cellular distress control. *Mol. Cell Biochem.* 2007 Nov;305(1-2):235-53.

[2] Forman HJ. Signal transduction and reactive species. *Free Radic. Biol. Med.* 2009 Nov 1;47(9):1237-8.

[3] Shlomai J. Redox control of protein-DNA interactions: from molecular mechanisms to significance in signal transduction, gene expression, and DNA replication. *Antioxid. Redox. Signal.* 2010 Nov 1;13(9):1429-76.

[4] Winterbourn CC, Hampton MB. Thiol chemistry and specificity in redox signaling. *Free Radic. Biol. Med.* 2008 Sep 1;45(5):549-61.

[5] Kovtun Y, Chiu WL, Tena G, Sheen J. Functional analysis of oxidative stress-activated mitogen-activated protein kinase cascade in plants. *Proc. Natl. Acad. Sci. USA*. 2000 Mar 14;97(6):2940-5.

[6] Ufer C, Wang CC, Borchert A, Heydeck D, Kuhn H. Redox control in mammalian embryo development. *Antioxid. Redox. Signal*. 2010 Sep 15;13(6):833-75.

[7] Sundar IK, Caito S, Yao H, Rahman I. Oxidative stress, thiol redox signaling methods in epigenetics. *Methods Enzymol*. 2010;474:213-44.

[8] Rada B, Leto TL. Oxidative innate immune defenses by Nox/Duox family NADPH oxidases. *Contrib. Microbiol*. 2008;15:164-87.

[9] Vozenin-Brotons MC, Sivan V, Gault N, Renard C, Geffrotin C, Delanian S, et al. Antifibrotic action of Cu/Zn SOD is mediated by TGF-beta1 repression and phenotypic reversion of myofibroblasts. *Free Radic. Biol. Med.* 2001 Jan 1;30(1):30-42.

[10] Flamm ES, Demopoulos HB, Seligman ML, Poser RG, Ransohoff J. Free radicals in cerebral ischemia. *Stroke.* 1978 Sep-Oct;9(5):445-7.

[11] Barzilai A. The contribution of the DNA damage response to neuronal viability. *Antioxid. Redox. Signal*. 2007 Feb;9(2):211-8.

[12] Fraser PA. The role of free radical generation in increasing cerebrovascular permeability. *Free Radic. Biol. Med.* 2011 Jun 12;51(5):967-77.

[13] Gupta SC, Hevia D, Patchva S, Park B, Koh W, Aggarwal BB. Upsides and downsides of reactive oxygen species for cancer: the roles of reactive oxygen species in tumorigenesis, prevention, and therapy. *Antioxid. Redox. Signal*. 2012 Jun 1;16(11):1295-322.

[14] Diaz B, Courtneidge SA. Redox signaling at invasive microdomains in cancer cells. *Free Radic. Biol. Med.* 2012 Jan 15;52(2):247-56.

[15] Stadtman ER. Protein oxidation and aging. *Science*. 1992 Aug 28;257(5074):1220-4.

[16] Liu J, Head E, Gharib AM, Yuan W, Ingersoll RT, Hagen TM, et al. Memory loss in old rats is associated with brain mitochondrial decay and RNA/DNA oxidation: partial reversal by feeding acetyl-L-carnitine and/or R-alpha -lipoic acid. *Proc. Natl. Acad. Sci. USA*. 2002 Feb 19;99(4):2356-61.

[17] Liu Y, Fiskum G, Schubert D. Generation of reactive oxygen species by the mitochondrial electron transport chain. *J. Neurochem*. 2002 Mar;80(5):780-7.

[18] Vanden Hoek TL, Becker LB, Shao Z, Li C, Schumacker PT. Reactive oxygen species released from mitochondria during brief hypoxia induce preconditioning in cardiomyocytes. *J. Biol. Chem*. 1998 Jul 17;273(29):18092-8.

[19] Hong H, Zeng JS, Kreulen DL, Kaufman DI, Chen AF. Atorvastatin protects against cerebral infarction via inhibition of NADPH oxidase-derived superoxide in ischemic stroke. *Am. J. Physiol. Heart Circ. Physiol*. 2006 Nov;291(5):H2210-5.

[20] Kahles T, Luedike P, Endres M, Galla HJ, Steinmetz H, Busse R, et al. NADPH oxidase plays a central role in blood-brain barrier damage in experimental stroke. *Stroke*. 2007 Nov;38(11):3000-6.

[21] Culcasi M, Rockenbauer A, Mercier A, Clement JL, Pietri S. The line asymmetry of electron spin resonance spectra as a tool to determine the cis:trans ratio for spin-trapping adducts of chiral pyrrolines N-oxides: the mechanism of formation of hydroxyl radical adducts of EMPO, DEPMPO, and DIPPMPO in the ischemic-reperfused rat liver. *Free Radic. Biol. Med.* 2006 May 1;40(9):1524-38.

[22] Yao H, Shu Y, Wang J, Brinkman BC, Haddad GG. Factors influencing cell fate in the infarct rim. *J. Neurochem.* 2007 Mar;100(5):1224-33.

[23] Yao H, Sun X, Gu X, Wang J, Haddad GG. Cell death in an ischemic infarct rim model. *J. Neurochem.* 2007 Nov;103(4):1644-53.

[24] Pamenter ME, Ali SS, Tang Q, Finley JC, Gu XQ, Dugan LL, et al. An in vitro ischemic penumbral mimic perfusate increases NADPH oxidase-mediated superoxide production in cultured hippocampal neurons. *Brain Res.* 2012 May 3;1452:165-72.

[25] Pamenter ME, Perkins GA, McGinness AK, Gu XQ, Ellisman MH, Haddad GG. Autophagy and apoptosis are differentially induced in neurons and astrocytes treated with an in vitro mimic of the ischemic penumbra. *PLoS One.* 2012;7(12):e51469.

[26] Han D, Williams E, Cadenas E. Mitochondrial respiratory chain-dependent generation of superoxide anion and its release into the intermembrane space. *Biochem. J.* 2001 Jan 15;353(Pt 2):411-6.

[27] Stolze K, Udilova N, Nohl H. Spin trapping of lipid radicals with DEPMPO-derived spin traps: detection of superoxide, alkyl and alkoxyl radicals in aqueous and lipid phase. *Free Radic. Biol. Med.* 2000 Nov 15;29(10):1005-14.

[28] Ali SS, Young JW, Wallace CK, Gresack J, Jeste DV, Geyer MA, et al. Initial evidence linking synaptic superoxide production with poor short-term memory in aged mice. *Brain Res.* 2011 Jan 12;1368:65-70.

[29] Dikalov SI, Harrison DG. Methods for Detection of Mitochondrial and Cellular Reactive Oxygen Species. *Antioxid. Redox. Signal.* 2012 Oct 19.

[30] Maeda H. Which are you watching, an individual reactive oxygen species or total oxidative stress? *Ann. N. Y. Acad. Sci.* 2008;1130:149-56.

[31] Gomes A, Fernandes E, Lima JL. Fluorescence probes used for detection of reactive oxygen species. *J. Biochem. Biophys. Methods.* 2005 Dec 31;65(2-3):45-80.

[32] Ali SS, Hsiao M, Zhao HW, Dugan LL, Haddad GG, Zhou D. Hypoxia-adaptation involves mitochondrial metabolic depression and decreased ROS leakage. *PLoS One.* 2012;7(5):e36801.

[33] Ali SS, Xiong C, Lucero J, Behrens MM, Dugan LL, Quick KL. Gender differences in free radical homeostasis during aging: shorter-lived female C57BL6 mice have increased oxidative stress. *Aging Cell.* 2006 Dec;5(6):565-74.

[34] Gabbita SP, Butterfield DA, Hensley K, Shaw W, Carney JM. Aging and caloric restriction affect mitochondrial respiration and lipid membrane status: an electron paramagnetic resonance investigation. *Free Radic. Biol. Med.* 1997;23(2):191-201.

[35] Ali SS, Marcondes MC, Bajova H, Dugan LL, Conti B. Metabolic depression and increased reactive oxygen species production by isolated mitochondria at moderately lower temperatures. *J. Biol. Chem.* 2010 Oct 15;285(42):32522-8.

[36] Douglas RM, Ryu J, Kanaan A, Del Carmen Rivero M, Dugan LL, Haddad GG, et al. Neuronal death during combined intermittent hypoxia/hypercapnia is due to mitochondrial dysfunction. *Am. J. Physiol. Cell Physiol.* 2010 Jun;298(6):C1594-602.

[37] Behrens MM, Ali SS, Dugan LL. Interleukin-6 mediates the increase in NADPH-oxidase in the ketamine model of schizophrenia. *J. Neurosci.* 2008 Dec 17;28(51):13957-66.

[38] Ali SS, Hardt JI, Dugan LL. SOD activity of carboxyfullerenes predicts their neuroprotective efficacy: a structure-activity study. *Nanomedicine.* 2008 Dec;4(4):283-94.

[39] Sosa V, Moline T, Somoza R, Paciucci R, Kondoh H, ME LL. Oxidative stress and cancer: an overview. *Ageing Res. Rev*. 2013 Jan;12(1):376-90.

[40] Waris G, Ahsan H. Reactive oxygen species: role in the development of cancer and various chronic conditions. *J. Carcinog*. 2006;5:14.

[41] Kovacic P, Jacintho JD. Mechanisms of carcinogenesis: focus on oxidative stress and electron transfer. *Curr. Med. Chem*. 2001 Jun;8(7):773-96.

[42] Afzal S, Jensen SA, Sorensen JB, Henriksen T, Weimann A, Poulsen HE. Oxidative damage to guanine nucleosides following combination chemotherapy with 5-fluorouracil and oxaliplatin. *Cancer Chemother Pharmacol*. 2012 Feb;69(2):301-7.

[43] Pamenter ME, Richards MD, Buck LT. Anoxia-induced changes in reactive oxygen species and cyclic nucleotides in the painted turtle. *J. Comp. Physiol.* B. 2007 May;177(4):473-81.

In: Free Radicals
Editor: Bill Stone

ISBN: 978-1-63117-177-2

Chapter X

Role of Antioxidants in Cancer Onset and Development

Vanessa Fuchs-Tarlovsky, PhD, MD, RD*[*1] and Jessica Calderon-Cuevas, MD[2]
[1]Oncology Servicie.
Hospital General de Mexico, and American Brithis Cowdray Medical Center, Oncology Center, Mexico City, Mexico
[2]Hospital ABC, Mexico City, Mexico. Universidad Anahuac, School of Medicine, Mexico City, Mexico

Abstract

Under normal circumstances, there is a steady balance between the production of oxygen derived free radicals and destruction by the antioxidant system. If there is any imbalance between the levels of pro-oxidants and antioxidants defenses, there is a chance that DNA damage could ensue leading to cancer development. Oxidative stress results in severe and constant damage to cellular structures and has been linked to many diseases, including cancer.

Reactive oxygen species (ROS) are formed in human cells as a consequence of aerobic respiration. Despite multiple conserved redox modulating systems, a given proportion of ROS continuously escape from the mitochondrial respiratory chain, being sufficiently potent to damage cells in various ways, including numerous carcinogenic DNA mutations. Oxidative stress resulting from an imbalanced ratio between ROS production and detoxification may also disturb physiological signal transduction, leading to chain reactions in lipid layers, and damage to multiple DNA repair enzymes.

Increased levels of free radicals and low levels of antioxidants have been observed in malignant tissue. Moreover, there is evidence supporting the role of ROS or free radicals such as oxygen singlet, superoxide anions, hydrogen peroxide and hydroxyl radical in the etiology of cancer. Certain aldehydes such as malondialdehyde (MDA), the end product of lipid peroxidation arising from free radical degeneration of polyunsaturated fatty acids

* Emal:vanessafuchs@hotmail.com

can cause cross linking in lipids, proteins and nucleic acids leading to cellular damage. We as humans are naturally equipped with antioxidant defenses enzymes such as superoxide dismutase (SOD) and catalase (CAT), which can protect against cellular and molecular damage.

The association of decreased cancer risk with sufficient intake of cruciferous vegetables that contain selenium, and some antioxidant vitamins is stronger than that reported for fruits and vegetables, because an active constituent in cruciferous is sulforaphane, which induces (via activation of the Nrf2/Keap1 system) phase 2 enzymes that protect against carcinogens and oxidants. Other nutrients, like vitamin C (ascorbic acid) are thought to have antioxidant functions in living systems. In this chapter we will overview some of the situations that leads to the imbalance that generates mutations causing cancer development.

Abbreviations

(5hmC)	5-hydroxymethylcytosine
(AIDS)	Acquired immunodeficiency síndrome
(BHT)	Butylated hydroxytoluene
(CAA)	Cancer-associated adipocytes
(CAT)	Catalase
(COPD)	Chronic obstructive respiratory disease
(CVD)	Cardiovascular disease
(DDR)	DNA-damage response
(EGCG)	Epigallocatechin-3-gallate
(FRAP)	The ferric reducing antioxidant potential
(IDDM)	Insulin-dependent diabetes mellitus
(IGF-I)	Insulin-like growth factor 1
(MDA)	Malondialdehyde
(NAC)	N-acetylcysteine
(NAO)	Natural anti-oxidant
(ORAC)	Oxygen radical absorbance capacity
(PSA)	Prostate-specific antigen
(ROS)	Reactive oxygen species
(SOD)	Superoxide dismutase
(TAC)	Total Antioxidant Capacity
(TPTZ–Fe3+)	Ferric–tripyridyltriazine complex
(TRAMP)	Transgenic Adenocarcinoma of the Mouse Prostate
(TRAP)	Total radical-trapping antioxidant parameters.

Introduction

Oxidative stress is a key component in linking environmental toxicity to the multistage carcinogenic process. Reactive oxygen species (ROS) are generated in response to both endogenous and exogenous stimuli. To counterbalance ROS-mediated injury, an endogenous antioxidant defense system exists: however, when oxidation exceeds the control mechanisms, oxidative stress arises. Chronic and cumulative oxidative stress induces deleterious modifications to a variety of macromolecular components such as DNA, lipids, and proteins that can lead to the development of chronic diseases [1].

There is enough new evidence indicating the importance of understanding the mechanisms of homeostatic control of total antioxidant capacity (TAC) in plasma and tissues and its modification during oxidative stress development. In table 1 we will define some important terms that will be mentioned many times in this chapter [2].

Oxidative stress is defined as a process in which the dynamic redox balance between oxidants and antioxidants is intensely shifted towards oxidative potentials. Hence, plasma redox status, defined as the sum of the reducing and oxidizing equivalents present in the fluid, is the result of the interaction of many different compounds and systemic metabolic processes [2].

Total Antioxidant Capacity (TAC) is the measure of the moles of a given free radical scavenged by a test solution. The term antioxidant activity should be restricted to characterize the rate constant of single antioxidants against a given oxidant [2].

The ferric reducing antioxidant potential (FRAP) assay measures the 'reducing power', the ability of plasma samples to reduce the colorless ferric–tripyridyltriazine complex (TPTZ–$Fe3+$) to its ferrous colored form (TPTZ–$Fe2+$). The total radical-trapping antioxidant parameters (TRAP) assay measures the 'chain-breaking' antioxidant capacity of plasma. The oxygen radical absorbance capacity (ORAC) assay is based on the same chemical principle as the TRAP assay [2].

The Fluo-Lip assay measures the 'chain breaking' antioxidant potential of plasma. It is based on the same concept (protection of a substrate afforded by plasma against peroxyl radical) as the TRAP and ORAC methods, with the main difference of being performed in a lipophilic environment. Thus, Fluo-Lip responds more efficiently to lipophilic antioxidants and this feature makes it complementary to TRAP [2].

Diet has an important role in regulating plasma redox status, being the main external contributor to the body defenses against oxidative insult. One of the first among these 'acute' studies was performed by Serafini et al. [2,3] who successfully demonstrated that tea and red wine, respectively, are capable of increasing plasma TAC after their consumption. These studies were called acute because they demonstrated these changes immediately after the consumption of the tea or wine. After these studies, many other groups demonstrated a similar ability for other wine derivatives, fruit juices, and even solid foods like onions, lettuce and chocolate. In fact, foods rich in antioxidants are able to increase plasma TAC immediately after their consumption. The kinetics of TAC observed is almost always the same, with a peak value around the first or the second hour after consumption and a metabolic decrease in about 4–5 h [3].

Results from 'chronic' studies, which means that the changes were observed at times after the consumption of the products and not immediately after consuming them, are far less homogeneous, for example, Bub et al., did not find any significant difference in TAC after several weeks of supplementation with spinach products or tomato and carrot juices, while single carotenoids like lutein, zeaxanthine, α - and β -carotene were significantly increased in lipoprotcins [4]. Similar results were obtained by Pellegrini and co-workers on healthy subjects using tomato purée, where no increased plasma TAC values were observed while lycopene and β -carotene results were significantly higher when consumed with tomato purees [5].

Table 1. Terms definitions

Concept	Abreviation	Definition	Limitations	Methods for Mesauring
Antioxidant Activity	aox	Is the rate constant of single antioxidants against a given oxidant, and it is just one of the aspects that contribute to determine TAC.	They are methods that are done for research purposes only; they are not done routinely or in daily bases.	Plasma Enzymes like Superoxide Dismutase, Catalse and peroxidase.
Oxidative Stress	-	Process in which the dynamic redox balance between oxidants and antioxidants is intensely shifted towards oxidative potentials.	They are methods that are done for research purposes only; they are not done routinely or in daily bases.	MDA Free Carbonyles Dityrosines.
Plasma Reduction and oxidation Status	Plasma Redox Status	Is the sum of the reducing and oxidizing equivalents present in the fluid, is the result of the interaction of many different compounds and systemic metabolic processes.	-	-
The Total Antioxidant Capacity	TAC	Is the measure of the moles of a given free radical scavenged by a test solution.	Is the result of many variables such as redox potentials of the compounds present in the matrix, cumulative and synergistic interaction, kind of stress, nature of the oxidizing substrate and antioxidant localization.	- FRAP -TRAP -ORAC -Fluo Lip -TEAC
The ferric reducing antioxidant potential	FRAP	Measures the 'reducing power' – the ability of plasma samples to reduce the colourless ferric–tripyridyltriazine complex (TPTZ–Fe3+) to its ferrous coloured form (TPTZ–Fe2+).	It is a simple and highly reproducible spectrophotometric assay using Fe(II) as a standard. The assay does not work at physiological conditions (pH of 3.6) and does not measure the contribution of liposoluble antioxidants and thiols.	Absorbance (595 nm).
The total radical-trapping antioxidant parameters	TRAP	Measures the 'chain-breaking' antioxidant capacity of plasma – its ability to scavenge peroxyl radicals.	TRAP is based on the protection afforded by plasma against the decay of a fluorescent target, the protein R-phycoerythrin (R-PE), during a chemically generated peroxidation reaction. The plasma in the reactive medium gives a lag time directly related to the amount and activity of its antioxidants. TRAP is particularly suitable for assessing TAC of plasma samples but is not appropriate for direct measurement of TAC of liposoluble antioxidants.	R-PE, R-phycoerythrin Fluorescence (ex 495 nm, em 575 nm)

Concept	Abreviation	Definition	Limitations	Methods for Mesauring
The oxygen radical absorbance capacity	ORAC	Is based on the same chemical principle as the TRAP assay, but plasma TAC is measured as the area under the curve (AUC) of fluorescence during time.	Since the quantification quantification of plasma TAC is obtained by the measurement of AUC, the main drawback of this method is the interference given by protein. Protein contribution to plasma TAC can be as high as 86% of the total value. TAC of liposoluble antioxidants cannot be directly measured even for ORAC assay.	β-PE Fluorescence (ex 495 nm, em 575 nm)
Fluo Lip Assay	Fluo-Lip	Measures the 'chain breaking'antioxidant potential of plasma.	It is based on the same concept as the TRAP and ORAC methods, with the main difference of being performed in a lipophilic environment. Thus, Fluo-Lip responds more efficiently to lipophilic antioxidants and this feature makes it complementary to TRAP. However, the main drawback of this method is the loss of vitamin C during the sample preparation.	DPHPC, 1-palmitoyl-2-((2-(4-(6-phenyl-trans-1,3,5-hexatrienyl)phenyl) ethyl)carbonyl)-sn-glycero-3-phosphocholine) (LDL-VLDL) Fluorescence (ex 354 nm, em 430)
Trolox equivalent antioxidant capacity	TEAC	Is based on the formation of ferrylmyoglobin radical (from reaction of metmyoglobin with H_2O_2) which may then react with ABTS to produce the ABTS•+ radical cation. The accumulation of ABTS•+ can be inhibited to an extent proportional to the TAC.	Biases against this method are the influence of plasma dilution and the nonphysiological conditions of analysis. In fact, the peroxidase process does not mimic radical formation in vivo and the assay uses a non-physiological radical.	ABTS•+, 2,2′-azinobis-(3-ethylbenzothiazoline-6-sulphonate). Absorbance (734 nm)

Conversely, Lee and colleagues observed an increment in plasma TAC after 7 days of consuming tomato products with extra virgin olive oil. Roberts et al., observed a notable increase in TAC as well as in plasma levels of ascorbic acid and carotenoids after consumption of fruits and vegetables [6].

When milk is added to tea and/or chocolate it strongly reduces the ability of these foods to boost plasma TAC. However, one contrasting finding came from Unilever's research group showing that addition of milk did not modify the increments of plasma TAC observed after drinking lyophilized tea [7].

When analyzing this situation in *in vitro* studies, TAC, antimutagenic activity and catechin levels in jejunal dialysates, obtained after adding some green and black tea in a gastrointestinal model, were considerably reduced in the presence of milk or other dietary components. The TAC of a mixture of flavonoids and proteins is less than the sum of the TAC of flavonoid and protein separately [8].

It is stated that TAC levels in humans has a genetic component. The magnitude of this genetic contribution to TAC was shown to be dependent on smoking status. This work proposes an intriguing and specific role played by a specific DNA trait that can be, selectively down- or upregulated by the environment, diet or other unknown stimuli [8].

TAC and Oxidative Stress-Related Diseases

Oxidative stress is involved in the development of several degenerative diseases. In different studies, serum TAC has been assessed in subjects affected by these pathologies and it was found that higher levels of oxidation are directly related with their onset or complications [9]. Sofic and colleagues observed a clear reduction of TAC in patients with diabetic polyneuropathy, anorexia nervosa, AIDS-related encephalopathy and cardiomyopathy [9].

Oxidative stress has been associated with the development of numerous chronic diseases such as type 2 diabetes, cardiovascular disease (CVD), osteoporosis, and cancer. Endogenous production of free radicals occurs during normal physiological processes, such as aerobic metabolism, oxidation of biological molecules, and enzymatic activity. There are some environmental factors such as ultraviolet radiation, air pollution, and cigarette smoking that may also contribute to the accumulation of free radicals in the body. Free radicals in large amounts can damage tissues and promote the upregulation of disease-related pathways such as inflammation. Modulating oxidative stress by dietary supplementation with antioxidant micronutrients such as vitamins C and E or phytochemicals, such as different carotenoids, may help prevent or delay the development of certain diseases. However, research on antioxidant supplementation and disease has not been consistent to some of its findings, which may be due, in part, to inter individual genetic variations [2]. Polymorphisms in genes coding for endogenous antioxidant enzymes or proteins responsible for the absorption, transport, distribution, or metabolism of dietary antioxidants have been shown to affect antioxidant status and response to supplementation. These genetic variants may also interact with environmental factors, such as diet, to determine an individual's overall antioxidant status [10].

Plasma TRAP values were in agreement with the stage of coronary heart disease. The lowest TAC values were related to patients with an episode of acute myocardial infarction, while higher values were associated with patients with unstable angina, stable angina and control subjects [11]. Plasma TAC values in insulin-dependent diabetes mellitus (IDDM) patients were lower when compared with healthy controls. Moreover, TAC appeared to be often correlated with diabetic complications, such as cardiovascular diseases and neuropathy [12].

Evidence regarding the association between TAC and cancer is very limited. Plasma TAC levels were lower in lung cancer patients compared with matched controls [13]. Increased serum levels of TAC were associated with reductions in breast cancer risk in a case-controlled study [14]. An increasing intake of diet TAC through plant food was inversely associated with risk of gastric cancer [8]. The 'TAC concept' might represent a resourceful and valuable tool to monitor redox status both *in vivo* and in epidemiological studies.

TAC in body fluids is directly related to antioxidant levels in plasma, free radical production and, as suggested by recent findings, under genetic control [15]. Moreover, environment, sex, age, hormones, life-style and dietary factors are potentially candidates involved in the oxidation process [2].

Cancer Generation, Progression and Promotion

Oxidative Stress and Inflammation Plays an Important Role in Cancer Development

Halliwell, in a recent review article clearly states when answering the question "does the oxidative stress that is likely to occur as a result of the tissue damage play any role at all in disease pathology?" The answer was a firm yes for cancer [16]. Lesions to DNA trigger the DNA-damage response (DDR), a complex, multi-branched cell-intrinsic process targeted to DNA repair, or elimination of the damaged cells by apoptosis. DDR aims at reducing permanence of mutated cells, decreasing the risk of tumor development: the more stringent the response, the lower the likelihood that sub-lethally damaged, unrepaired cells survive and proliferate [16].

Antioxidant enzymes such as superoxide dismutase play many complex roles in tumor development, after initially preventing the initial DNA damage. Likewise, it is emerging that dietary antioxidants help control tumor onset and progression by preventing DNA damage, a situation that opens a novel and promising frontier to anticancer therapy [17].

Oxidative stress and inflammation are involved in lung cancer pathophysiology. In a recent study by Barreiro et al., investigators found that regardless of the presence of an underlying respiratory condition like chronic obstructive respiratory disease (COPD), situations like protein oxidation, oxidative damaged DNA, and inflammation are remarkably increased in the normal airways and blood of patients with lung cancer [18].

Numerous studies with chemical carcinogens have shown that the effects on the initiation, promotion, and progression of carcinogenesis are initiated via the generation of oxygen and other free-radical intermediates. Substances like polyphenols possess potent anti-oxidant properties, including the scavenging of oxygen radicals, nitric oxide, and lipid radicals and this situation has many effects including anti-oxidation, modulation of carcinogen metabolism, inhibition of cellular proliferation, induction of apoptosis, and cell-cycle arrest.

Investigations related to the association of fruit and vegetable intake and prostatic cancer risk in men less than 65 years of age showed that the consumption of large amounts of vegetables particularly cruciferous was associated with a reduced risk of prostate cancer. Some of these studies are epidemiological where there were fewer incidences of certain diseases where certain food product was consumed more often [19]. Almost all the well-designed controlled clinical trials have shown that alpha-tocopherol (the prime lipid-soluble antioxidant) did not prevent prostate cancer or any other cancer [20].

In epidemiological studies the lower incidence of prostatic cancer in Asians was linked with the presence of isoflavonoids derived from soy that are consumed on a daily bases, and also found that at high concentrations in prostatic fluids. In other investigations authors found that a high consumption of foods containing soy resulted in elevated concentrations of phytoestrogens, including genistein in plasma, urine, and prostatic fluid [19,21]. And it was also proved that soybean phytochemicals, including genistein, inhibited *in vivo* growth of prostatic cancer tumors [22,23]. Some other investigations demonstrated that dietary administration of genistein (500 mg/kg/day) significantly reduced the percentages of TRAMP (Transgenic Adenocarcinoma of the Mouse Prostate) in male mice [24].

Natural anti-oxidant (NAO), a mixture of polyphenols and flavonoids isolated from spinach leaves, is an effective free-radical scavenger and inhibitor of the lipoxygenase enzyme and NAO that can easily be used in mice because it is water-soluble and stable at high temperatures and lacks toxicity (LD50 of NAO in mice is 1,500 mg/kg) [25]. The administration of NAO has shown to be superior as an anti-oxidant in both *in vitro* and *in vivo* models (dermal, oral, and IP administration) that of the well-known anti-oxidants vitamin E and butylated hydroxytoluene (BHT). The beneficial effect of NAO was related to its anti-oxidative functions, as well as its anti-inflammatory actions [25].

Green tea has been shown to exert chemopreventive effects against tumourigenesis and tumor growth in various rodent organs. These effects were attributed to the biochemical and pharmacological activities of polyphenolic constituents, most notably epigallocatechin-3-gallate (EGCG) [26]. Japanese and Chinese populations, who regularly consume green tea, have the lowest incidences of prostate cancer in the world [27].

N-acetylcysteine (NAC), an analogue and precursor of reduced glutathione, was found to lower the incidence of neoplastic and preneoplastic lesions induced by several chemical carcinogens in rodents. These lesions included lung adenomas, bladder carcinoma, skin papilloma, colon carcinoma, and mammary adenocarcinoma. Oral administration of NAC (0.025–4 g/kg) revealed anticarcinogenic activity and a dose related delay in formation of primary tumors [28,29].

Prostate cancer is an excellent candidate for disease chemoprevention because it is typically diagnosed in elderly men and a delay in neoplastic development achieved through pharmacological or nutritional intervention could result in a substantially reduction prostate cancer mortality.

In another study the effect of tomato sauce-based pasta dishes on human patients was compared to that of the other randomly selected prostate cancer patients. The results showed that this lycopene rich-containing diet was effective in reducing DNA oxidative damage in the prostate, as well as the serum levels of prostate-specific antigen (PSA), a member of the kallikrein related peptidase family and secreted by the epithelial cells of the prostate gland. This compound was present in small quantities in the serum of healthy men but often elevated in the presence of prostate cancer [30].

Saturated fats have been associated with advanced prostate cancer risk. The results obtained by Wechter et al., in the TRAMP model suggested that metastatic potential or invasiveness of the cancer was considerably diminished by a combination of E-7869 (R-flurnipropen, a nonsteroidal anti-inflammatory drug) and a lower saturated-fat content of the diet [31].

Antioxidants Can Be Effective in Treating Prostate Cancer in the TRAMP Mouse Model

Aged TRAMP mice are oxidatively stressed and following treatment with NAO or NAC, the level of lipid hydroperoxides/H_2O_2 returned to normal when measured in plasma samples collected from wild-type and TRAMP mice at 2 interim sacrifice intervals and termination of the study. The significant reduction of the hydro peroxides/H2O2 levels in blood by NAO may contribute to its effectiveness in the reduction of the severity of prostatic hyperplasia. NAO was effective in reducing hydroperoxides/H2O2 in TRAMPs only when oxidative stress occurred, but not basal hydroperoxide/H2O2 levels. The exact molecular pathways that contribute to higher plasma levels of ROS in TRAMP mice are unknown and deserve further investigation [30]. Gupta et al., showed that oral administration of green tea in drinking water (500 mg/kg/day) caused a significant inhibition of the development, progression, and metastasis of prostatic cancer to distant organ sites. Oral infusion of green tea polyphenols on TRAMP mice caused significant inhibition of serum IGF-I and restoration of serum IGFBP-3 levels [32].

Importance of 5-Hydroxymethylcytosine (5hmC)

It has been recently shown that the levels of 5-hydroxymethylcytosine (5hmC) are strongly reduced relative to the corresponding normal tissue surrounding the tumor. 5hmC is the most abundant of the peroxidation products and it is referred to as a sixth DNA base. This product is obtained in an enzymatic pathway that involves oxidation and ten-eleven translocations called TET1, TET2, TET3. Using liquid chromatography-mass spectrometry, anti-5hmC antibody-based immuno-dot blots and immunohistochemistry, Pfeifer et al., demonstrated tumor-associated reduction of 5hmC levels for cancers of the lung, brain, breast, liver, kidney, prostate, intestine, uterus and melanoma during treatment [33]. Other investigators confirmed this observation by showing loss of 5hmC in different types of solid tumors. Moreover, reintroduction of TET2 (one of the mutated genes that contain translocations commonly seen in human myeloid malignancies) has been shown to restore 5hmC levels and decrease metastatic potential of melanoma cells. When some co-immuno-stained tissue sections with antibodies against 5hmC and against the Ki67 antigen was observed, authors found that 5hmC and Ki67 are almost never present simultaneously in a single cell [34].

When combined both immunohistochemical analysis of 5hmC loss and the presence of Ki67-positive cells it can be used as a biomarker for cancer diagnosis. The lack of or strong reduction of 5hmC in tumors suggests that proliferating cells lose 5-hydroxymethylcisteine (5hmC). In most cases, the bulk tumor mass is depleted of 5hmC even when Ki67-positive cells are rare, suggesting that these tumor cells have had a past history of proliferation leading to loss of 5hmC, which is then not re-established [34].

Another recently explored topic is related to adipose tissue and its apparent influence on tumor development. Obese individuals have a higher risk of developing certain cancers (endometrial, esophageal, and renal cell cancer). However, the risk of developing other cancers such as melanoma, rectal, and ovarian seems to be not related with body mass [35]. Obesity is characterized by impaired adipose tissue function, leading to adipocyte hypertrophy, inflammation, hypoxia and induced angiogenesis, extracellular matrix remodeling and fibrosis as well as additional stress responses. Recent data implicates systemic and paracrine factors secreted from adipose tissue during the obese state, promoting cancer development and progression [36]. Adipocyte mediated conversion from androgen to estrogen contributes to the development of certain cancers types including endometrial that is significantly more frequent in obese women than in lean individuals [35].

Moreover, many tumor types (gastric, breast, colon, renal, and ovarian) grow in the anatomical surroundings of adipose tissue. During their interaction with cancer cells, adipocytes dedifferentiate into pre-adipocytes or are reprogrammed into cancer-associated adipocytes (CAA) [37]. CAA secretes adipokines, which stimulate the adhesion, migration, and invasion of tumor cells. Cancer cells and CAA exchange metabolites. Specifically, CAA release fatty acids through lipolysis, which are then transferred to cancer cells for energy production through β-oxidation. The abundant availability of lipids helps the tumor to progress and grow without control. Given that adipocytes are a major source of adipokines and energy for the cancer cell, to be able to understand the mechanisms involved may be the clue for new cancer therapies. [35].

Alteration of lipid metabolism is related nowadays with the proliferation of cancer cells, the changes of expression and activity of lipid metabolizing enzymes are directly regulated by the activity of oncogenic signals. The dependence of tumor cells on the dysregulated lipid metabolism suggests that proteins involved in this process are excellent chemotherapeutic targets for cancer treatment. There are currently several drugs under development or in clinical trials that are based on specifically targeting the altered lipid metabolic pathways in cancer cells. Further understanding of dysregulated lipid metabolism and its associated signaling pathways will help us to better design efficient cancer therapeutic strategy [38].

Conclusion

Oxidative stress has been linked to chronic diseases like cancer. The need for enough dietary antioxidants or in case the individual needs are not covered by diet alone, antioxidant supplements is becoming clearly more important now that there is a better understanding the underlying mechanisms (as detailed above) that explain this situation. There are many foods, besides fruit and vegetables, which contain antioxidants in sufficient quantities to be able to inhibit the changes that oxidative stress generates. However, diet has changed so much in recent years that many people do not consume enough of these antioxidant rich foods.

It is imperative to improve nutritional habits to be able to prevent these chronic diseases, especially cancer, which if not diagnosed in time, can be lethal, killing thousands of young productive people every year. It is not only important to have good general nutritional habits, but also to follow personalized diets when one has an oncologic disease, as there are many nutrients whose beneficial properties are specific to certain types of cancer, and that may contribute to slow disease progression and improve time and quality of life.

References

[1] Fuchs-Tarlovsky V. Role of antioxidants in cancer therapy. *Nutrition*. 2013,29(1):15-21.

[2] Serafini M, Del Rio D. Understanding the association between dietary antioxidants, redox status and disease: is the Total Antioxidant Capacity the right tool?. *Redox. Report*. 2004; 9 (3): 145-152.

[3] Serafini M, Ghiselli A, Ferro-Luzzi A. Red wine, tea, and antioxidants. *Lancet.*1994: 344:626.

[4] Bub A, Waltz B, Abrahamse L et al., Moderate intervention with caroteniod-rich vegetable products reduces lipid peroxidation in men. *J. Nutr*. 2000; 130:2200-2206.

[5] Pellegrini N, Riso P, Porrini M. Tomato consumption does not affect the total antioxidant capacity of plasma. *Nutrition*. 2000; 16: 268-271.

[6] Lee A, Thurham DI, Chopra M. Consumption of tomato products with olive oil but no sunflower oil increases the antioxidant activity of plasma. *Free Radic. Biol. Med.* 2000; 29:1051-1055.

[7] Leenen R, Roodenburg AJ, Tijburg LB et al., A single dose of tea with or without milk increases plasma antioxidant activity in humans. *Eur. J. Clin. Nutr*. 2000;54(1):87-92.

[8] Serfani M, Bellocco R, Wolk A et al., Total antioxidant potential of fruit and vegetables and risk of gastric cancer. *Gastroentrology*. 2002; 123:985-991.

[9] Sofic E, Rustembergovic A, Kreoyer G, Cao G. Serum antioxidant capacity in neurological, psychiatric, renal diseases and cardiomyopathy. *J. Neural Transm*. 2002; 109: 711-719.

[10] Da Costa LA, Garcia-Bailo B, Badawi A et al., Genetic determinants of dietary antioxidant status . *Prog. Mol. Biol. Transl. Sci.* 2012;108:179-200.

[11] Niculescu L, Stancu C, Sima A, et al., The total peroxyl radical trapping potential in serum- an assay to define the stage of atherosclerosis. *J. Cell Mol. Med.* 2001: 5(3): 285-94.

[12] Vessby J, Basu S, Mohsen R, Berne C, Vessby B. Oxidative stress and antioxidant status in type 1 diabetes mellitus. *J. Intern Med.* 2002; 251: 69–76.

[13] Erhola M, Nieminen MM, Kellokump-Lehtinen P et al., Plasma peroxyl radical trapping capacity in lung cancer patients: a case control study. *Free Radic. Res*. 1997; 26:439-447.

[14] Ching S, Ingram D, Hahnel R et al., Serum levels of micronutrients, antioxidants and total antioxidant status predict risk of breast cancer in a case control study. *J. Nutr.* 2002; 132:303-306.

[15] Ghiselli A, Serafini M, Natella F, et al., Total antioxidant capacity as a tool to assess redox status: critical view and experimental data. *Free Radic. Biol. Med.* 2000; 29:1106-1114.

[16] Halliwell B. Free radicals and antioxidants: updating a personal view. *Nutrition Reviews.* 2011;70(5):257-265.

[17] Caputo F, Vegliante R, Ghibelli L. Redox modulation of the DNA damage response. *Biochem. Pharmacol.* 2012; 84(10):1292-306.

[18] Barreiro E, Fermoselle C, Mateu-Jimenez M et al., Oxidative stress and inflammation in the normal airways and blood of patients with lung cancer and COPD. *Free Radic. Biol. Med.* 2003 ;(10.1016).

[19] Morton MS, Chan PS, Cheng C, et al., Lignans and isoflavonoids in plasma and prostatic fluid in men: Samples from Portugal, Hong Kong, and the United Kingdom. *Prostate.* 1997; 32:122-128.

[20] Yang CS, Suh N, Kong AN. Does vitamin E prevent or promote cancer?. *Cancer Prev. Res.* (Phila). 2012 May: 5(5):701-5.

[21] Zhang S, Wang Y, Chen Z et al., Genistein enhances the efficacy of cabazitaxel chemotherapy in metastatic castration-resistant prostate cancer cells. *Prostate.* 2013 ;10.(1002) :22705.

[22] Schleicher RL, Lamartiniere CA, Zheng M, Zhang. The inhibitory effect of genistein on the growth and metastasis of a transplantable rat accessory sex gland carcinoma. *Cancer Lett.* 2009; 136: 195–201.

[23] Zhou JR, Gugger ET, Tanaka T, Guo Y, Blackburn GL, Clinton SK . Soybean phytochemicals inhibit the growth of transplantable human prostate carcinoma and tumor angiogenesis in mice. *J. Nutr.* 2009 129: 1628–1635.

[24] Mentor-Marcel R, Lamartiniere CA, Eltoum IE et al., Geinstein in the diet reduces the incidence of poorly differentiated prostatic adenocarcinoma in transgenic mice (TRAMP). *Cancer Res.* 2001; 61:6777-6782.

[25] Grossman S, Reznik R, Tamari T. New plant water soluble antioxidant (NAO) from spinach. Frontiers of reactive oxygen Species in Biology and Medicine, Asada K, Toshikawa T (eds). Amsterdam: Elsevier Science BV;1994.

[26] Yang F, de Villiers WJ, McClain CJ et al., Green tea polyphenols block endotoxin-induced tumor necrosis factor-production and lethality in a murine model. *J. Nutr.* 1998; 128:2334-2340.

[27] Denis L, Morton MS, Griffiths K. et al., Diet has a preventive role in prostatic disease. *Eur. Urol.* 1999; 35: 377-387.

[28] De Flora S, Astengo M, Serra D et al., Inhibition of urethan-induced lung tumors in mice by dietary N-acetylcysteine. *Cancer Lett.* 1986; 32:235-241.

[29] De Flora S, Cesarone CF, Balansky RM, et al., Chemopreventive properties and mechanisms of N-acetylcysteine. The experimental background. *J. Cell Biochem. Suppl.* 1995; 22:33-41.

[30] Nyska A, Suttie A, Baskshi S, et al., Slowing Tumorigenic Progression in TRAMP Mice and Prostatic Carcinoma Cell Lines Using Natural Anti-Oxidant from Spinach,

NAO-A comparative study of three Anti-Oxidants. *Toxicologic Pathology* .2003; 31(1): 33-51.

[31] Wechter WJ, Leipold DD, Murray ED Jr, et al., E-7869 (R-flurbiprofen) inhibits progression of prostate cancer in the TRAMP mouse. *Canc. Res.* 2000; 60:2203-2208.

[32] Gupta S, Hastak K, Ahmad N et al., Inhibition of prostate carcinogenesis in TRAMP mice by oral infusion of green tea polyphenols. *Proc. Natl. Acad. Sci.* 2001; 98:10350-10355.

[33] Pfeifer G, Kadam S, Seung-Gi J. 5-hydroxymetylcytosine and its potential roles in development and cancer. *Epigenetics Chromatin*. 2013; 6:10.

[34] Jin SG, Jiang Y, Qiu R, Rauch TA, Wang Y, Schackert G, Krex D, Lu Q, Pfeifer GP. 5-Hydroxymethylcytosine is strongly depleted in human cancers but its levels do not correlate with IDH1 mutations. *Cancer Res*. 2011; 6:7360–7365.

[35] Nieman KM, Romero IL, Van Houten B, et al., Adipose Tissue and adipocytes support tumorigenesis and metástasis. *Biochem. Biophys. Acta* .2013; pii: S1388-1981(13)00057-7.

[36] Hefetz-Stela S, Scherer PE. Adipocytes: impact on tumor growth and potential sites for therapeutic intervention. *Pharmacol Ther*. 2013; 138(2):197-210.

[37] Nieman KM, Kenny HA, Penicka CV et al., Adipocytes promote ovarian cancer metastasis and provide energy for rapid tumor growth. *Nat. Med.* 2011; 17(11):1498-503.

[38] Zang F, Du G. Dysregulated lipid metabolism in cancer. *World J. Biol. Chem*. 2012; 3(8):167-74.

EDITOR CONTACT INFORMATION

Dr. Bill Stone
Professor and Director of Pediatric Research
East Tennessee State University,
Department of Pediatrics
Johnson City, TN 37614
Tel: 423-439-8762
Email: stone@etsu.edu

Index

A

B

D

E

F

G

H

I

J

K

L

M

N

O

P

Q

R

S

T

U

V

W

X

Y

Z